Diagnostic Tests in NEUROLOGY

Diagnostic Tests in **NEUROLOGY**

Paul M. Matthews, M.D., D.Phil.
Former Chief Resident
Montreal Neurological Hospital
Montreal, Quebec, Canada

Douglas L. Arnold, M.D., F.R.C.P.(C.)
Assistant Professor
Department of Neurology and Neurosurgery
McGill University Faculty of Medicine
Staff Neurologist
Montreal Neurological Hospital
Montreal, Quebec, Canada

With Contributions by

Stirling Carpenter, M.D.

Norman K. So, M.B., B.Chir., M.R.C.P.

Donatella Tampieri, M.D.

Andrew N. Wilner, M.D.

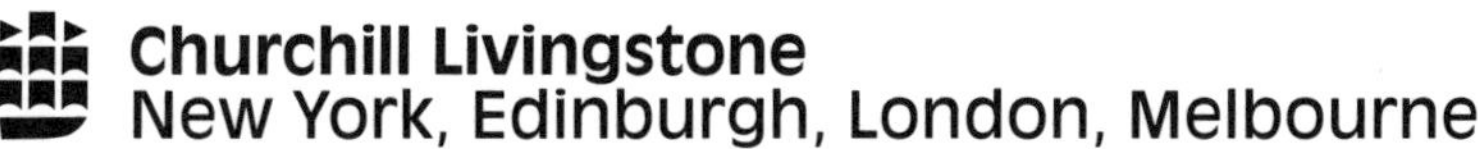

Library of Congress Cataloging-in-Publication Data
Diagnostic tests in neurology / edited by Paul M. Matthews, Douglas L.
Arnold
p. cm.
Includes bibliographical references.
Includes index.
ISBN 0-443-08621-4
1. Nervous system—Diseases—Diagnosis. 2. Neurologic
examination. 3. Diagnosis, Laboratory. I. Matthews, Paul M.
II. Arnold, Douglas L., date.
[DNLM: 1. Nervous System Diseases—diagnosis. WL 141 D536]
RC348.D53 1991
616.8'0475—dc20
DNLM/DLC
for Library of Congress 90-2416
CIP

Distributed in the United Kingdom by Churchill Livingstone, Robert Stevenson House, 1–3 Baxter's Place, Leith Walk, Edinburgh EH1 3AF, and by associated companies, branches, and representatives throughout the world.

Acquisitions Editor: *Robert A. Hurley*
Copy Editor: *Marian Ryan*
Production Designer: *Marci Jordan*
Production Supervisor: *Christina Hippeli*

Printed in the United States of America

First published in 1991

CONTRIBUTORS

Douglas L. Arnold, M.D., F.R.C.P.(C.)

Assistant Professor, Department of Neurology and Neurosurgery, McGill University Faculty of Medicine; Staff Neurologist, Montreal Neurological Hospital, Montreal, Quebec, Canada

Stirling Carpenter, M.D.

Professor, Department of Neurology and Neurosurgery and Department of Pathology, McGill University Faculty of Medicine; Chief, Department of Neuropathology, Montreal Neurological Hospital, Montreal, Quebec, Canada

Paul M. Matthews, M.D., D.Phil.

Former Chief Resident, Montreal Neurological Hospital, Montreal, Quebec, Canada

Norman K. So, M.B., B.Chir., M.R.C.P.

Staff Neurologist, Department of Neurology, Cleveland Clinic Foundation, Cleveland, Ohio

Donatella Tampieri, M.D.

Assistant Professor, Department of Neuroradiology, McGill University Faculty of Medicine; Staff Neurologist, Montreal Neurological Hospital, Montreal, Quebec, Canada

Andrew N. Wilner, M.D.

Medical Consultant, Department of Neurodiagnostic Services, Carolinas Medical Center; Staff Neurologist, Carolina Neurological Clinic, P.A., Charlotte, North Carolina

PREFACE

This book is intended as an introduction to the major tests currently used in general adult clinical neurology. Part I discusses principles and applications of those tests that are relatively specific to neurologic diagnosis. Part II briefly outlines a wider range of tests, which are organized in terms of their uses for evaluation of common neurologic syndromes. The material in Part II is intended to be of use in the emergency room and on the ward as strategies for evaluation are initially planned.

We have tried to keep the material at the level required for a junior neurology resident. However, we hope it also will be more generally useful for others responsible for neurologic evaluation of patients and interpretation of neurologic tests.

Diagnostic Tests in Neurology is not intended in any way to be a textbook of neurology. Rather, it focuses on a relatively narrow topic: the use of diagnostic tests in neurologic evaluations. Tests can be important, but their usefulness depends on the care taken in obtaining the clinical history, performing a careful neurologic examination, and formulating a thoughtful and complete differential diagnosis. With this in mind, we want to emphasize that the material–particularly that in Part II–is intended to stimulate thought, not to be used as a "cookbook" for neurologic evaluation.

Many people have helped in producing this book. Particularly important have been Catherine and Benjamin Matthews and Sharyn Mannix, who have somehow managed to continue living with us during this and concurrent projects. The good ideas in the book were likely borrowed from our colleagues at the Montreal Neurological Institute. (We probably got the bad ideas largely by not paying enough attention to what our colleagues were saying!) Specific thanks must go to Catherine Allaire, who helped with the research, and to Drs. Aube, Francis, and Stewart, for critically reading sections of Part II. We are also grateful to Irene Sauchuk and Barbara Whitson, who uncomplainingly typed the manuscript.

We are grateful to the many people at Churchill Livingstone who have helped bring the book to press. Joan Morrison got us started. Robert Hurley kept us going and remained calm as deadline after deadline passed without a completed manuscript. Finally, Marian Ryan and Jacqueline Gibbons helped us put the book into final form.

Paul M. Matthews, M.D., D. Phil.
Douglas L. Arnold, M.D., F.R.C.P.(C.)

CONTENTS

Part I

Fundamental Principles and Applications

The first section of this book is meant to provide a practical introduction to the major laboratory tests that are particularly important for workup of neurologic problems. Effort is made in each chapter to provide some insight into the principles behind the tests, although we tried to keep the emphasis practical. Understanding the way the tests work allows better appreciation for the range of questions that can be usefully addressed. Perhaps more important, understanding how results are generated may encourage an appreciation of the nature of the artifacts and errors in interpretation that can be associated with each test. References are provided at the end of the chapters to direct the reader to more detailed discussions.

Considerable emphasis has been placed in recent years on using quantitative estimates of sensitivity and specificity to guide the application of tests in general medicine. We also feel that it is important to consider sensitivity and specificity in ordering tests. However, quantitative methods seem to be poorly suited to practice of a specialty such as neurology, in which consultations are often requested specifically for consideration of unusual diagnostic possibilities that are too uncommon or too variable in their presentations to allow explicit analysis of test performance characteristics. Many of the tests (e.g., radiologic tests) described also allow variable thresholds for interpretation of abnormalities. Specificity and sensitivity may change over wide ranges in such cases, depending on the clinical likelihood of the abnormality. For these reasons, little emphasis is given to quantitative estimation of these parameters in the following chapters.

READINGS

McNeil BJ, Keller E, Adelstein SJ: Primer on certain elements of medical decision making. N Engl J Med 293:211, 1975

Sox H (ed): Common Diagnostic Tests: Use and Interpretation. American College of Physicians, Philadelphia, 1987

LUMBAR PUNCTURE AND EXAMINATION OF CEREBROSPINAL FLUID 1

The lumbar puncture is the most generally useful neurologic test. In certain circumstances (e.g., CNS infection, carcinomatous meningitis, subarachnoid hemorrhage), examination is diagnostic. In many others (e.g., polyneuropathies, multiple sclerosis) it complements the clinical presentation to confirm the diagnosis. It has the further advantages of being rapid, safe, and inexpensive. It is one test in which all neurologists should become expert, both in execution and interpretation.

CEREBROSPINAL FLUID

The CSF surrounds structures of the CNS in the subarachnoid space (Fig. 1-1). It is secreted by the choroid plexus in the lateral, third, and fourth ventricles. The total volume of CSF in an adult is about 120 cm^3, of which 25 cm^3 is in the ventricles. It flows from the sites of production in the ventricles to the subarachnoid space around the brain and spinal cord via the foramina of Magendie and Luschka.

Fluid freely moves through the subarachnoid space. It is absorbed by arachnoid granulations, aggregations of tiny nipple-shaped processes of arachnoid tissue along the venous sinuses. They are particularly abundant along the superior sagittal sinus.

When considering the significance of removal of small amounts (10 to 15 cm^3) of CSF for diagnostic purposes, it is reassuring to note that about 500 ml of CSF is secreted per day (0.4 cm^3/min). The half-time for complete CSF renewal is only about 4.5 hours.

CSF is secreted from the choroid plexus by energy-dependent processes. The active secretory mechanisms allow the CNS to be maintained

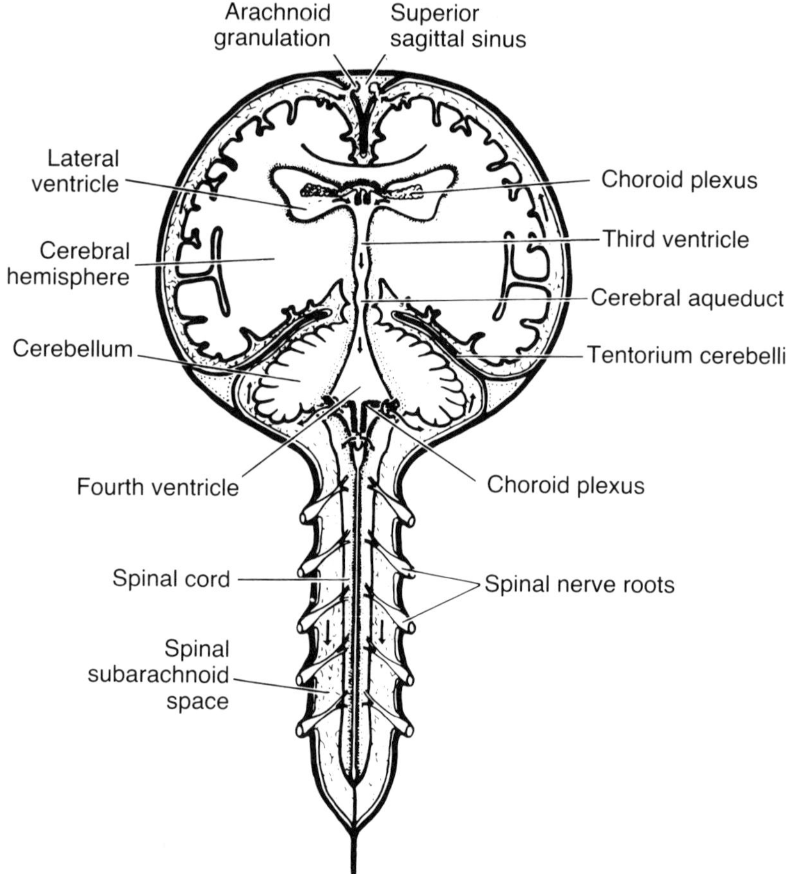

Fig. 1-1. CSF pathways in humans. (From Millen et al., 1962, with permission.)

as a specialized environment in the body. CSF composition is different in several respects from that of plasma (Table 1-1). Differences between CSF and plasma are also maintained by the selective permeability of the cerebral vasculature. However, the vessels are freely permeable to water, and therefore plasma and CSF osmolarities are equal.

The so-called blood-brain barrier is not a simple mechanical barrier.

Table 1-1. Typical Composition of Normal Lumbar Cerebrospinal Fluid and Serum

	Cerebrospinal Fluid	Serum
Osmolality	295 mOsm/L	295 mOsm/L
Sodium	138 mM	138 mM
Chloride	119 mM	102 mM
pH	7.33	7.41 (arterial)
CO_2 tension	6.1 kPa	5.3 kPa
Glucose	3.4 mM	5.0 mM
Total protein	0.35 g/L	70 g/L
Albumin	0.23 g/L	42 g/L
IgG	0.03 g/L	10 g/L

(Data from Fishman, 1980.)

Multiple mechanisms contribute to the maintenance of CSF composition. Foremost are the active transport processes involved in CSF formation mentioned previously, but anatomic factors are also important. Unlike the walls of most vessels in the body, the endothelial cells in the walls of cerebral vessels are joined by tight junctions. Diffusion from the capillary lumen to the extravascular space is facilitated by vesicular transport within endothelial cells. Transport within endothelial cells appears to be uniquely selective in cerebral vessels.

In pathologic states, the blood-brain barrier may break down, altering the composition of CSF in important ways. This process can occur with changes in more than one element of the barrier. Increased and less selective vesicular transport is probably the most important. This has been seen with sustained hypertension, after convulsive seizures, or after hypoxia or ischemic episodes. The prominent breakdown of the blood-brain barrier around vessels of tumors results from the tumor neovascularization involving endothelial cells having different transport properties from those of normal vessels. Opening of tight endothelial junctions can also occur (e.g., in the hyperosmolar state after mannitol administration—a mechanism that has been used to increase the delivery of chemotherapeutic agents to brain tumors).

LUMBAR PUNCTURE

Sampling of the CSF can be helpful in evaluating any of the tremendous range of neurologic problems that involve inflammation, infection, hemorrhage, or degeneration of the CNS. Specific indications include diag-

Table 1-2. Contraindications to Lumbar Puncture

Absolute
Lumbar epidural abscess or other infection over the site of entry
Relative
Increased ICP
Suspected brain abscess or other focal mass lesion
Anticoagulation
Coagulopathy
Thrombocytopenia (<40,000 platelets/mm^3)
Severe scoliosis

nosis of suspected CNS infection, subarachnoid hemorrhage (in the absence of clear subarachnoid blood on computed tomography [CT]), infectious polyneuritis (Guillain-Barré syndrome), demyelinating disease (multiple sclerosis [MS]), and carcinomatosis meningitis. Measurement of opening pressure and trial drainage of CSF or infusion tests have been used for evaluation of normal pressure hydrocephalus. The lumbar puncture (LP) can also be used therapeutically, for example, in intrathecal delivery of antibiotics or chemotherapeutic agents.

Contraindications to Lumbar Puncture

Probably the only absolute contraindication to LP is a lumbar infection, such as an epidural abscess, that prevents access to the subarachnoid space without tracking the needle through purulent areas (Table 1-2). A mass lesion and suspected or known intracranial hypertension should be considered a major relative contraindication. The potentially most dangerous situations are found with space-occupying lesions or where edema is massive and rapid in onset. The risk of herniation depends on location of the mass lesion as well as size, degree of edema, and rate of onset. A patient with a mass lesion who undergoes LP should be observed closely for at least 6 to 12 hours for signs of impending herniation. The capability for rapid intubation and hyperventilation should be present and an intravenous line running. Mannitol for intravenous administration should be available.

Other important relative contraindications to LP are coagulopathies and thrombocytopenia, conditions that predispose to local hemorrhagic complications. Ideally at least 6 hours should elapse after discontinuing heparin before performing an LP to allow normalization of the patient's partial thromboplastin time (PTT). A further 3 to 4 hours post-LP is necessary for local hemostasis before reinitiating heparin therapy. With warfarin (Coumadin) the patient can be reversed with vitamin K if the situation is not urgent and further oral anticoagulant therapy is not immediately anticipated. For cases requiring more rapid action, 4 to 6 units of fresh-frozen intravenous (IV) plasma should restore the 25 percent of normal coagulation factor activity necessary to normalize clotting activity in an adult. Thrombocytopenia below about 40,000/mm^3 (or higher levels if platelets are dysfunctional) should be treated with platelet transfusion before the LP. In the absence of antibodies against the platelets or splenic sequestration, each unit of platelets should increase the total count by about 6,000/mm^3.

Severe scoliosis should be considered a relative contraindication to LP without radiologic guidance.

Anatomy Relevant to the Lumbar Puncture

The lumbar puncture involves placing a needle into the subarachnoid space guided only by surface anatomy and the anticipated relative positions of structures in the spinal column. Understanding the local anatomy will make this procedure much easier to perform (Fig. 1-2).

The spinal cord is in the vertebral canal formed by the vertebral arch dorsally and the vertebral body. The arch is formed by the pedicles and the articular and spinous processes. The latter are readily palpated and mark the midline of the spinal canal. The spinal needle is usually directed between adjacent spinous processes to perforate the dural sac near the midline.

The ligamentum flavum, a thick, longitudinal, fibrous band, runs along the dorsal aspect of the vertebral canal. The vertebral bodies mark the ventral side of the spinal canal. A rich venous plexus lies in the anterior aspect of the vertebral canal.

The spinal cord and cauda equina within the vertebral canal are enveloped by three membranes: the dura, arachnoid, and pia mater. The latter is closely adherent to the cord and roots. The former two are normally kept closely apposed by CSF filling the subarachnoid space. CSF is obtained by penetration of the subarachnoid space after the needle passes into the posterior vertebral canal. Penetration should be below L2 (the rostral end of the spinal cord), where only lumbosacral roots are in the dural sac.

A Step-by-step Approach to Lumbar Puncture

There are many ways to perform lumbar puncture. We will present an approach that has worked well for us. We will also try to explain the rationale behind many of the suggestions.

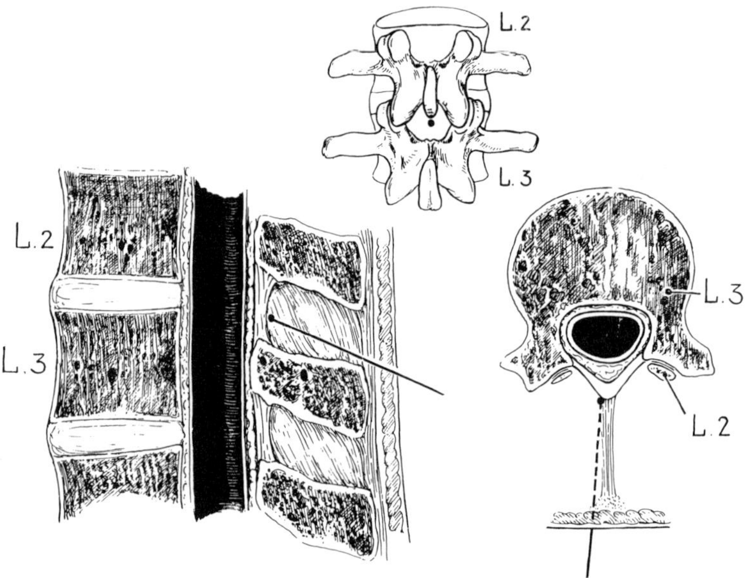

Fig. 1-2. Correct angulation of the needle for a lumbar puncture in an average subject. The skin is punctured at about the midline and the needle is directed rostrally by about 15 degrees. (From Macintosh et al., 1973, with permission.)

Step 1

Check coagulation parameters and the platelet count. Explain the indications and procedure to the patient and obtain consent. Check the optic discs to rule out papilledema and for the presence of venous pulsations. Although papilledema is an unreliable sign, if venous pulsations are present there is little possibility of increased intracranial pressure, for which special precautions should be taken (see preceding). When focal deficits are present or consciousness is impaired, a CT scan should be obtained before the LP.

Step 2

Draw serum glucose. The relationship between serum and CSF glucose concentrations is dynamic. The 1 to 2 hours needed for equilibration (see following) may be important to bear in mind around mealtimes, particularly in elderly patients or others with poor control of serum glucose concentration. The CSF glucose concentration must always be interpreted relative to serum glucose concentration: CSF glucose concentration in the normal range with an elevated serum glucose concentration may represent hypoglycorrhachia.

Step 3

Place the patient in the lateral recumbent position with the patient's back facing you. The lower back should be perpendicular to the mattress of the bed. A pillow between the knees will help avoid rotation of the hips and spine. Flex the hips and have the patient curl into the fetal position to open the space between adjacent lumbar spinous processes.

Step 4

Identify the superior iliac crests. An imaginary line drawn between them intersects the upper L4 vertebral body. Entrance of the spinal needle between L2–L3 or L3–L4 is usually safe as the spinal cord extends no further than the L2 vertebral body in adults; in children it extends lower.

Step 5

Organize materials for the procedure on a sterile field in easy reach. With sterile technique drape and cleanse the area. In washing, use circular movements from the center outward to minimize the risk of contaminating the entrance site with organisms from nonsterile areas of skin.

Step 6

Check the spinal needle and its stylet. Prepare the manometer. Open four tubes for CSF collection. Draw up 15 cm^3 1 percent Xylocaine in a syringe with a fine-gauge needle for local anesthesia. All of this can be accomplished while the antiseptic cleaning solution is left in place to kill bacteria.

Step 7

Remove any excess of the antiseptic cleaning solution with an alcohol-soaked swab. Identify the chosen interspace again. Bracket the spinous processes with fingers of the nondominant hand to mark the spot where the characteristic depression over the space between spinous process is

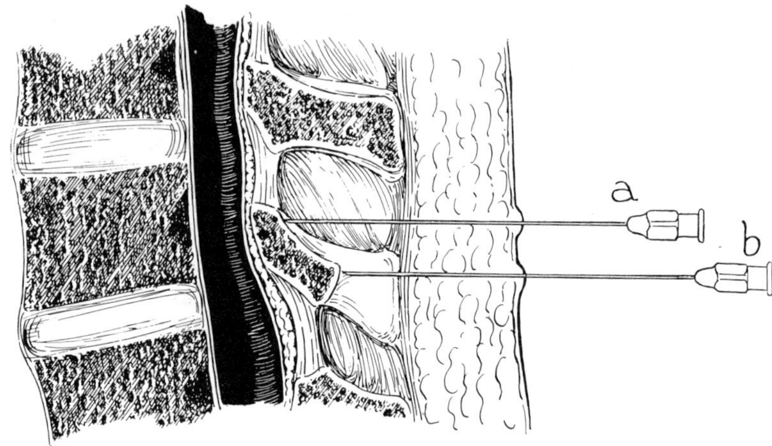

Fig. 1-3. The posterior surface of the lamina of a lumbar vertebra slopes downward and backward. If the needle encounters bone at a shallow depth, it impinges on the lower border of the lamina; if the obstruction is deep, it impinges on the upper border. (From Macintosh et al., 1973, with permission.)

felt. Locally infiltrate Xylocaine intradermally and over the periosteum below. Wait about a minute for anesthesia to develop.

Step 8

Insert the 20- to 22-gauge spinal needle at the chosen point. Once through the tough epidermis, the thumb and forefingers of the dominant hand can be used to advance the shank while those of the other hand support and direct the needle at the skin. The needle should be directed roughly toward the umbilicus, about 10 to 15 degrees cephalad (Fig. 1-3). Because the patient's back is perpendicular to the bed, the needle should be directed parallel with the surface of the mattress. The bevel of the needle should be positioned upward so that the needle will slide *between* longitudinal fibers of dura rather than cutting them.

In elderly patients, the ligamentum flavum may be calcified, but it is never so solid that it cannot be readily penetrated. In contrast, bone gives a dense, firm resistance and irritation of the periosteum is uncomfortable.

If bone is encountered at a shallow depth, it is probably the spinous process of the superior vertebra. The needle should be then almost completely removed and inserted more caudad. If bone is encountered deep, it is most likely to be at the inferior vertebra, and the needle should be partially withdrawn and redirected more cephalad, at least initially. A sudden shooting pain in the legs indicates that a root has been hit, which is almost always a sign that the needle has entered the spinal canal too far laterally. The needle should be withdrawn and redirected away from the affected side to find the midline.

Step 9

A well-directed needle will slide easily through overlying tissue and give a firm, soft resistance at the ligamentum flavum, followed by a slight sudden release of resistance ("pop") as the dura and arachnoid membrane are penetrated.

At frequent points as the needle is inserted, stop and remove the stylet to look for CSF flow, indicating that the needle has entered the subarachnoid space. Once fluid begins to return, advance a further 1 to 2 mm after replacing the stylet.

No fluid may flow despite being in the subarachnoid space if a nerve root or a film of arachnoid is obstructing the needle tip. Rotating the needle tip 90 degrees should free it.

A "dry tap" can also result if CSF pressure is too low to distend the lumbar cistern. Repeating the procedure with the patient seated upright can solve this problem. The patient should then be leaning forward to maximize the separation between the lumbar spinous processes. The needle should again be directed to the midline, about 10 to 15 degrees cephalad relative to the curvature of the spine at the interspace about to be entered. The only disadvantage of this approach is that precise measurement of CSF pressure relative to the torcular herophili is not possible.

Most traumatic taps are caused by penetration of the extensive venous plexus on the ventral wall of the canal. This problem can be avoided by pushing the needle ventrally very slowly, removing the stylet to check for CSF flow every 2 mm or so after reaching the ligamentum flavum.

Step 10

When CSF is flowing, attach the manometer. Note the fluid color and opening pressure. When the fluid level in the manometer has stabilized, small pressure waves with each heart beat (2 to 5 mmH_2O) and respiration (4 to 10 mmH_2O) should be apparent. If the opening pressure is high, ensure that the patient is relaxed. Elevation of central venous pressure with abdominal compression from anxiety and the awkward position of the patient during an LP are the most common causes of increased opening pressure. Pressures of 20 to 25 cmH_2O should not be accepted as abnormal until at least 5 minutes have elapsed and the anxious patient has been calmed.

Step 11

Collect CSF serially in four tubes, noting the order of collection. The first few drops are often bloody, even in a carefully performed tap, so we always discard them.

At least 2 cm^3 should be collected in tubes 1, 3, and 4 and 5 cm^3 in tube 2. However, it is always wise to collect enough CSF to allow several cubic centimeters to be saved for an unanticipated test. There is no correlation between the incidence of post-LP headache and the amount of fluid removed in diagnostic taps.

If the CSF is bloody, note whether the fluid clears as more is collected, suggesting a traumatic tap, or whether the fluid is xanthochromic, suggesting less recent hemorrhage.

Getting talc from the gloves into the CSF should be avoided as the particles can cause some confusion when the cell count is performed. Avoid direct contact with the mouths of the collection tubes or placing a finger directly over the end of the open spinal needle—the stylet will stop CSF flow just as effectively.

Step 12

When all CSF is collected, remove the needle with a steady motion. Apply local pressure with a sterile gauze for as long as several minutes, depending on the amount of bleeding.

Step 13

It is generally advised that the patient remain supine for an extended period after LP to minimize the risk of a post-LP headache. This may facilitate sealing of the dural tear caused by the LP needle. We generally ask the patient to lie prone for at least 1 hour and supine for another 3 to 4 hours. Some data suggest that the incidence of LP headaches is lowest for those who lie prone. This position slightly reduces hydraulic pressure at the site of entrance in the dural sac and may promote local pooling of blood for a coagulant seal. However, the efficacy of any maneuvers to prevent headache *after* the dural hole is made is uncertain (see *Post-Lumbar Puncture Headache*).

Step 14

The following tests should be routinely considered:

Tube 1, cell count (1 to 2 cm^3) (for comparison with tube 4 if tap is bloody)

Tube 2, protein and glucose, oligoclonal bands, serology, and other biochemical tests as needed (5 to 7 cm^3)

Tube 3, microbiologic stains and cultures (3 to 5 cm^3)

Tube 4, cell count and extra CSF (3 to 5 cm^3)

Large quantities of CSF are needed for culture of organisms such as fungi that are present in low titers. Although fluid may be transferred into other tubes after collection, it is best to leave the sample for microbiology unopened, minimizing risks of contamination.

Situations are occasionally encountered in which the LP is technically extremely difficult because of obesity, a history of back surgery or severe arachnoiditis, scoliosis, or other factors. Although with enough time and patience from both doctor and patient most LPs can be performed, there are reasons it is unwise to traumatize the patient with repeated unsuccessful attempts if the situation is not urgent. Use of fluoroscopic guidance for the needle may be desirable; we have found this to be a much underused option.

A needle inserted far lateral to the midline or a cisternal tap is possible when the traditional approach is contraindicated (e.g., when there is an overlying infection in the lumbar region). These techniques should only be performed by skilled personnel, usually under radiologic guidance. Note that the composition of CSF in the basal cisterns differs significantly from that in the lumbar sac.

Complications of Lumbar Puncture

LP generally has few risks, but they should be discussed with the patient before performing the procedure (Table 1-3). The most frequent and troublesome complications are post-LP headache and local back pain.

Headache

In our practice, perhaps 1 in 10 patients develops post-LP headache. The headaches are characteristically frontal and are relieved by lying supine. Neck ache is not uncommon. Occasionally postural nausea, vomiting, tinnitis, cold sweats, and blocking of the ears may also be noted. Head-

Table 1-3. Complications of Lumbar Puncture

Post-LP headache
Local backache
Herniation of uncus or cerebellar tonsils
Infection (vertebral osteomyelitis, meningitis, or epidural abscesses)
Subarachnoid or spinal subdural hemorrhage
Diplopia with cranial nerve VI palsy
Dermoid formation

aches are more likely to occur in younger and female patients. The onset may occur within 15 minutes of the LP or as late as 4 days after, although onset within 12 to 24 hours is most usual. They frequently persist for 4 to 7 days, but may resolve earlier or last as long as 2 weeks.

Presumably the headaches arise from traction on the meninges and pain-sensitive blood vessels, with leak of CSF from the torn dura at the LP site. It must be reemphasized that they are *not* related to the amount of CSF removed at the time of the LP; they may be related to the size of the hole made in the dura, however. Headaches are clearly more common with the use of larger gauge needles. Skilled neurologists have reported a very low incidence of headaches with use of 24- to 26-guage spinal needles (a syringe is needed for aspiration of CSF).

It is not certain that lying flat after LP actually prevents post-LP headache. It has been suggested that this practice may merely delay onset; however, lying flat unequivocally relieves an established headache.

Local Backache

Local backache may arise from root irritation and trauma to the periosteum, local extravasation of CSF or blood, minor damage to the annulus fibrosus, or frank disc herniation. Extravasation of CSF can be minimized by using a narrow-gauge needle and penetrating the dura only once. If the spinal needle is inserted slowly and near the midline, roots encountered should slide away easily. Advancing slowly with frequent checking for CSF flow after penetration of the ligamentum flavum will prevent penetration of ventral veins.

Infection

Infections can occur with inadequate attention to sterile technique or by tracking the needle through purulent areas. Meningitis should begin to develop within 12 hours of the LP. More indolent infections, such as vertebral osteomyelitis or an epidural abscess, may also occur.

Herniation

Herniation of the uncus or cerebellar tonsils is certainly the most dramatic complication. Herniation occurs when free communication of CSF and rapid equilibration of CSF pressure throughout the subarachnoid space is impaired. Consequently, the risk of herniation is particularly high with posterior fossa masses if meningeal inflammation or a mass has obstructed usual pathways of CSF flow.

Hemorrhage

Although most local bleeding is not clinically significant, a traumatic tap can complicate interpretation of later LPs by residual xanthochromia. It usually occurs when the needle is pushed too far and encounters the venous plexus on the ventral aspect of the canal. Bleeding can also result from trauma to the small radicular vessels of the cauda equina. Large amounts of bleeding into the subarachnoid space can cause arachnoiditis. More immediately threatening hemorrhagic complications are found in anticoagulated patients or those with coagulopathies. Spinal subdural hemorrhage can cause cauda equina cord compression.

Diplopia

A relatively rare complication is diplopia secondary to an abducens nerve palsy. The mechanism is presumably stretching of the nerve over the petrous bone as CSF leakage from the lumbar cistern pulls intracranial structures downward.

Dermoid Tumor

Even more unusual is late formation of a dermoid tumor in the subarachnoid space from epidermal cells deposited during an LP. However, this is one reason it is important to keep the stylet in place as the spinal needle is advanced through the skin.

EXAMINATION OF THE CEREBROSPINAL FLUID

Observations made at the time of LP and accurate determination of glucose concentration are extremely important. Most clinical decisions can be made on the basis of the appearance, opening pressure, cell count, and

CSF/serum glucose concentration ratio. Total protein often adds further information. Gram stain and cultures are critical when infections are suspected. Other tests are more useful for refining diagnoses than for guiding immediate therapy (e.g., oligoclonal bands and serologic tests).

Appearance

The appearance of the CSF is best appreciated by viewing it next to a tube of water in strong, white light against a white background. Normal CSF is clear. In pathologic states the fluid may be yellow, bloody, xanthochromic, or purulent. The yellow color arises from chromogens in proteins. As a rule, elevation of the total protein to greater than 1.0 g/L is necessary for a significant color change. It is important to distinguish the resulting appearance from that of xanthochromia. Highly proteinaceous CSF foams easily with stiff bubbles that persist. Adding acid or heating the CSF precipitates denatured protein in thick, white clumps.

CSF is tinged pink from blood when there are more than about 500 red blood cells (RBC)/cm^3. Intact RBC imply a fresh hemorrhage: erythrocytes lyse after only about 1 to 2 hours in CSF. Hemolysis releases hemoglobin, which also colors CSF red, but is easily distinguished from fresh blood because it does not sediment with centrifugation.

As elsewhere in the body, free hemoglobin is first oxidized to methemoglobin and ultimately degraded to bilirubin. This causes a progressive color change from red to brown to yellow (xanthochromia). The amount of free oxyhemoglobin is maximal in the first few days after a bleed and disappears within about 1 week (Fig. 1-4). Bilirubin begins to be produced within about 2 days and persists for 2 to 3 weeks, thus providing a relatively prolonged marker for hemorrhage. Sensitive tests for bilirubin should be routinely available in the clinical laboratory. Because these tests are so sensitive, however, it is impossible to distinguish between a recent minor hemorrhage from an aneurysm (a warning bleed), for example, and that from a traumatic tap. Thus, CSF from the *first* tap in cases of suspected hemorrhage is critical, as xanthochromia on subsequent taps can result from an initial traumatic tap. Large amounts of methemoglobin are seen only when isolated pockets of blood have been present for some time, as in subdural hemorrhages, cysts, or intracerebral hematomas.

CSF appears purulent with a leukocytosis of 1,000 cells/ml or more. A hazy yellow appearance is seen with cell counts greater than 200 cells/ml. Relatively low cell counts (50 to 100 cells/ml) can also be appreciated because of the so-called Tyndall effect, which causes CSF to sparkle when light from individual cells is refracted if the tube is viewed perpendicular to a strong beam of light. Unfortunately, it is not possible to distinguish between talc, dust, and leukocytes by visual examination alone.

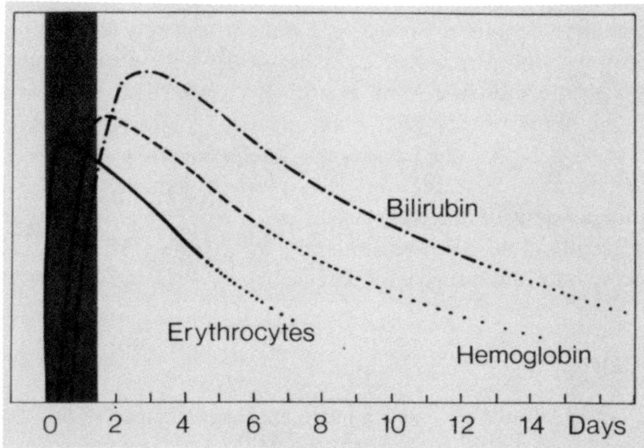

Fig. 1-4. Pigmentary changes in CSF after subarachnoid hemorrhage. During the first day, RBC count peaks and then gradually falls over the next week. Hemoglobin released from lysed RBCs begins to appear between 4 and 10 hours, giving a pinkish hue to the centrifuged CSF. After 9 to 15 hours, a yellow color from bilirubin begins to appear. Bilirubin can be detected for 2 weeks or more in the CSF (From Fishman, 1980, with permission.)

Opening Pressure

Opening pressure is determined by the pressure in the torcular herophili and any additional hydrostatic pressure exerted by the column of CSF from that level; thus it depends on position. With the patient recumbent, normal CSF pressure is between 8 and 20 cmH_2O in the lumbar sac, the cisterna magna, and the ventricles. When the patient is sitting, lumbar CSF pressure rises by 10 to 30 cmH_2O. This amount represents only a fraction of the theoretical hydrostatic pressure that would be exerted in a rigid tube because of compliance of the structures of the CNS. Using this position causes pressure in the cisterna magnum to fall to 0 cmH_2O and causes that in the ventricles to actually be negative.

If there is no obstruction in the subarachnoid space, hydrostatic pressure changes will be transmitted throughout the CSF space. Because the cranial vault is rigid, intracranial pressure (ICP) increases with increases in the volume within the cranial vault. Increased CSF production (e.g., papilloma) or decreased absorption (e.g., venous thrombosis), intracranial masses (e.g., blood, tumor, or abscess), cerebral edema, or blood will also increase ICP. The most common cause of increased ICP is transiently elevated central venous pressure as a patient tenses abdominal muscles. Increased intracranial pressure can also occur with other conditions associated with changes in central venous pressure (e.g., congestive heart failure). One should recall that many agents that lower systemic blood pressure (e.g., Ca-channel blockers) actually increase CSF pressure by causing intracranial vasodilation. However, in general, CSF pressure is largely independent of arterial pressure.

Pathologically low CSF pressures may arise from CSF block with mass lesions or severe inflammatory processes.

Cell Count

The cell count should always be performed personally by the examining physician. It is essential to perform the cell count as soon as possible, at least within 1 to 2 hours, after an LP. With delay, cell lysis, precipitation, and fibrin formation may change the cell count significantly.

The cell count involves determining the number of RBC, leukocytes, or other cells per unit volume. The relative proportion of the different classes of leukocytes is also important. The cell count is performed using a counting chamber under the microscope. A typical counting chamber has a precisely defined grid of 3×3 mm at its base and a depth of 0.1 mm to give a total volume of 0.9 mm^3. After a drop of CSF is added to the chamber, the cells are counted and the number is corrected to be expressed as cells per cubic milliliter. It is helpful to routinely mix the CSF with a precisely known amount of crystal violet in a micropipette before counting. Leukocytes take up this vital dye, allowing them to be more easily identified and facilitating differentiation of the different classes of leukocytes. The dilution of CSF by dye must be taken into account when expressing the final cell count.

Because CSF lyses red cells, the latter are seen only with fresh hemorrhages: after traumatic taps, subarachnoid hemorrhages, intraparenchymal hemorrhages with migration of RBC, or venous occlusion with venous congestion and secondary leak of cells. In a modern hospital, a CT scan is usually readily available and gross subarachnoid hemorrhage is easily diagnosed. However, small bleeds are often diagnosed only by LP.

If relatively small numbers of red cells are found ($<1{,}000/mm^3$) the major concern is to distinguish subarachnoid hemorrhage from a traumatic tap. A number of clues may be used. The most important relies on the observation the the damaged vessel usually seals rapidly after a traumatic tap. The red cell count in the first tube in such cases is higher than that

Table 1-4. Neutrophilic—Low Glucose CSF Profile

Meningitis
Bacterial
Acute syphilitic
Viral (early, occasionally with mumps or LCM)
Amebic
Chemical
Parameningeal infections
Cerebral abscess
Embolic cerebral infarction secondary to bacterial endocarditis
Idiopathic meningeal inflammation
Mollaret's meningitis (early)
Behçet syndrome
Spinal arachnoiditis

LCM, lymphocytic choriomeningitis.
(Modified from Swartz and O'Hanley, 1987, with permission.)

in the last tube. In contrast, roughly equal amounts of blood should be present in all tubes with subarachnoid hemorrhage. It is helpful to centrifuge the specimen: immediately after a traumatic tap the supernatant CSF should be clear, whereas if the blood represents prior hemorrhage (greater than a few hours old), the CSF will be pink or xanthochromic. It may take 1 to 2 hours for a small amount of blood released in the cranial subarachnoid space to diffuse to the lumbar cistern.

The white blood cell (WBC) count rises with inflammation. Leukocytes migrate from capillaries by the process of *emperipolesis* in which the whole

Table 1-5. Lymphocytic—Normal Glucose CSF Profile

Meningitis or meningoencephalitis
Viral
Partially treated bacterial
Neurosyphilis (acute or subacute, meningovascular, general paresis)
Fungal (early)
Tuberculosis (early)
Carcinomatous
Chemical
Brain abscess
Parameningeal infections
Vasculitides
Systemic Lupus Erythematosus
Granulomatous
Spinal arachnoiditis

(Modified from Swartz et al., 1987, with permission.)

Table 1-6. Lymphocytic—Low Glucose CSF Profile

Meningitis
Partially treated bacterial
Tuberculous
Fungal
Syphilitic (acute or subacute)
Viral (occasionally mumps and lymphocytic choriomeningitis and rarely with echovirus)
Listeria (monocytes)
Leptospirosis
Carcinomatous
Rheumatoid
Parasitic disease
Meningeal sarcoidosis
Vasculitides
Subarachnoid hemorrhage
Brain abscess

(Modified from Swartz et al., 1987, with permission.)

cell is engulfed by the endothelial membrane to form a giant vesicle. The normal upper limit for the leukocyte count is about 4 to 5/mm^3, with perhaps only one polymorphonuclear cell/mm^3. A mild leukocytosis (5 to 20 WBC/mm^3) is abnormal but nonspecific. The usual inflammatory reaction seen after myelography, spinal anesthesia, hemorrhage, or infarction may be of this order.

Much more dramatic responses are seen with CNS infections. Acute bacterial meningitis tends to be associated with a greater inflammatory response than aseptic meningitis. Most bacterial infections should be associated with cell counts greater than 1,000 WBC/mm^3 (early or partially treated bacterial meningitis can have lower cell counts, though). Cell counts this high are rare with aseptic meningitides. When the cell count is exceptionally high (5,000 to 10,000 leukocytes/cm^3), the possibility of rupture of a cerebral or perimeningeal abscess should be considered; often such a rupture is associated with a particularly abrupt clinical presentation.

The differential count may provide a clue to the etiology of the inflammation. In general, elevated *polymorphonuclear leukocytes* are seen with bacterial and mycobacterial infections (Table 1-4). Increased numbers of *lymphocytes* are associated with chronic infections (e.g., chronic meningitis and even septic emboli in endocarditis), partially treated bacterial infections, viral infections, noninfectious inflammatory processes (e.g., acute flare of MS), and fungal infections (Tables 1-5, 1-6). A monocytosis is seen with chronic inflammation and with *Listeria monocytogenes* meningitis. *Eosinophils* are relatively rare and seen with helminthic infections

Table 1-7. Situations Associated with CSF Eosinophilia

- Infection
  - Parasitic
    - *Taenia solium* (cysticercosis)
    - *Angiostrongylus cantonensis* (eosinophilic meningitis)
    - *Ascaris*
    - *Echinococcus granulosus*
    - *Trichinella spiralis*
  - Fungal
    - *Coccidioides immitis*
  - Treponemal
    - *Treponema pallidum* (neurosyphilis)
  - Mycobacterial
    - *Mycobacterium tuberculosis*
  - Viral
    - Lymphocytic choriomeningitis
    - Coxsackie
- Chemical
  - Myelography
  - Foreign body reaction
- Malignancy
  - Lymphoma
  - Leukemia
- Demyelinating Disease
  - Multiple sclerosis
  - SSPE

(Adapted from Koberski, 1979, with permission.)

and other parasitic diseases, including cystiscercosis and occasionally with TB meningitis, neurosyphilis, CNS lymphoma, and foreign body reaction (Table 1-7).

Glucose

Glucose concentration in CSF varies throughout the CNS, with concentrations falling as the fluid proceeds from ventricular to cisternal to lumbar subarachnoid spaces. The normal CSF/serum glucose concentration ratio in the lumbar sac is >0.6 after sufficient time to allow full equilibration between concentrations in the vascular and CSF compartments. Under normal conditions, approximately 2 hours are needed for equilibration. Thus, the CSF/serum glucose concentration ratio can fall transiently postprandially. Glucose moves from blood to the CSF by facilitated diffusion via saturable membrane transporters. With high serum glucose concentrations (>25 mm), saturation of transporters can occur, lowering the relative CSF glucose.

Low CSF glucose concentration will be present with hypoglycemia, but the normal ratio of CSF/serum glucose concentration should be maintained. *Hypoglycorrhachia* refers to a depression of the concentration ratio. It is found to varying degrees with most meningeal inflammatory processes. Acute bacterial, tuberculous, fungal, and carcinomatous meningitis almost always leads to a low CSF glucose concentration. Less dramatic decreases can frequently be found with meningeal sarcoidosis, parasitic infections (e.g., cysticerosis and trichinosis), or chemical meningitis. Vasculitic inflammations, such as cerebral lupus or rheumatoid meningitis, may lower CSF glucose. Viral meningitis with mumps, lymphocytic choriomeningitis, or herpes simplex may produce mild to moderate decreases.

Subarachnoid hemorrhage also causes hypoglycorrhacia. The mechanisms causing hypoglycorrhacia in these pathologic states are not clear. Three possibly important factors involve both decreased delivery and increased metabolism. The first is increased cortical glucose metabolism. Some have hypothesized that unidentified factors involved in inflammation may stimulate cortical glucose uptake. A second factor may be the extra glucose uptake by inflammatory leukocytes. Given their metabolic rates, however, this is generally seen as much less significant. Finally, there may be impairment of glucose diffusion into the CSF. This mechanism may be particularly important in accounting for the decreased CSF glucose concentration after subarachnoid hemorrhage. CSF glucose concentration may remain depressed as long as 2 to 3 weeks after resolution of the cellular inflammatory response after acute meningitis.

Total Protein

CSF protein concentration rises with breakdown of the blood-brain barrier, slowed reabsorption, or increased local synthesis of immunoglobulins. Breakdown of the blood-brain barrier may occur with inflammation, ischemia, trauma, or tumor neovascularization. Slowed reabsorption can occur in situations associated with very high CSF protein concentration, such as bacterial meningitis or subarachnoid hemorrhage.

The normal concentration of protein in the lumbar cistern is 0.20 to 0.45 g/L, whereas it is at the highest concentration in the subarachnoid space. The CSF protein concentration increases progressively in areas more distal from sites of synthesis: normal concentrations in ventricular CSF are <0.15 g/L; cisternal CSF, <0.30 g/L; and lumbar CSF, <0.45 g/L. Thus increased CSF circulation, for example after an LP, may lead to relatively lower or even falsely normal values for total protein in the lumbar CSF.

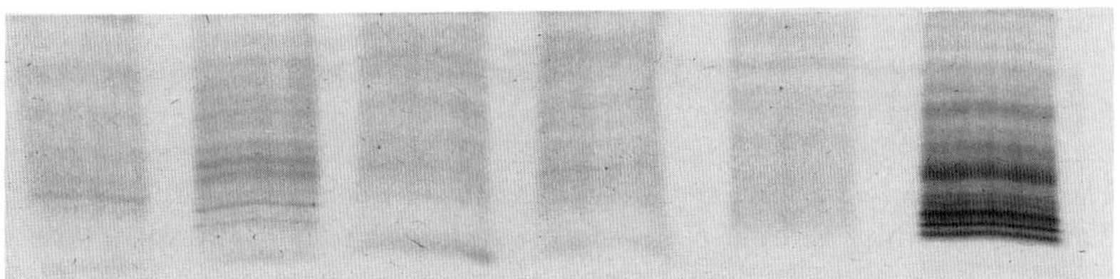

Fig. 1-5. Isoelectric focusing of CSF samples. Lanes are numbered from left. Lanes 1 through 4 are from patients with MS. Lane 5 is from a patient after a cerebrovascular accident. Lane 6 is from a patient with SSPE. Lanes 2 and 6 are clearly positive, whereas lanes 3 and 4 show three faint bands. Lane 1 shows a single band. The patterns in lanes 1, 3, and 4 illustrate the difficulty of reporting a result as positive or negative in many cases (Courtesy of Dr. G. Francis).

Electrophoresis and immunoelectrophoresis are used for qualitative and quantitative estimation of CSF proteins. In normal CSF, about 70 percent of the total protein is albumin and at most 12 percent gamma globulins (Table 1-1). The protein arises primarily from serum proteins selectively transported into the CSF. Increases in CSF immunoglobulins, therefore, may reflect systemic dysimmune states as well as local synthesis. When CSF immunoglobulins are elevated, the serum concentrations should always be checked simultaneously.

The immunoglobulin (Ig) fraction may be increased even if the total protein is within normal limits. Elevated CSF IgG is found in active multiple sclerosis and acute inflammatory polyradiculopathy. It may be found also with intracranial tumors and most other inflammatory CNS diseases, including encephalitis, meningitis, neurosyphilis, arachnoiditis, and subacute sclerosing panencephalitis (SSPE) to name only a few.

The rate of Ig synthesis in the CSF can be estimated as the CSF IgG index. Studies of MS patients have suggested that this index is a significantly more sensitive marker of local CNS immunoglobulin synthesis than the Ig concentration alone. A normal CSF index ranges from 0 to 0.77, where:

$$\text{CSF Ig index} = (\text{IgG}_{\text{CSF}} \times [\text{albumin}]_{\text{serum}}/([\text{albumin}]_{\text{CSF}} \times \text{IgG}_{\text{serum}})$$

Polyclonal immunoglobulins migrate in a diffuse band on an agarose gel with electrophoresis. Monoclonal immunoglobulins form discrete bands on the gel within the area of gamma globulin migration (Fig. 1-5). Because it is thought that each clone of B cells gives rise to a specific immunoglobulin, such oligoclonal bands must arise from only a few clones of cells.

CNS production is confirmed by establishing that discrete bands present in the CSF are not present in the serum. Oligoclonal bands have been most important in the diagnosis of multiple sclerosis: approximately 80 percent of patients with clinically definite MS have CSF oligoclonal bands. They are found in a variety of other conditions, however, including inflammatory polyneuropathies, neurosyphilis, cryptococcal meningitis, SSPE, and even cerebral infarction.

Microbiology

The most important point about microbiologic studies of CSF is that the yield of cultures increases with the number of organisms incubated and their viability at the time of culture. This means that the volume of CSF sent to microbiology and the rate at which it is transported and processed by the laboratory critically affect the diagnostic usefulness of the test. Large volumes of CSF are particularly important for fungal cultures because the density of these organisms in CSF is almost always very low. In evaluating a patient with chronic meningitis, CSF volumes as large as 15 to 20 cm^3 should be considered almost the minimum amount that should be sent for microbiologic examination.

The second point lies in the importance of the Gram stain in acute bacterial meningitis. The Gram stain takes no more than 5 minutes, has high sensitivity, and is extremely specific. Appropriate antibiotic therapy can often be chosen immediately after this test. Administering partial antibiotic treatment before the tap can alter bacterial membranes and significantly reduce the sensitivity, but the examination is always worthwhile.

In addition to culture, Gram stain, acid-fast bacillus (AFB) smear for tuberculosis, and the India ink smear for *Cryptococcus*, there are a variety of serology tests for viral, bacterial, and fungal antigens, the availability of which varies among laboratories.

Cytology

Cytologic examination of CSF allows identification of atypical cells present only in small numbers. It is most helpful for diagnosis of CNS neoplasms, particularly those with leptomeningeal involvement. Cytopathologic observation of malignant cells is not very sensitive, but is relatively specific. The examination may provide useful clues in other situations, as well, although in non-neoplastic disease cytopathologic evaluations are frequently too sensitive and nonspecific in defining abnormalities.

Only between 0.5 and 2.0 cm^3 of CSF are needed. The cells present are concentrated by one of three methods: membrane filtration, gravity sedimentation, or cytocentrifugation. The former is most popular and generally has the highest rate of cell recovery (between 70 and 80 percent). Not all histologic studies can be performed with each technique, so in specific cases one of the other, less efficient methods of concentration may be used.

A standard investigation involves preparation of a modified Papanicolou (Pap) smear. The Pap smear allows identification of gross cytoplasmic and nuclear cytologic characteristics. Normal CSF contains a few lymphocytes and macrophages, occasional cells from the choroid plexus, and cuboidal ependymal cells shed from the ventricular walls. Contaminants from skin and subcutaneous tissue and starch particles from gloves may also be found.

Inflammatory processes cause a leukocytosis, but may also be associated with diagnostic cytologic characteristics. The details of interpretation are beyond the scope of the present discussion, but a few examples will illustrate some of the uses of the method. Lymphocytes released in response to viral infections may show prominent nucleoli (potentially leading to confusion with neoplastic cells). Herpes simplex encephalitis can lead to formation of large intranuclear inclusions in lymphocytes or ependymal cells that may be diagnostic. In *Cryptococcus* infections the free yeast form may be recognized or seen intracellularly in macrophages.

Hemorrhage into the subarachnoid space will lead to the presence of macrophages distended by vacuoles. The macrophages are filled initially with erythrocytes and their lipid breakdown products and, later, hemosiderin. In various storage disorders, such as Tay-Sachs, foamy macrophages are filled with the inappropriately accumulating substance.

Identification of neoplastic cells is based on recognition of cytologic patterns associated with malignancy. The reliability of cytologic diagnosis of neoplasia increases with the number of signs of malignancy recognized. Reports are frequently phrased according to a simple classification system:

1. No evidence of malignancy
2. Atypical cells without signs of malignancy
3. Suspected malignancy
4. Definite malignancy

Malignant transformation is marked by characteristic changes in the structure of the cell and its staining properties. The ratio of nuclear to cytoplasmic volumes increases. Nuclei may show a markedly inhomogeneous chromatin, accommodate multiple nucleoli, and show considerable polymorphism between cells. With higher grade tumors, more fre-

Table 1-8. Typical Findings in Acute CNS Infections

Disease	Opening Pressure	Cell Count	Cell Type	Total Protein	Glucose
Viral					
Viral meningitis	N or ↑	+−++++[a]	P (early), L	N−+++	N[b]
Viral encephalitis	N or ↑	N−++++	P (early), L, RBC[c]	N−+++	N or ↓
Poliomyelitis	N or ↑	+−++++[d]	P (early)	N−++	N
Herpes zoster	N	+−++++	L	N−++	N
Bacterial					
Bacterial meningitis (untreated)	↑	+++−++++	N[e]	+−++++	↓
Brain abscess	↑	+−++++[f]	P	+−+++	↓
Myobacterial					
Tuberculous meningitis	↑	++−++++	L, M, some P	N−+++	↓[g]
Spirochetal[h]					
Leptospirosis[i]					
Initial stage	N	+−+++	P	N	N
Secondary stage	N	++−++++	L, P	N−++	N−[1]

[a] Very high counts suggest LCM.
[b] May be slightly reduced with mumps and LCM.
[c] RBC and xanthochromia characteristic of herpes simples or other necrotizing encephalitis.
[d] Cell count falls with time: acutely (preparalytic), about 200/mm^3; at 1 week, about 50/mm^3; at 1 mo, about 5/mm^3.
[e] Monocytes predominate with *Listeria monocytogenes* infections.
[f] Cell counts may be extremely high with rupture into ventricle.
[g] Characteristically low.
[h] See Table 1-9.
[i] Data from Gsell, 1978.

Values represent the majority of patients presenting, but not all.

Total protein (g/l)

0.45–0.75	+
0.75–1.00	+ +
1.01–5.00	+ + +
>5.01	+ + + +

Cell count (cells/mm^3)

5–25	+
26–50	+ +
51–150	+ + +
>151	+ + + +

Cell type

- L = Lymphocytes
- M = Monocytes
- P = Polymorphonuclear leukocytes
- E = Eosinophils
- RBC = Red blood cells

N = normal range

(Data from Fishman, 1980, except where otherwise noted.)

quent mitoses may be seen. More specific is that the mitoses appear abnormal, with three or more poles or showing atypical chromosomes. The cytoplasm may become more basophilic with increased RNA content. Specific types of tumors may show distinct patterns (e.g., cytoplasmic signet-ring inclusions in epithelial cell tumors).

A major application of CSF cytology is in evaluation for CNS spread of the acute leukemias and lymphomas that frequently diffusely seed the subarachnoid space. Specific antisera directed against B and T cells can be used for immunophenotypic characterization of leukocytes. Although general inflammatory states bring a mixed B- and T-cell response, T cells predominate. In contrast, malignancies usually involve proliferation of abnormal B-cell clones.

Immunohistochemical staining involves incubation, first with specific primary rabbit antiserum directed against either human B- or T-cell markers with the test slide, then with goat-anti-rabbit Ig (the bridge), and finally with a rabbit-anti-goat, peroxidase-linked antibody. When this preparation is treated with hydrogen peroxide and diaminobenzene, a colored precipitate is formed. The major problem with this technique is that sufficient CSF must be obtained for enough slides to be prepared to establish adequate controls. It should be noted that, with leukemias in which neoplastic cells are present in the peripheral blood, contamination of CSF by a traumatic tap can lead to false-positive results.

It is important to appreciate that the sensitivity of CSF examination for neoplasia is poor unless there is leptomeningeal involvement. One of the larger series (Glass et al., 1979) reports negative CSF studies in 98 percent (65/66) of patients without leptomeningeal spread, whereas 33 percent (5/15) of studies were positive with signs of focal meningeal disease, and 66 percent (25/38) were positive with signs of multifocal dissemination. Carcinomas of the lung and breast, melanomas, and carcinoma of the stomach are the metastatic tumors most likely to cause meningeal carcinomatosis.

CSF ABNORMALITIES IN DISEASE: GENERAL PRINCIPLES

The characteristics of CSF described earlier are each influenced by too many factors to allow for specific guidelines for interpretation of CSF abnormalities. Brief discussions of findings in specific disease processes follow. Further information is available in Tables 1-4 to 1-12.

Table 1-9. Typical Findings in Neurosyphilis

Disease	Opening Pressure	Cell Count[a]	Cell Type[a]	Total Protein[a]
Early	N	N–+ +	L	N or ↑
Latent	N	N	N	N
Subacute				
Syphilitic meningitis	N or ↑	+ – + + + +	L, M	N or ↑
Meningovascular	N or ↑	+ – + + +	M	N or ↑
General paresis	N	+ – + + +	M	↑
Tabetic	N	N– + +	M	N or ↑

[a] See footnote to Table 1-8 for explanation of abbreviations.
(Data from Fishman, 1980.)

Cerebrovascular Disease

Cerebrovascular ischemic or hemorrhagic events are associated with breakdown of the blood-brain barrier (grossly in hemorrhagic lesions) and a secondary inflammatory reaction to extravasated blood and necrotic tissue. After a large hemorrhage or ischemic event leading to cytotoxic edema, an early increase in opening pressure may occur. Increases in ICP are also seen with secondary obstruction of CSF outflow as a consequence of blood in the CSF.

Early after a hemorrhagic cerebrovascular accident (CVA), the ratio of WBC/RBC is similar to that in blood, but slowly a mild leukocytosis may develop with lymphocyte and monocyte predominance. Xanthochromia will be present from the first few hours after hemorrhage and will last for 3 to 4 weeks (see Fig. 1-3).

Subarachnoid hemorrhage is associated with decreased CSF glucose. However, despite increased CSF glycolytic rates in areas surrounding ischemic lesions, CSF glucose concentration is not depressed in uncomplicated ischemic lesions. CSF protein concentration will also be markedly elevated with hemorrhage due to extravasated blood. It is generally normal or only mildly elevated with ischemic events.

Central Nervous System Infection

Acute Meningitis

The diagnostic importance of early CSF examination for determining therapy in cases of suspected meningitis cannot be overemphasized. With untreated bacterial meningitis, the organism may be identified by gram stain in as many as 80 percent of cases and later recovered in culture in

Table 1-10. Typical CSF Findings in Chronic Infections of CNS[a]

Disease	Opening Pressure	Cell Count[b]	Cell Type[b]	Total Protein[b]	Glucose
Fungal					
Cryptococcus[c,d]	N or ↑	N–+ + + +	L, P	N–+ + +	↓
Coccidioidomycosis					
Early	↑	+ – + + +	P	N–+	N or ↓
Late	↓ or ↑	+ + + +	M, E[e]	+ + – + + + +	↓
Parasitic					
Toxoplasmosis[f]	N or ↑	N–+ +	M	+ – + + + +	N
Cysticerocosis	N or ↑	N–+ + + +	P, M, E	N–+ +	N or ↓

[a] See also Table 1-9. There is often significant variability in CSF manifestations of disease, depending on sites involved, the ability of the host to respond immunologically, and the stage of the infection.
[b] See footnote to Table 1-8 for explanation of abbreviations.
[c] CSF india ink-positive for spores.
[d] Data from Weenik and Bruyn, 1978.
[e] Occasional eosinophilia only.
[f] Data from Couvreur and Desmonts, 1978.
(Data from Fishman, 1980, except where otherwise noted.)

Table 1-11. CSF Findings in Noninfectious CNS Inflammatory Disorders

Disease	Cell Count[a]	Cell Type[a]	Total Protein[a]
Demylinating			
SSPE[b]	N	N	N–+ +
MS	+	L	N–+ +
Optic neuritis	+	M	N–+ +
GBS[c]	N	N	+ +–+ + + +
Vasculitides			
SLE	N–+ +	L, P[d]	N–+ +
Rheumatoid arthritis[e]	N	N	N
Giant cell arteritis			
Extracranial	N	N	N
Intracranial	N–+	L	N–+ + + +
Granulomatous angiitis	+–+ + + +	L	N–+ + + +
Idiopathic			
Mollaret's meningitis	+ + + +	M, P	+–+ +
Behçet syndrome[f]	+–+ + +	L	N–+
Sarcoidosis[g]	N–+ +	M	N–+ + +
Chemical			
Meningitis	+ + +–+ + + +	P, L	+ +–+ + + +
Lumbar disc	N–+ +	L	N–+ +

[a] See footnote to Table 1-8 for explanation of abbreviations.
[b] Immunoglobulin-globulin fraction is elevated to 20–50% of total protein.
[c] In some cases a moderate pleocytosis may be observed later in the course of the disease. Maximal total protein concentration occurs between 4–14 days after onset. It is usually normal initially.
[d] Need to rule out opportunistic infection, especially when polymorphonuclear leukocytes are prominent.
[e] Elevated protein concentration may accompany arthritis in spinal arachnoiditis.
[f] Data from Alema, 1978.
[g] CSF glucose concentration usually decreased.
(Data from Fishman, 1980, except where otherwise noted.)

a somewhat greater percentage of cases. After partial treatment, the sensitivity of these tests falls, but can remain as high as 60 percent. Gram stains or cultures are rarely positive with a brain abscess unless it has ruptured into the CSF.

As early viral infections may present with a predominance of granulocytes (e.g., echovirus) and protein concentration elevations may be modest in bacterial meningitis, evaluation of CSF glucose often determines whether empiric antibiotic therapy is begun (Table 1-8). Occasionally, CSF glucose concentration is slightly reduced in mumps meningitis and lym-

Table 1-12. Typical Findings in Neoplastic Diseases

Disease	Opening Pressure	Cell Count[a]	Cell Type[a]	Total Protein[a]	Glucose
Intraparenchymal tumor	N or ↑	N–+ +	L[b]	N–+ + +[c]	N
Meningeal carcinomatosis	N or ↑	N–+ + + +	L, P[b]	N–+ + + +	N or ↓
Paraneoplastic syndromes					
Progressive multifocal leukoencephalopathy	N	N	N	N	N
Subacute cerebellar degeneration	N	N–+	M	N–+ +	N
Carcinomatous polyneuropathy	N	N	N	N–+ + +	N
Spinal cord tumor[d]	N or ↓[e]	N–+	M[b]	N–+ + + +	N

[a] See footnote to Table 1-8 for explanation of abbreviations.
[b] Malignant cells may be found with cytologic examination. See text.
[c] Higher values associated with the more vascular tumors that show greater breakdown of the blood-brain barrier.
[d] In general there is little difference between intramedullary and extradural tumors.
[e] Sign of spinal block obstructing CSF flow.
(Data from Fishman, 1980.)

phocytic choriomeningitis. Rarely, it is normal early in bacterial meningitis. The pleocytosis may actually continue to increase for the first 24 hours after the start of effective therapy for acute bacterial meningitis, but should begin to decrease significantly over the next 2 days. A persistent depression of CSF glucose for 2 weeks or more may be seen, despite a good clinical response to therapy.

Tuberculosis classically may have a distinctive presentation with low CSF glucose concentrations in association with lymphocytosis. Parasitic infections are notable for giving CSF eosinophilia, although this may be absent with solely parenchymal lesions. Also notable is the occasional presence of RBCs, presumably from microhemorrhages. RBCs are also seen in encephalitic processes.

Chronic Meningitis

The syndrome of chronic meningitis is defined on the basis of the chronic clinical course and signs of meningeal inflammation, particularly increased protein concentration and leukocytic pleocytosis. Infectious, neoplastic, vasculitic, and granulomatous processes, as well as chemical irritants may give rise to this syndrome. Consistent with the chronic course, the protein concentration elevation and cellularity are mild to moderate (Table 1-10). Most etiologies lead to lymphocytic predominance, although chemical irritation, systemic lupus erythematosus (SLE), and certain relatively unusual bacterial (*Actinomyces, Listeria,* and *Nocardia*) and fungal infections can be associated with a neutrophilic reaction. As mentioned earlier, large quantities of CSF and repeated cultures are needed to rule out infectious etiologies because of the indolent nature of these agents.

Neurosyphilis

The clinical manifestations of neurosyphilis are myriad: syphilitic meningitis, vascular syphilis, general paresis, and tabes dorsalis. An unreactive peripheral blood fluorescent treponemal antibody absorption (FTA-ABS) test excludes the possibility of neurosyphilis. Examination of the CSF is probably warranted in all patients not adequately treated who have positive serology, even with no neurologic signs or complaints. However, perhaps 20 percent of patients with neurosyphilis will have a normal CSF examination. Because of this fact, the severity of the condition, and the relatively few risks associated with treatment, many choose to treat all cases of suspected neurosyphilis, whether clearly active or not. Late tabes dorsalis may be associated with a normal CSF examination in the face of significant neurologic deficits, but these presumably arise from old, fixed lesions that will not be significantly affected by treatment.

Asymptomatic primary syphilis may be associated with mild CSF abnormalities but their significance is uncertain. In contrast, syphilitic meningitis is associated frequently with increased ICP, a marked lymphocytosis, and moderate hypoglycorrhachia. Chronic inflammation, usually with a monocytosis of under 150 to 200 cells/cm^3, mild to moderately increased total protein concentration, increased IgG, and a usually normal glucose concentration are seen in general paresis. The cellularity and increased total protein concentration are more modest in tabes dorsalis.

If neurosyphilis is treated without complications, repeat examinations every 6 months for 2 years or until the CSF is normal are recommended.

Bacterial Endocarditis

Septic emboli from bacterial endocarditis can lead to diverse abnormalities ranging from multiple focal abscesses to subarachnoid hemorrhages or solely ischemic lesions. CSF abnormalities are similarly diverse. Most commonly the CSF is normal, but (as implied by the clinical symptoms) it may be purulent with hypoglycorrhachia, and it may show signs of chronic inflammation or fresh blood, depending on the clinical syndrome.

Encephalitis

Common viral meningitides may also present with encephalitic signs, which are usually minor and fully reversible. Early recognition of the less common necrotizing encephalitides is important, as the most common, herpes simplex encephalitis, shows a good response to systemic antiviral therapy. The focal temporal lobe cerebritis causes mass effect and elevates CSF pressure. Even extensive parenchymatous disease may give rather low cell counts, usually between 50 and 100 cells/mm^3, consisting of predominantly lymphocytes after the initial phase. Most specific is the association of moderate lymphocytic pleocytosis with RBCs and xanthochromia. Total protein concentration is usually moderately elevated, but can be normal.

Central Demyelinating Disease

Central demyelinating processes may acutely give rise to a mild lymphocytic pleocytosis and moderately increased CSF protein concentration (Table 1-7). CSF in about one-third of patients presenting with active MS is characterized by mild elevation of protein and a mild lymphocytosis.

However, if there are more than 50 cells/mm^3, the diagnosis is unlikely. Positive oligoclonal bands and elevated CSF IgG (in the absence of a corresponding increase in serum IgG) are much more frequently found.

Polyneuritis

Characteristic of the acute idiopathic polyneuritis of the Guillain-Barré syndrome is the so-called albumino-cytologic dissociation, marked by minimal cellularity with a dramatic increase in CSF total protein concentration (Table 1-11). This may only be found a week or so after the onset of symptoms. It is hypothesized that permeability changes in the capillaries of the spinal roots are responsible for the increased total protein. This pattern is also found with other inflammatory processes involving dorsal root ganglia (e.g., herpes zoster). Chronic inflammatory polyneuropathies are usually associated with minimal pleocytosis and an increase in protein concentration.

Vasculitides

It is difficult to make many generalizations about CSF findings in the vasculitides except to emphasize that findings are nonspecific and that the presence of abnormalities is a relatively insensitive sign of active disease (Table 1-7). In general, hypersensitivity vasculitides that involve the small meningeal vessels may be more likely than the large vessel arteritides to produce an inflammatory profile in the CSF. The primarily meningeal inflammation in idiopathic processes, such as Behçet syndrome or Mollaret's meningitis, is apparent in the CSF.

Degenerative and Metabolic Diseases

Examination of the CSF is an important part of the workup for degenerative and metabolic diseases, primarily because it can rule out other etiologies of CNS dysfunction. The findings are almost never specific enough for diagnosis of these disorders.

Dementias of the Alzheimer's type and related disorders may result in a minimal elevation of CSF protein but otherwise normal CSF. In a small fraction of patients with Alzheimer's disease there is a mild monocytosis and in one-third of patients the protein is elevated. Specific proteins associated with different dementing processes may be able to be identified in CSF in the near future.

Cell counts exceeding 10 lymphocytes/mm^3 or total protein in excess of 1.0 g/L are almost never found in amyotrophic lateral sclerosis. Degenerative bony changes, such as lumbar disc disease or cervical spondylosis, may be associated with a meningeal chronic inflammatory response, but it is usually mild.

Diabetic sensory neuropathies involving sensory root ganglia can lead to marked elevations of total protein; two-thirds of patients may have protein concentrations between 0.5 and 2.25 g/L. However, positive oligoclonal bands or increased CSF IgG are not characteristic of diabetes. Significant cellularity also is not usual.

Hepatic encephalopathy is not associated with any specific finding in routine testing, although CSF protein may be elevated in comatose patients. In contrast, uremic encephalopathy is often associated with a moderate elevation of CSF protein concentration.

The CSF in toxic encephalopathies is generally unremarkable, except with lead, which causes diffuse cerebral edema. In addition to increased opening pressure, a moderate monocytic pleocytosis and elevated total protein concentration can be seen.

Neoplastic Disease

Examination of CSF is potentially risky and frequently unrewarding in evaluation of neoplastic diseases (Table 1-12). Mass effects can raise the opening pressure. Depending on the location of the mass lesion(s), this may lead to uncal herniation with the change in CSF hemodynamics following LP.

Parenchymatous lesions may increase CSF protein concentration with breakdown of the blood-brain barrier secondary to neovascularization. Xanthochromia from microhemorrhages or gross bleeding is also sometimes seen. Meningeal involvement is classically associated with hypoglycorrhachia, a mild pleocytosis, mild to moderately increased protein, and increased pressure. Increased protein concentration may also be the sole manifestation. Only in the case of meningeal carcinomatosis is the diagnostic yield of cytologic examination significant: carefully prepared Pap stains may show malignant cells in over two-thirds of cases. Paraneoplastic syndromes may be associated with increased total protein without cellularity.

Epilepsy and Migraine

Short-lived, mild pleocytosis may develop after generalized seizures. More profound changes suggest other processes in addition to the seizure. During migraine attacks, both increased cellularity and protein concentration have been noted, although this is certainly not generally true.

A Few Empiric Rules

As stated at the opening of this section, it is difficult to establish clear general guidelines for the interpretation of CSF findings because the parameters are rather nonspecific. However, the following rules apply to CSF interpretation.

1. As the volume of the cranial vault is limited, edema, masses, or chronic inflammation can *increase* the opening pressure. Increased central venous pressure with abdominal compression by tensed muscles in the anxious patient or secondary to congestive heart failure will also increase intracranial pressure. Conversely, obstruction of CSF flow in the spinal subarachnoid space will lead to *decreased* opening pressure.
2. Increase numbers *polymorphonuclear leukocytes* are associated with acute infections. *Lymphocytes* or *monocytes* are found with chronic infections. *Eosinophils* (relatively rarely seen) are associated with reactions to foreign bodies, tumors, or parasitic infections.
3. CSF glucose concentration is depressed by processes that cause meningeal inflammation, particularly when granulomatous, bacterial, or carcinomatous.
4. CSF total protein concentration is elevated by breakdown of the blood-brain barrier secondary to inflammation, trauma, or tumor neovascularization. Increased CSF immunoglobulin concentration, frequently with monoclonal species (oligoclonal bands) is seen in local inflammatory processes from autoimmune disease, infection, or tissue damage.

READINGS

Alema G: Behçet's disease. p. 475. In Vinkin PJ, Bruyn GN (eds): Handbook of Neurology. Vol. 34. Elsevier Science Publishing, Amsterdam, 1978

Bigner SH, Johnston WW: Cytopathology of the Central Nervous System. Masson, New York, 1983

Boss J, Thornton GF: Infectious Diseases of the Central Nervous System. Neurologic Clinics. Vol. 4, WB Saunders, Philadelphia, 1986

Cole M: Examination of the CSF. p. 29. In Toole JF (ed): Neurologic Diagnosis. FA Davis, Philadelphia, 1969

Couvreur J, Desmonts G: Toxoplasmosis. p. 115. In Vinkin PJ, Bruyn GN (eds): Handbook of Neurology. Vol. 35. Elsevier Science Publishing, Amsterdam, 1978

Fishman RA: Cerebrospinal Fluid in Disease of the Nervous System. WB Saunders, Philadelphia, 1980

Glass JP, Melamed M, Chernick NL, Posner JB: The meaning of positive CSF cytology. Neurology 29:1369, 1979

Gold E: Serologic and virus isolation studies of patients with varicella or herpes zoster infection. New Engl J Med 274:181, 1966

Gsell OR: Leptospirosis and relapsing fever. p. 395. In Vinkin PJ, Bruyn GN (eds): Handbook of Neurology. Vol. 33. Elsevier Science Publishing, Amsterdam, 1978

Koberski T: Eosinophilia in the cerebrospinal fluid. Ann Intern Med 91:70, 1979

Kolmel HW: Atlas of Cerebrospinal Fluid Cells. 2nd Ed. Springer-Verlag, New York, 1977

Korein J, Cravioto H, Leicach M: Reevaluation of the lumbar puncture: a study of 129 patients with papilledema and intracranial hypertension. Neurology 9:290, 1959

Latovski N, Abrams G, Clark C et al: Cerebral cystercerosis. Neurology 28:838, 1978

Macintosh R, Lee JA: Lumbar Puncture and Spinal Analgesia. 3rd Ed. Churchill Livingstone, Edinburgh, 1973

Maren TF: CSF, aqueous tumor, and endolymph. In Mountcastle VB (ed): Medical Physiology, Vol. II. CV Mosby, St Louis, pp. 1218, 1980

Marton KI, Gean AD: The spinal tap: a new look at an old test. Ann Intern Med 104:840, 1986

Mathies AW: Influenza meningitis. p. 53. In Vinkin PJ, Bruyn GN (eds): Handbook of Neurology. Vol. 33. Elsevier Science Publishing, Amsterdam, 1978

Millen JW, Woolam DHM: The Anatomy of the Cerebrospinal Fluid. Oxford University Press, London, 1962.

Petito F, Plum F: The lumbar puncture. New Engl J Med 290:225, 1974

Raymond JR, Raymond PA: Post-lumbar puncture headache: etiology and management. West J Med 148:551, 1988

Simon RP: Neurosyphilis. Arch Neurol 42:606, 1985

Swartz M, O'Hanley P: Central nervous system infections. pp. viii, 1. In Rubenstein E, Federman D (eds): Scientific American Medicine. Scientific American, New York, 1987

Weenik HR, Bruyn GW: Cryptococcus of the nervous system. p. 459. In Vinkin PJ, Bruyn GN (eds): Handbook of Neurology. Vol. 35. Elsevier Science Publishing, Amsterdam, 1978

ULTRASOUND TECHNIQUES FOR EVALUATING CEREBROVASCULAR DISEASE 2

Intra-arterial digital subtraction angiography (IA-DSA) still provides the best visualization of intracranial and extracranial vessels (see Ch. 3). Both large and small vessel disease can be studied. Vascular malformations can be defined. Information on flow in the larger vessels is also available from the sequence of changes in images collected serially after dye injection. Cardiac angiography and ventriculography provide similar information for cardiac vessels, define wall motion and valve function, and can identify abnormal structures such as vegetations, wall thrombi, and myxomas. However, these techniques are invasive, and carry significant potential morbidity. Thus, great interest has arisen in alternative noninvasive techniques to evaluate cerebrovascular disease.

There are several indirect methods of evaluating blood flow in the carotid arteries (e.g., supraorbital Doppler, phonangiography, and ocular plethysmography), but they are now largely of historic interest. Current routine techniques rely on ultrasound to define anatomy and flow characteristics of the common, internal, and external carotid arteries around the carotid bifurcation. B-mode ultrasound provides a two-dimensional image from which vessel patency and wall characteristics can be directly determined. Doppler studies complement this with measurements of blood flow velocity and turbulence. Duplex studies provide both B-mode and Doppler data simultaneously.

Echocardiography is the primary technique for direct identification of potential sources of cardiac emboli. M-mode ultrasound studies can be used to define valve dysfunction arising from vegetations with endocarditis or other abnormalities. However, in general, this is not the examination of choice for neurologic problems. B-mode echocardiography provides a two-dimensional image of the heart chambers, allowing study of wall motion and visualization of large thrombi. Valve motion can also be examined and surface characteristics demonstrated. Patent septal foramina can be seen or their presence inferred from tracing the course of echogenic bubbles introduced into the right side of the heart after intravenous injection.

Several years ago, intravenous digital subtraction angiography (IV-DSA) was introduced, in an effort to provide a noninvasive approach to visualization of the intracranial and intrathoracic vessels and the extracranial vessels of the posterior circulation. Unfortunately, image quality is much poorer than with IA-DSA. Even with optimal studies, medium- and small-sized vessels cannot be visualized well. In addition, important information about hemodynamics acquired by observation of the time course of vessel filling in selective IA-DSA is lost. Large dye loads are needed, which increases patient morbidity. There is now no role for this technique.

The latest approach to cerebrovascular imaging is magnetic resonance angiography (MRI). This exciting technique potentially offers visualization of both intracranial and extracranial medium and large vessels, at least limited quantitation of flow velocities, and tissue characterization of vessel wall abnormalities. However, MRI is just beginning to enter the clinical arena and will not be discussed further here.

After a brief review of the relevant pathologic features of cerebrovascular disease, we will discuss the clinical application of ultrasound techniques to its study in adult neurology.

PATHOLOGY OF CEREBROVASCULAR DISEASE

Thrombotic Disease

Most atherosclerotic cerebrovascular disease is extracranial. Hemodynamic stresses contribute to development of lesions: atherosclerosis is most pronounced around sites of turbulence in major arteries such as the internal carotid just distal to the bifurcation, the origins of the internal or common carotid arteries or the vertebral arteries, and the basilar artery. Smaller intracranial vessels are much less involved, possibly because of reduced wall stresses with lower perfusion pressures. However, in diabetics, Orientals, and blacks, disease of the siphon region of the middle cerebral artery (MCA) is more commonly found. Patients with long-standing hypertension, diabetes, or vasculitis may have small-vessel disease.

Atherosclerotic lesions can lead to distal hypoperfusion by narrowing vessel caliber. With mild to moderate stenosis, distal flow can be maintained by increases in perfusion pressure. The resistance to flow is inversely proportional to the vessel cross-sectional area. It is important to keep in mind that the latter is proportional to the *square* of the radius. Thus, a 25 percent progression (from 50 to 75 percent stenosis) results in greater than a 300 percent increase in resistance in blood flow. For the internal carotid, a residual lumen diameter of less than about 2 mm begins to become hemodynamically significant at normal perfusion pressures. Even larger lumens may result in impaired flow if two sites along the same vessel (e.g., at the carotid bifurcation and in the MCA siphon) are affected.

Embolic Disease

The atherosclerotic plaques that enlarge to form stenotic lesions also predipose to embolism (artery-to-artery). Platelets can be activated on the abnormal endothelial surfaces. Histologic characteristics of plaques reflect their potential for generating platelet or cholesterol emboli. Simple calcified plaques do not appear to generate platelet emboli frequently unless they have enlarged to the point of causing significant vessel stenosis and marked alterations in local blood flow. However, subintimal hemorrhages can occur that may dislodge calcified particles or cholesterol crystals as embolic showers. The resulting endothelial ulceration promotes formation of loosely adherent platelet aggregates. Local hemorrhage can also lead to formation of a mural thrombus in an ulcerated plaque.

Emboli also arise from the heart. Cardiac emboli may be responsible for as many as 15 to 30 percent of all ischemic strokes. Abnormal cardiac wall motion after a myocardial infarction (MI), during atrial fibrillation, or with a dilated cardiomyopathy allows local stasis of blood and thrombus formation. Mobile thrombi that extend into the ventricular chamber or thrombi on irregularly contracting segments of wall have a high probability of embolization. With atrial fibrillation, small thrombi tend to form in the atria, particularly the atrial appendage.

Valvular disease is a potential source of platelet, fibrin, or infected emboli. Valve motion abnormalities are frequently present before vegetations can be visualized. Artificial valve surfaces are particularly strong stimuli to platelet activation. Advanced rheumatic heart disease is also associated with a very high rate of systemic embolization, because several factors simultaneously present predispose to embolization: poor valve motion, an abnormal valve surface, atrial fibrillation, and the dilated cardiomyopathy.

An increased risk of emboli has been associated with idiopathic mitral valve prolapse (MVP). However, MVP can be demonstrated by echocardiography in as much as 20 percent of the female population, so clearly the overall risk is low. Calcific aortic stenosis is a similar problem among the elderly; it is common and occasionally the only abnormal finding in patients with stroke. Some studies have associated it with embolic stroke, but any causal relationship remains speculative.

Deep venous thromboses are rare causes of cerebral emboli. They can give rise to paradoxic emboli, so-called because right-sided emboli should normally be trapped in the microvasculature of the pulmonary circulation. A patent foramen ovale can provide a right-to-left shunt for such an embolus. Such shunts can be intermittent. In a significant percentage of otherwise normal individuals, the foramen ovale is closed by a loose flap of tissue kept in place only by the pressure differential between the right and left atria. When the pressure differential is transiently reversed (for example, with the pulmonary hypertension following a pulmonary embolus), the foramen ovale opens, establishing a path for emboli to the brain.

PRINCIPLES OF ULTRASOUND EXAMINATIONS

Studying Morphology with Ultrasound

Both carotid duplex and echocardiography instruments use ultrasound (frequencies of 4 to 8 MHz, well above the threshold of human hearing) to generate an image. The sound waves are transmitted only through compressible media. At interfaces between two different tissues, a portion of the incident beam is reflected, giving rise to an echo. The amount reflected increases as differences in acoustic impedance (a physical property related to density) between the two media increases. Ultrasound energy is also randomly dissipated into the medium.

An image is generated by correlation of signals in a sequence of transmitted pulses with the corresponding echoes. As the time required for a reflected signal to return to the detector is proportional to the distance traveled, the position of a reflecting surface (which is the interface between two tissues or other conducting media) relative to the ultrasound probe can be determined. The generated image, therefore, represents outlines of interfaces within the volume studied.

An M-mode ultrasound image is a one-dimensional plot of acoustic reflectance from interfaces at different depths in a sample as a function of time. When sampling over a cardiac valve, it gives good information on valve motion. It can be used also to define linear dimensions across the

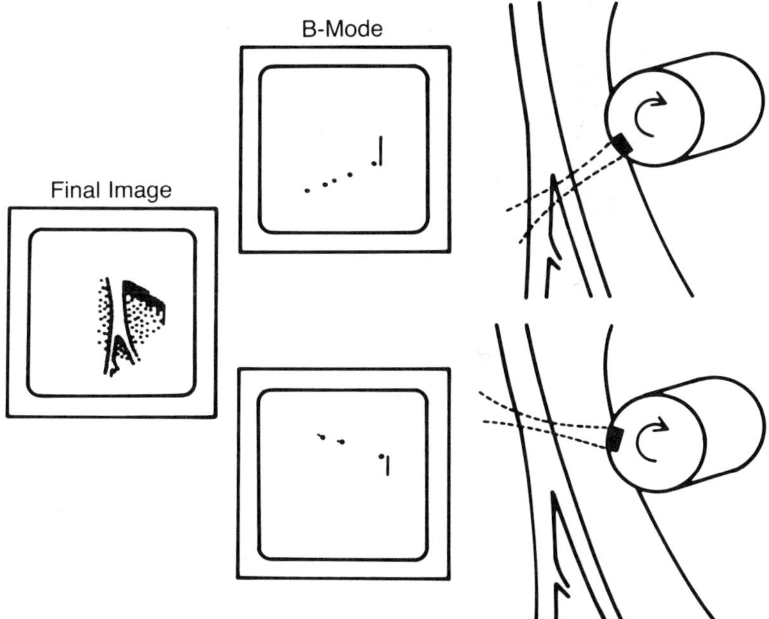

Fig. 2-1. Ultrasonic B-mode scanning. The position and orientation of the incident ultrasound beam, along with the echo return time, are used to place echo signals in their representative anatomic positions on the display. (From Zweibel, 1986, with permission.)

heart chambers. However, with the general availability of two-dimensional B-mode scanning, M-mode scanning is generally of little use in neurologic investigations.

B-mode ultrasound scanning develops an image by segmental scanning over an approximately 120-degree arc, using a rotating or fixed array of tiny piezoelectric crystals to generate ultrasound signals (Fig. 2-1). Sweep repetition times are rapid and a video image is maintained through each scan period, allowing a real-time image to be presented. The image is fan-shaped, as the ultrasound beams are linearly divergent from the probe (Fig. 2-2). Resolution and contrast fall off at the limits of the image as the ultrasound energy is dissipated.

Penetration of the ultrasound beam is determined by both the number and nature of the reflecting interfaces and energy dissipation. In a given

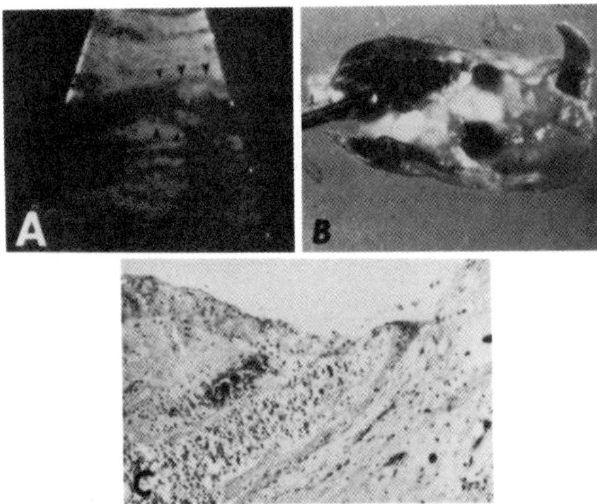

Fig. 2-2. Differences in acoustic impedence among normal vessel walls, flowing blood, consolidating hemorrhage, fibrin deposits, and calcifications allows the histology of vessel wall abnormalities to be inferred from the B-mode scan. In this example from a diseased carotid later studied after endartectomy: **(A)** an ultrasonogram of a lesion with heterogeneous plaque; **(B)** gross specimen of the same lesion, which shows a large, recent intraplaque hemorrhage (pointer); and **(C)** a photomicrograph from the same plaque showing acute hemorrhage (hematoxylin and eosin, ×125). (From Reilly, et al., 1983, with permission.)

sample, penetration decreases as the scanning frequency increases. Lower frequencies (<5 MHz) are used when deeper penetration is required (e.g., for studies of cardiac valve and wall motion). Higher frequencies (>7 MHz) are used for examinations of the more superficial carotid arteries. An advantage of higher frequencies is that they allow increased linear resolution.

One important cause of poor penetration and low signal intensity is shadowing, which occurs when the major proportion of the transmitted signal is returned by a highly reflecting interface superficial to the area of interest (Fig. 2-3). Calcium in bone or vessel wall plaques may cause shadowing. Shadowing may make it impossible to measure precisely the residual lumen diameter at the site of a calcified, stenosing plaque, for example. An intervening poorly conducting medium, such as air (which conducts ultrasound relatively poorly), will reduce penetration. Thus echocardiographic studies on patients with hyperinflated lungs from chronic obstructive pulmonary disease (COPD) are often of poor quality.

The intensity of the reflected signal at the probe changes with the angle of the incident beam with respect to the reflecting surface. It is greatest when the beam is perpendicular (90 degrees) to the plane of the reflecting surface. This fact must be taken into account when assessing variations in echogenicity across an image.

Imaging Carotid Arteries with Ultrasound

Although imaging of large intracerebral vessels is now possible, the most important role of ultrasound techniques in cerebrovascular disease is still in evaluating the extracranial carotid arteries. Useful images of the common carotid artery from the clavicle to the level of the bifurcation and the origins of the internal and external carotid arteries to as high as the angle of the jaw may be obtained.

A technically good study demands patient cooperation. The patient lies with shoulders relaxed and head gently extended away in slight flexion to maximize access to the area over the arteries. The technician obtains images in real time as the probe is positioned over the course of the artery in the neck. An acoustic gel is placed between the transducer and skin.

The reliability of an examination depends on operator skill and anatomic features of the vessel examined. Localization is the initial problem. Unequivocal identification of vessels is best achieved with a longitudinal image that includes the common carotid and the bifurcation. Expansion at the carotid bulb may distinguish the internal carotid from the external carotid.

Transverse images through areas of suspected stenosis usually best define any narrowing. Because the diseased lumen is not a perfect circle, at least two views in different planes are needed to estimate residual lumen diameters (Fig. 2-3). Good measurements cannot always be made. In obese patients, those with limited neck mobility, or those unable to cooperate for other reasons, it may be technically impossible to obtain images from the required orientations. Tortuous vessels may be impossible to appropriately align within the image.

The echogenic character of the vessel wall may provide clues about the histology of wall lesions (Fig. 2-2). Normal arterial walls yield two echogenic bands from the outer face of the adventitia and inner face of the intima. The luminal surface of the intima should be echo-free and merge with the hypoechogenic lumen of flowing blood.

Fibrofatty plaques of uncomplicated atherosclerosis are only faintly echogenic, particularly when small. Thrombus resting on a plaque also has an acoustic impedance similar to blood. Fibrous plaques are moderately echogenic and less likely to be missed.

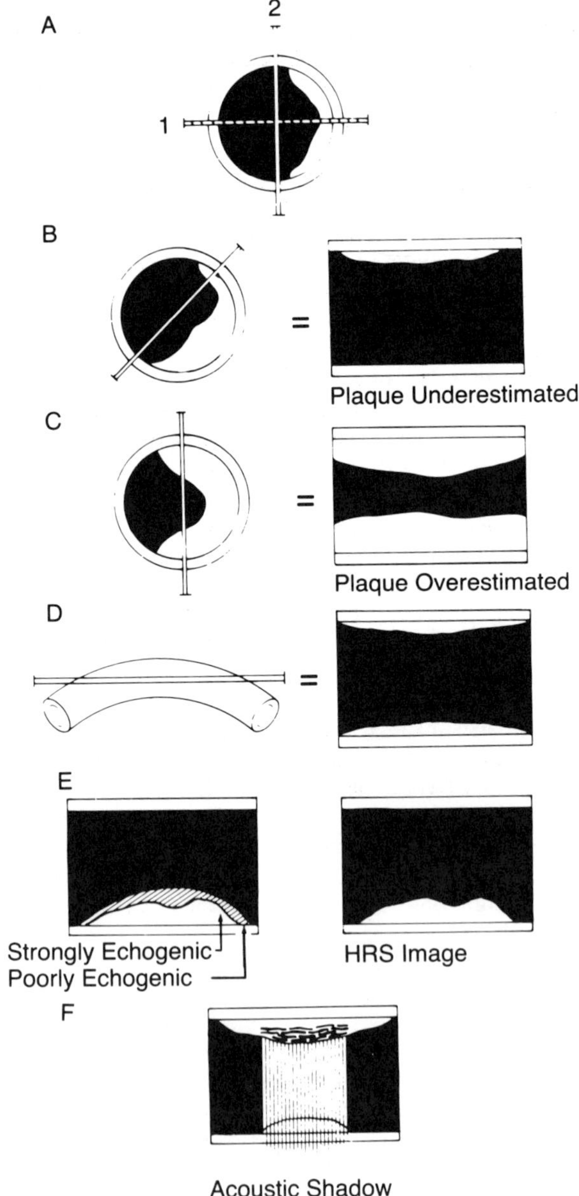
A
2
1
B
=
Plaque Underestimated
C
=
Plaque Overestimated
D
=
E
Strongly Echogenic
Poorly Echogenic
HRS Image
F
Acoustic Shadow

Calcifications in plaques are highly echogenic. Inhomogeneously echogenic calcified plaques with an inner hypodense layer may represent hemorrhagic plaques. Acute hemorrhage and plaque disruption is thought to be an important cause of artery-to-artery embolic disease. Hypoechoic regions along a plaque may represent ulcerations or thrombus within an ulcerated area. However, variations in the echoes from along the wall may also represent artifacts, particularly if a variation is visible in only one plane of view.

The sensitivity of modern B-mode ultrasound instruments for identifying plaques has been a point of debate. It is probably largely determined by operator skill, and in the best hands, sensitivity is probably excellent.

B-mode ultrasound is relatively sensitive to significant stenosis in the areas that can be visualized. The major problem is that, with high-grade stenosis, which usually arises from calcified lesions at the site of occlusion, signal alterations and shadowing by large plaques may impair resolution sufficiently to make it impossible to define the small residual lumen. In consequence, high-grade stenosis may be misinterpreted as total occlusion. Distinction between occlusion and high-grade stenosis is clinically important; therefore, when ultrasound suggests total occlusion in a symptomatic patient, angiography is usually indicated.

Evaluation of Flow with Doppler Studies

Information obtained on blood flow within the vessel is complementary to that obtained from B-mode studies. It can be particularly helpful if total occlusion is suspected on the basis of the B-mode examination. Flow information can be obtained from ultrasound studies using the Doppler effect.

If the reflecting surface is stationary, the frequency of the reflected ultrasound beam is unchanged from that of the incident beam. However, if the reflecting surface is moving with respect to the ultrasound source,

Fig. 2-3. Sources of error in B-mode ultrasound plaque diagnosis: **(A)** Longitudinal images along line 1 will demonstrate the plaque deposit, but longitudinal sections along line 2 will not; **(B)** a longitudinal section along the line shown will underestimate the severity of the plaque; **(C)** longitudinal sections along this line will overestimate plaque severity; **(D)** longitudinal sections through a curving vessel may suggest the presence of plaque when none is present, since portions of the vessel are not imaged directly along the vessel diameter; **(E)** plaque severity may be underestimated when strongly echogenic plaque is not seen; and **(F)** acoustic shadowing may obscure plaque. (From Zweibel et al., 1983, with permission.)

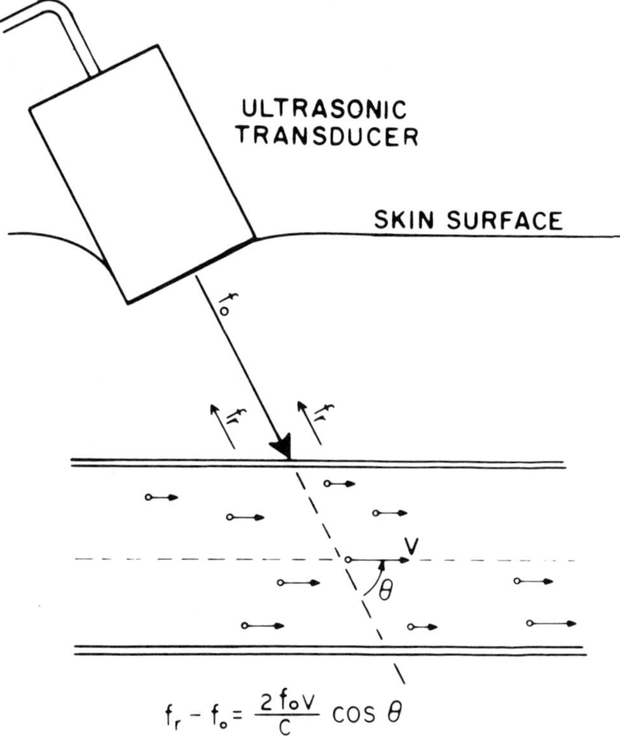

Fig. 2-4. Arrangement for obtaining Doppler signals from blood. The frequency of the beam reflected from moving red cells (f_r) is shifted from that of the incident beam (f_o). The amount of the so-called Doppler shift ($f_r - f_o$) is proportional to the velocity of the flowing blood (V) for a given angle of the transducer with respect to the direction of flow (θ). The speed of sound in the medium (c) is a physical constant. (From Zweibel, 1986, with permission.)

the frequency of the reflected sound will be shifted in frequency by the Doppler effect (Fig. 2-4). The frequency of the reflected beam increases with movement toward the source and decreases for movement away from it. The magnitude of this frequency shift (the so-called Doppler shift) is proportional to the relative velocities of the source and the reflecting surface. It also varies with the angle of the incident beam relative to the direction of movement: it is maximal when the two are parallel and drops

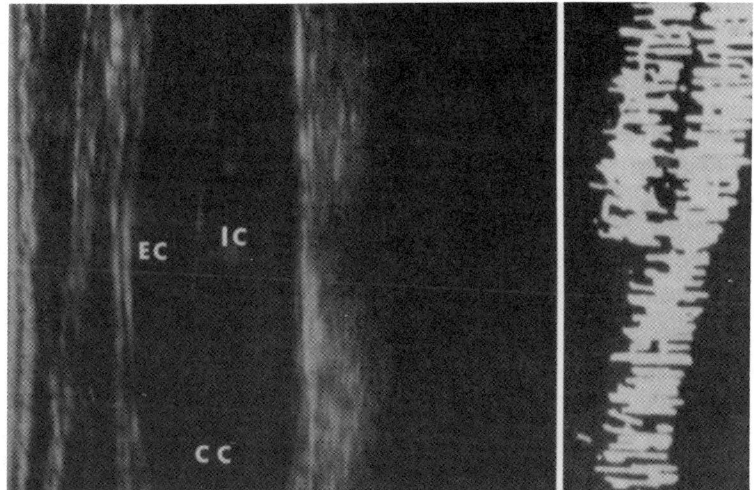

Fig. 2-5. **(A)** Longitudinal B-mode and **(B)** Doppler images of the common carotid bifurcation. EC, external carotid; IC, internal carotid; CC, common carotid. (From Ackerman, 1983, with permission.)

to zero when the incident beam is exactly perpendicular to the direction of motion. Thus, if the angle between the direction of motion and the incident beam is known, the relative velocity of movement can be accurately calculated from any frequency shift.

Red blood cells (RBC), the membranes of which have a different acoustic impedance from serum, are good ultrasound reflecting surfaces in whole blood. The proportion of an incident beam reflected by flowing blood is directly proportional to the hematocrit. A continuous wave ultrasound source and a receiver that filters out sound at the transmitted frequency can be used to generate a signal that arises only from ultrasound reflected from moving surfaces (e.g., RBC) (Fig. 2-5). This can be used qualitatively to identify flowing blood.

In practice, it is more useful combine flow and spatial information. This can be accomplished by combining a pulse train generator with a receiver to record the Doppler shift as a function of the time of the echo relative to the transmitted pulse. The echo time defines linear position with respect to the probe. The Doppler shift defines flow of the red cells with respect to the transmitter at that point. A simple flow-imaging Doppler device links a continuous-wave or pulsed Doppler probe to a flexible mechanical arm, the position of which, with respect to the plane of the neck, can be correlated with the intensity of the Doppler signal in the echo. This allows a spatially oriented, qualitative flow image of the carotid circulation to be developed. Range-gating, which permits echoes to be recorded only after a specified echo delay interval, allows selection of flow at a defined depth. This may eliminate unwanted contributions from overlying veins. However, these images are crude, time-consuming to generate, and of very limited use by themselves.

Quantitative information on flow velocities within a vessel is much more valuable. Flow velocities in a normal vessel vary across the lumen and change with the size of the lumen. Fluid near the vessel wall moves slowly, whereas fluid in the lumen center moves most rapidly. In larger vessels, flow has a blunt profile in which most of the fluid moves at about the same, rapid velocity as that in the center. In contrast, a small or stenotic vessel has only a small proportion of relatively rapidly moving fluid at the center of the lumen, with the largest proportion slowed by close proximity to the walls. Vessel wall irregularities or extreme narrowing create high velocity, turbulent flow. Turbulent flow is characterized by a broad range of velocities and directions of flow.

Thus the Doppler signal from a vessel consists of signals with a range of amplitudes and frequencies, corresponding to the different volumes of the fluid moving with different velocities. The data can be analyzed in plots of Doppler shift frequency as a function of signal amplitude (spectral analysis). Spectral analysis of the Doppler signal from the full vessel lumen can be used to infer the degree of local vessel stenosis.

The cardiac cycle causes flow in the carotids to be pulsatile. Analysis of pulsatile flow characteristics allows inferences to be made concerning lumen diameters distal and proximal to the sites of examination (Fig. 2-6), based on the general principle that the difference between maximum and minimum flow rates in a pulsatile system is increased as the resistance to flow rises. The normal internal carotid artery is a high-volume, low-resistance system. The pulsatile flow shows a broad, smooth systolic peak with diastolic flow equivalent to as much as one-third of peak systolic flow. In contrast, in the external carotid, where distal resistance is high, the systolic peak is sharper and the diastolic flow rate is relatively slower.

Narrowing of vessels will generate an abnormal signal pattern through the cardiac cycle. With increasing stenosis just proximal to the point of observation, peak systolic flows may increase and show a greater dispersion of frequencies and lower diastolic flow rates. Obstruction distal to the point of observation will lead primarily to slowing of the diastolic flow velocities. Obstruction of flow much more proximal to the heart than

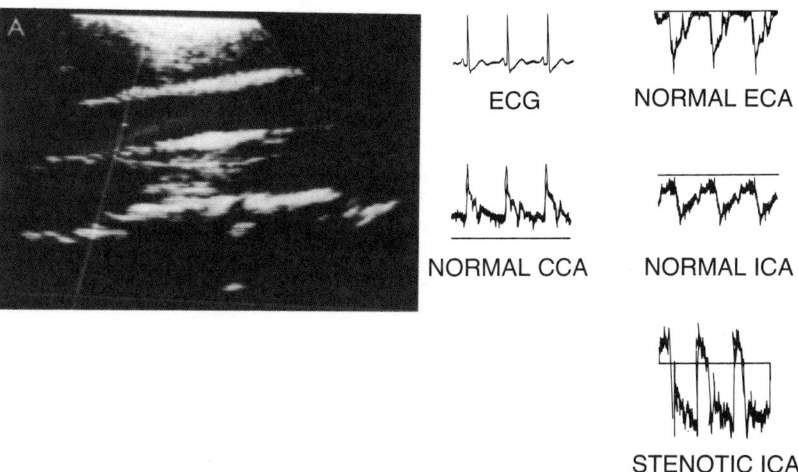

Fig. 2-6. Records obtained with a duplex ultrasound system, illustrating pulsed echo sector scan image combined with range-gated Doppler signal detection. **(A)** Sector scan image of a normal common carotid artery. The direction of the Doppler beam across the artery is toward the base of the neck, at the left side of the figure, and is indicated by the dotted line, with a horizontal tick representing the position of the sampling volume within the common carotid, about halfway between the anterior and posterior wall. **(B)** On the left, artist's reproductions of a Doppler range-gated directional ultrasound time display from a normal common carotid artery, with simultaneous ECG (above) and Doppler velocity plot (below). The solid line represents zero flow. Flow toward the transducer is displayed above that line (beam directed caudad as in Fig. A). On the right, reproductions of signals from normal external and internal carotid arteries, and from flow just distal to an internal carotid stenosis, are shown for comparison (beam directed cephalad, predominant flow away from the transducer). Flow in the external carotid is usually minimal in diastole, as shown here, whereas blood flow in the internal carotid is readily detectable throughout diastole. With the sampling volume placed in the jet just distal to an internal carotid stenosis, high velocity flow is apparent. Note that the greatly increased signal amplitude from the high velocity flow produces "aliasing" (spurious indication of flow toward the transducer) due to technical limitations of the instrument. (From Lees et al., 1982, with permission.)

the observation point will give pulsatile waveforms with lower, wider, and more slowly peaking systolic flow rates. The flow patterns also depend on the position in the lumen chosen for study: generally, flow at the lumen center is most informative.

Doppler studies are more useful than B-mode studies for defining hemodynamically significant stenosis, although the degree of stenosis is inferred rather than directly measured. Important limitations of Doppler studies are their insensitivity to nonstenosing plaques and their dependence on systemic hemodynamic state. Just as with B-mode imaging, the distinction between high-grade stenosis and total occlusion cannot be made reliably.

Duplex Doppler Studies: Vessel Anatomy and Flow

Duplex Doppler instrumentation combines capabilities for high resolution B-mode imaging with those for localized Doppler flow velocity measurement. The combination of flow and anatomic information, particularly for wall irregularities, makes duplex Doppler more sensitive and specific for clinically significant carotid lesions than either Doppler or B-mode ultrasound alone. Its importance also lies in its safety and low cost relative to invasive studies. Sensitivity for stenosis is high, so duplex studies may reasonably be used as a screening test for carotid disease. There is less likelihood of misinterpreting high-grade stenosis as complete occlusion, but occlusion must still be confirmed angiographically for symptomatic patients. Duplex Doppler is ideally suited to situations that demand serial follow-up of carotid lesions (e.g., in patients with severe but subcritical stenosis, or postendarterectomy).

CARDIAC ECHOCARDIOGRAPHY

Many echocardiographically definable abnormalities of the cardiac valves are associated to some degree with embolic stroke. In some patients, such as those with rheumatic mitral valve stenosis or vegetations of bacterial endocarditis, the risk of stroke is clearly high. In others, such as patients with calcific aortic stenosis or MVP, the increased risk is relatively small and the clinical significance of such findings in stroke patients must be interpreted cautiously.

The resolution of echocardiography limits it to visualization of lesions that are at least millimeters in diameter. As most lesions in bacterial endocarditis are smaller, the sensitivity of the test is low for diagnosis of this disease. However, visualization of lesions may correlate to some degree with their embolic potential: the risk of embolic stroke is probably higher for patients with vegetations large enough to be seen with echocardiography.

Sensitivity is also a problem in searching for emboli from mural thrombi associated with atrial fibrillation. Most commonly such emboli form in the atrial appendage, an area poorly visualized by echocardiography. In addition, the thrombi are small. The diagnosis, therefore, is usually established on the basis of ECG and clinical findings.

Echocardiography is more useful for detecting ventricular wall thrombi, which most frequently occur in patients with acute myocardial infarction. Echocardiographic studies have correlated large, freely moving thrombi projecting into the ventricle with higher embolic potential. The mural thrombi with high embolic potential that develop in dilated cardiomyopathies are usually too small to be visualized directly.

Paradoxic emboli should be considered in patients without clear cardiac risk factors or fixed cerebrovascular disease. They may follow deep venous thrombosis if there is a right-to-left shunt, either through the lungs (e.g., pulmonary arteriovenous malformation) or heart (e.g., atrial septal defect). However, any interatrial septum lies along the axis of the ultrasound beam in the standard four-chamber and short-axis views of the heart and, therefore, is not visualized well by echocardiography. In order to increase sensitivity, a contrast-echo study can be performed. Saline containing small echogenic bubbles is injected into an anticubital vein with simultaneous echocardiography of the heart. The bubbles are then easily followed from the right side of the heart, and into the chambers of the left in the presence of a septal defect. In the absence of a cardiac right-to-left shunt, the bubbles will not be seen in the chambers of the left side. However, a negative study does not rule out an intermittent patent septal defect, which opens with transient increases in right-sided pressures (e.g., after a pulmonary embolus).

When should an ECG be ordered? The diagnostic yield is low in an unselected population of middle-aged or elderly patients with transient ischemic attacks or recent cerebral infarcts. Because the prevalence of cardiac disease contributing to stroke in this population is relatively low, the predictive value of the study is poor. Selection of that subgroup of patients who have clinical evidence of cardiac disease (cardiomegaly, ECG changes consistent with myocardial infarction (MI), atrial fibrillation, prosthetic valves, or conduction abnormalities) increases the predictive value significantly. As an example, the theoretic predictive value of such selection can be particularly appreciated for an acute anterior MI. Assuming the sensitivity and specificity for ventricular mural thrombi may be as high as 95 and 85 percent, respectively, and given that the prevalence of mural thrombi after anterior MI is about 30 percent, the predictive value of a routine test is about 75 percent. This is high enough to provoke a change in patient management (e.g., anticoagulation). However, in a different setting, if the prevalence of mural thrombi decreases even to 20 percent, the predictive value falls to 50 percent (i.e., the theoretic predictive value of flipping a coin!)

In young people with stroke, the overall prevalence of cardiac emboli disease is higher than in older adults, perhaps even approaching 30 percent. Thus all younger patients with suspected embolic stroke, in the absence of a clear etiology, should undergo echocardiographic examinations.

READINGS

Ackerman RH: Non-invasive diagnosis of carotid disease in the era of digital subtraction angiography. p. 263. In Barnett HJM (ed): Neurologic Clinics. Vol. 1. No. 1. WB Saunders, Philadelphia, 1983

Cerebral Embolism Task Force: Cardiogenic brain embolism. Arch Neurol 43:71, 1986

Greenland P, Knopman DS, Mikell FL, et al: Echocardiography in diagnostic assessment of stroke. Ann Intern Med 95:51, 1981

Haugland JM, Asinger RW, Mikell FL, et al: Embolic potential of left ventricular thrombi detected by two-dimensional echocardiography. Circulation 70:588, 1984

Lees RS, Myers GS: Non-invasive diagnosis of arterial disease. Adv Intern Med 27:475, 1982

Morganroth J, Parisi A, Pohorst G: Non-invasive Cardiac Imaging. Year Book Medical Publishers, Chicago, 1983

Reilly LM, Lusby RJ, Hughes L, et al: Carotid plaque histology using real-time ultrasonography: clinical and therapeutic complications. Am J Surg 146:188, 1983

Zweibel WJ, Austin CW, Sackett JF, et al: Correlation of high-resolution, B-mode and continuous-wave Doppler sonography with arteriography in the diagnosis of carotid stenosis. Radiology 149(2):523, 1983

Zweibel WJ (ed): Introduction to Vascular Ultrasonography. Ed. 2. Grune & Stratton, Orlando, FL, 1986

IMAGING STUDIES OF THE CENTRAL NERVOUS SYSTEM 3

Donatella Tampieri

GENERAL PRINCIPLES OF COMPUTED TOMOGRAPHY AND MAGNETIC RESONANCE IMAGING

Both computed tomography (CT) and magnetic resonance imaging (MRI) produce digitized images. The image for each, therefore, has a matrix representation, and each pixel (the single unit of the matrix) has a numeric value that is converted into a white-gray scale.

In CT, the pixel value is a measure of the attenuation of the incident x-ray beam by the tissue. The degree of x-ray attenuation is proportional to the electron density of the tissue. Thus CT is most sensitive to structures of higher electron density such as bone (calcium-containing) and blood (iron-containing).

In MRI, a radiofrequency (RF) pulse is applied to excite the protons of the tissue (usually primarily those of water, except in fatty tissue such as the diploë where lipid protons are abundant), and the protons emit in consequence a radiofrequency signal, the intensity of which is proportional to the number that are excited by the applied RF pulse. Each pixel, therefore, is a representation of the intensity of the signals from protons within the tissue examined after a given RF pulse.

After each RF pulse, protons in the sample need a finite period to return to a state from which they can be excited again. The time needed is governed by the T_1-relaxation rate. It is different for protons in different compounds (e.g., fat and water) or for water protons in different environments (e.g., free or protein bound in a cell). The intensity of the signal emitted after a RF pulse also decays because of processes that promote randomization (and thus destructive interference) of signals from individual protons. This randomization tendency is expressed in terms of the T_2-relaxation rate. Differences in T_1- and T_2-relaxation rates between different tissues caused by differences in physical state and chemical composition generate contrast in MRI. Because protons are most abundant in soft tissues (which are predominantly either water or fat), MRI is most sensitive to soft tissue lesions and least sensitive for evaluation of calcified material such as bone.

Note that because contrast is generated in such different ways, CT and MRI have different terminologies. For CT the terms *hypodense, isodense* or *hyperdense* are used to describe a given area of tissue in comparison with the normal parenchyma. The terms *hypointense, isointense,* and *hyperintense* are used in MRI to describe the appearance of a given area of tissue in comparison with the normal parenchyma.

Whereas the CT image is acquired in a standard way, different techniques may be used for MRI. Different techniques can generate different relative contrasts from the same tissues. The appearance of the image (as well as acquisition time and resolution) also depends on the strength of the magnetic field used. We will not enter into the technical details of the different MRI acquisition techniques, but refer the reader to more specific publications (see readings list).

The most common MR signal acquisition technique is the spin-echo (SE) method. Either T_1- (short interpulse delay [TR] and short spin-echo time [TE]) or T_2- (long interpulse delay [TR] and long spin echo time [TE]) weighted images can be produced. As the names imply, contrast in the former depends most on differences in T_1-relaxation times, whereas contrast in the latter depends most on differences in T_2-relaxation times. So-called proton density images can also be produced with sequences having relatively long TR and short TE.

Each tissue (under the same conditions and examined with the same applied field strength) is characterized by constant T_1- and T_2- relaxation time values. It is helpful to memorize the relative T_1 and T_2 values for two common tissues, such as CSF and fat. At the magnetic field strength of 1.5 Tesla, the CSF has long T_1- and T_2-relaxation times and, therefore, appears hypointense in T_1-weighted and hyperintense in T_2-weighted images. Fat has a short T_1 and a relatively short T_2 and appears hyperintense in T_1-weighted and isointense in T_2-weighted images.

NORMAL ANATOMY OF THE BRAIN AS DEFINED BY CT AND MRI

Figures 3-1 to 3-3 represent images of the normal brain, obtained from similar levels, using CT and MRI. Clinically important anatomic structures are identified.

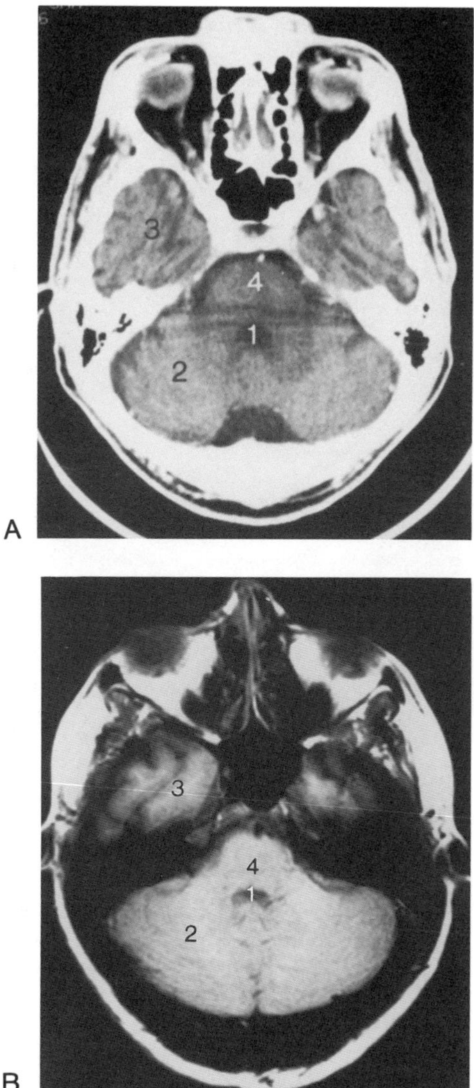

Fig. 3-1. Clinical anatomy of the normal human brain. Views in the axial plane are displayed caudally to rostrally in Figs. A–H. Comparison of **(A)** CT and **(B)** MRI (1.5 T, TR 450 msec, TE 30 msec). 1, Fourth ventricle; 2, cerebellar hemisphere; 3, temporal lobe; 4, pons cerebri. (*Figure Continues.*)

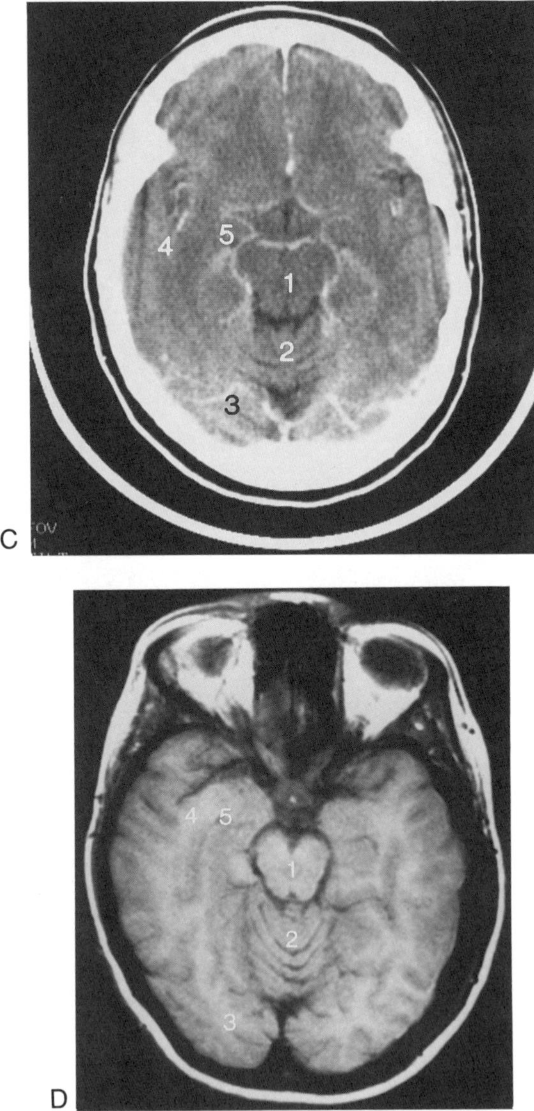

Fig. 3-1 (*Continued*). Comparison of (**C**) CT and (**D**) MRI (1.5 T, TR 450 msec, TE 30 msec). View in the axial plane. 1, midbrain; 2, vermis; 3, occipital lobe; 4, temporal lobe; 5, temporal horn. (*Figure Continues.*)

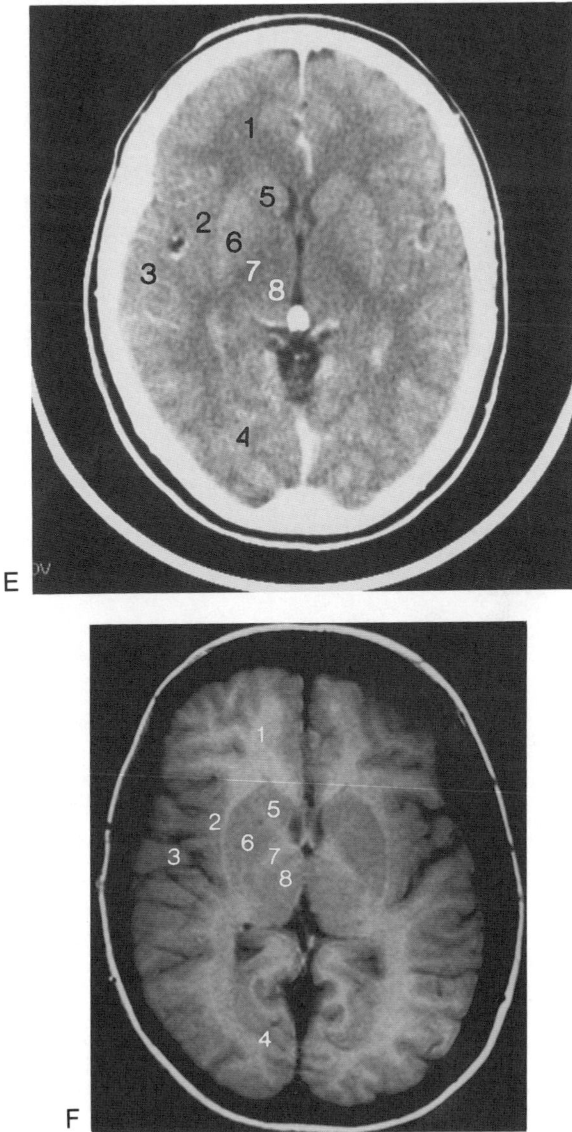

Fig. 3-1 (*Continued*). Comparison of **(E)** CT and **(F)** MRI (1.5 T, TR 450 msec, TE 30 msec). View in the axial plane. 1, frontal lobe; 2, insula; 3, temporal lobe; 4, occipital lobe; 5, head of the caudate nucleus; 6, lentiform nucleus; 7, internal capsule; 8, thalamus. (*Figure Continues.*)

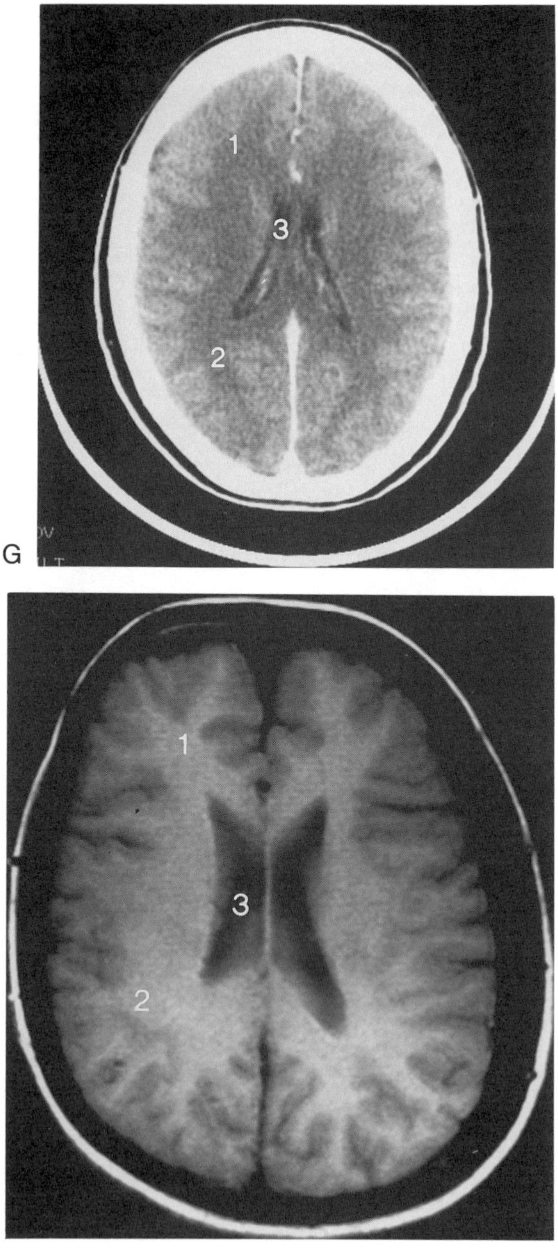

Fig. 3-1 (*Continued*). Comparison of **(G)** CT and **(H)** MRI (1.5 T, TR 450 msec, TE 30 msec). View in the axial plane. 1, frontal lobe; 2, parietal lobe; 3, lateral ventricle.

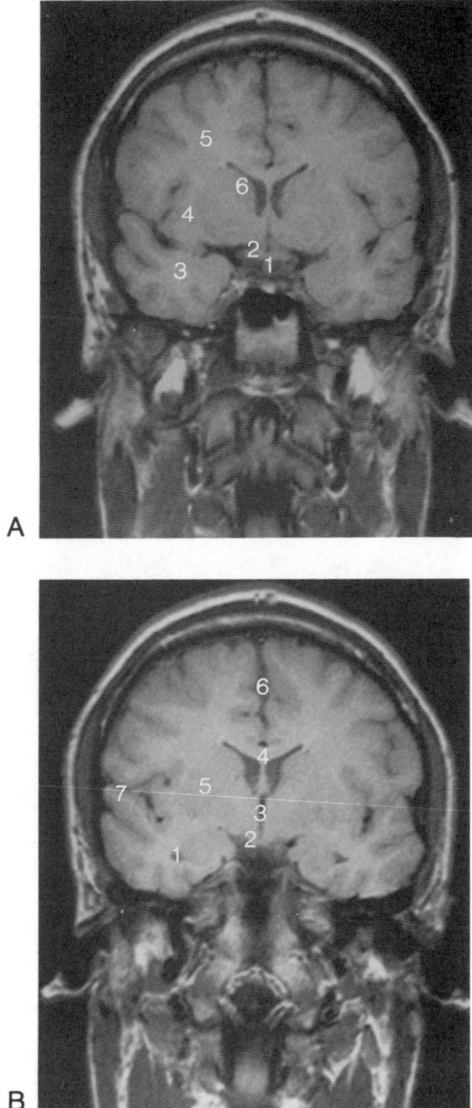

Fig. 3-2. Clinical anatomy of the normal human brain. Views in the coronal plane are displayed anteriorly to posteriorly in Figs. A–D. **(A)** MRI (1.5 T, TR 450 msec, TE 30 msec). 1, pituitary stalk; 2, optic chiasm; 3, temporal lobe; 4, insula; 5, frontal lobe; 6, head of caudate nucleus. **(B)** MRI. View in the coronal plane. 1, temporal horn; 2, mamillary body; 3, third ventricle; 4, corpus callosum; 5, lentiform nucleus; 6, interhemispheric fissure; 7, sylvian fissure. (*Figure Continues.*)

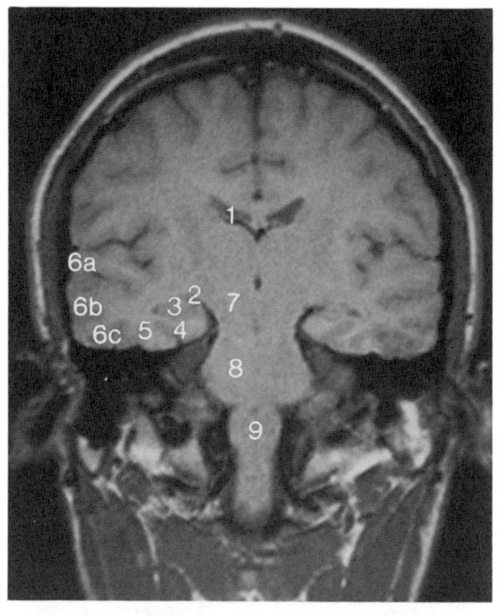

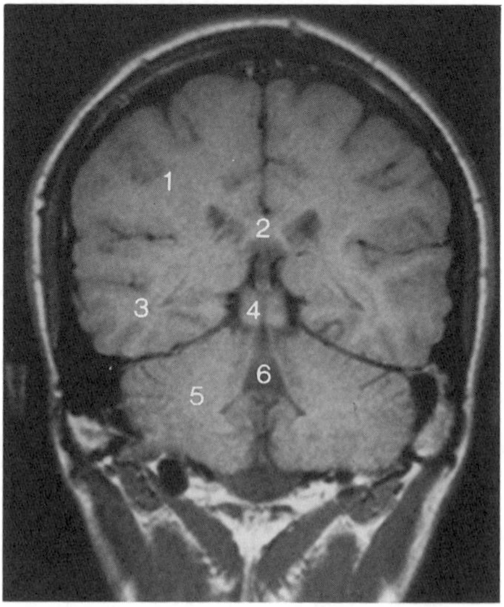

D

Fig. 3-2 *(Continued).* **(C)** MRI (1.5 T, TR 450 msec, TE 30 msec). View in the coronal plane. 1, atrium of the lateral ventricle; 2, choroidal fissures; 3, hippocampal gyrus; 4, parahippocampal gyrus; 5, fusiform gyrus; 6, temporal gyri: (a) superior, (b) middle, and (c) inferior; 7, midbrain; 8, pons cerebri; 9, medulla oblongata. **(D)** MRI. View in the coronal plane. 1, parietal lobe; 2, splenium of the corpus callosum; 3, temporal lobe; 4, quadrigeminal plate; 5, cerebellar hemisphere; 6, fourth ventricle.

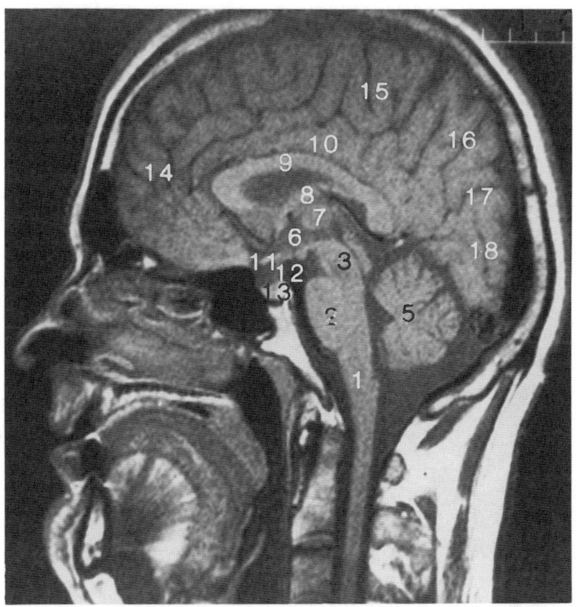

Fig. 3-3. Clinical anatomy of the normal human brain. MRI (1.5 T, TR 250 msec, TE 30 msec) in the sagittal plane. 1, medulla oblongata; 2, pons cerebri; 3, midbrain; 4, fourth ventricle; 5, vermis of cerebellum; 6, third ventricle; 7, massa intermedia; 8, fornix; 9, corpus callosum; 10, gyrus cinguli, 11, optic chiasma; 12, pituitary stalk; 13, pituitary gland; 14, frontal lobe; 15, paracentral lobule; 16, pre-cuneus; 17, parieto-occipital fissure; 18, cuneus.

PATHOLOGY OF THE BRAIN AS DEFINED BY CT AND MRI

Trauma

CT is the examination of choice in the evaluation of trauma patients, as it allows simultaneous assessment of the brain parenchyma and skull. We will review the major situations commonly encountered, giving some illustrative examples.

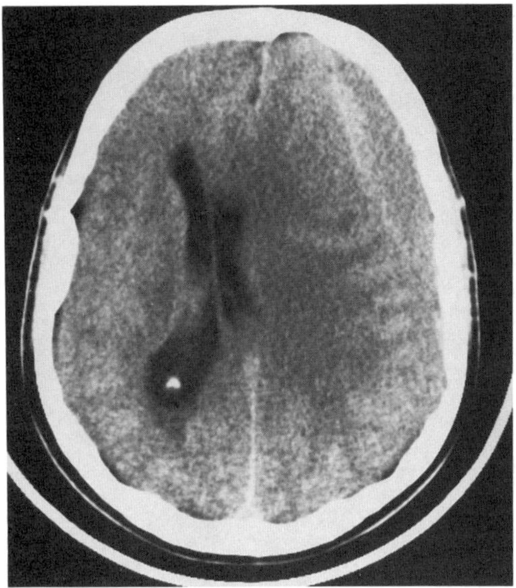

Fig. 3-4. Plain CT scan of the head. Subacute subdural hematoma, causing compression of the left cerebral hemisphere and lateral ventricle and shift of the midline structures to the right. Note the isodense appearance (relative to brain parenchyma) of the hematoma in the subacute phase. The enlargement of the right lateral ventricle suggests herniation below the falx cerebri.

Brain Contusions

A brain contusion can be focal or diffuse (concussion). The CT appearance of focal contusions is as an ill-defined, hypodense corticosubcortical area showing a loss of the white-gray matter differentiation without any major mass effect. These changes are consistent with acute focal edema. Brain contusions are usually located at the same level as the skin laceration and are not necessarily associated with skull fractures. Diffuse swelling of the brain can also result from major trauma: CT shows a diffuse hypodensity of the white matter consistent with diffuse edema. Mass effect will reduce the size of lateral ventricles and the subarachnoid spaces.

Hemorrhagic Contusions

The hemorrhagic component of a contusion manifests as multiple areas of corticosubcortical hyperdensity consistent with hemorrhagic petechiae. The most common locations are the frontobasal regions in the rectus or orbital gyri and the temporal pole. In major trauma, one may observe contre-coup hemorrhages caused by the rapid displacement of the brain within the cranial cavity, which results in a second hemorrhagic contusion located opposite to the site of trauma.

Hematomas

Self-contained collections of blood can be localized within the parenchyma, or in the subdural extradural spaces. *Intraparenchymal hematomas* accompanying trauma are usually related only to major trauma. A lesion appears as a well-defined, hyperdense area, usually surrounded by some hypodensity from reactive edema. The lesion may cause mass effect (depending on its size) and thus displacement and compression of the midline structures and the ventricular system.

Subdural hematomas usually have a concave-convex shape because of the easy detachment of the arachnoid from the dura, the latter being strongly adherent to the inner table of the skull. Subdural hematomas can be acute, subacute, or chronic and each type has a distinctive CT appearance. *Acute subdural hematomas* (within 3 days) appear completely hyperdense because of the high electron-density of fresh blood. In the *subacute phase* (from about 3 days through 2 to 3 weeks) (Fig. 3-4) the blood becomes isodense with brain parenchyma and, therefore, the diagnosis may be difficult. For example, in cases of bilateral subacute isodense subdural hematomas, the midline structures are not displaced because the mass effect is bilateral. Injection of contrast will allow visualization of the meninges and thus better definition of the extent of the hematomas. *Chronic hematomas* (beyond about 3 weeks) usually appear hypodense because of the altered electron density within the hematoma after degradation of the blood components (Fig. 3-5).

Extradural hematomas (Fig. 3-6) appear as well-defined hyperdense blood collections with a typical biconvex appearance, often located in close relationship to the branches of the middle meningeal artery and associated with cranial fractures. The biconvex shape of the hematoma results from the strong attachment of the dura to the inner table of the skull. Extradural hematomas in the posterior fossa, although rare, may occur. Therefore, CT of the head in trauma patients should always include slices covering all volumes from the base to the vertex of the skull.

Subarachnoid Hemorrhages

Blood within the subarachnoid spaces, ventricular system, or cistern is often present in trauma patients. *Subarachnoid blood* appears hyperdense in the CSF. If the history of trauma is not clear, the possibility of a ruptured

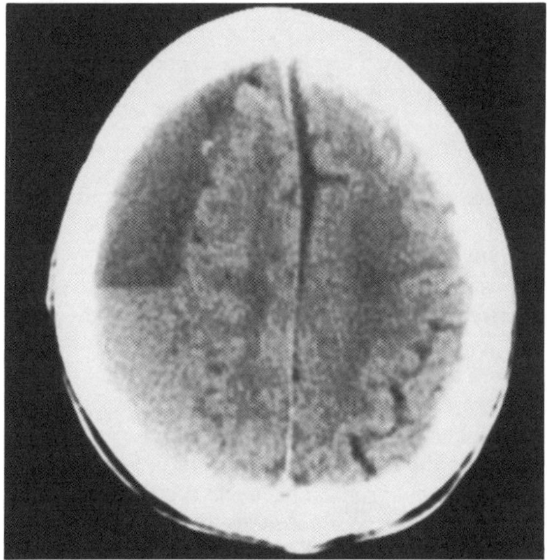

Fig. 3-5. Plain CT scan of the head. Chronic subdural hematoma over the right convexity with an area of more recent sudural hemorrhage. The subdural hematoma has the classic concave-convex appearance. The older, anterior portion of the hematoma is hypodense, while the posterior portion is iso- to hyperdense, consistent with more recent bleeding. Note also a small subdural collection of blood along the falx cerebri in the left frontal region.

aneurysm should be considered. Small subsequent hemorrhages may cause prominent symptoms (e.g., headache, vomiting), but not be apparent on CT.

Limitations of MRI in Head Trauma

The use of MRI for the examination of head trauma is limited, for practical reasons. Trauma patients are difficult to manage and often require respiratory support. Because patients have difficulty remaining still for the many minutes required, the quality of the MRI scans is often very poor. Furthermore, MRI does not detect blood well within the first 24 hours (see the next section).

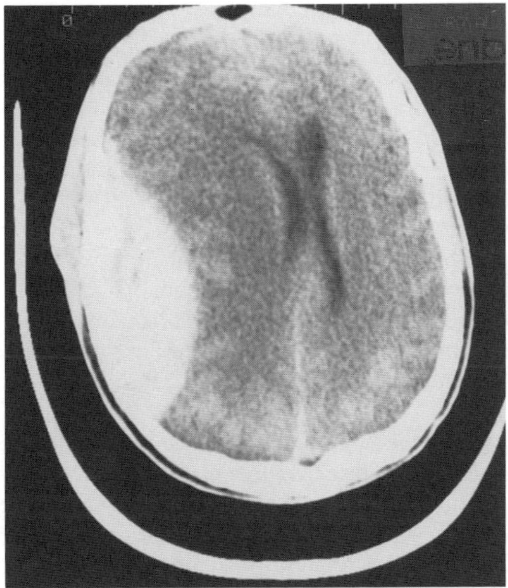

Fig. 3-6. Plain CT scan of the head. Acute extradural hematoma with typical biconvex shape in the right frontoparietal region. The hematoma is causing severe edema of the right hemisphere, compression of the lateral ventricles, and contralateral shift of the midline structures.

Vascular Disease

Intraparenchymal Hematomas

An intraparenchymal hematoma usually appears as a well-defined, hyperdense area on CT. Surrounding hypodensity from reactive edema evolves over 2 to 3 days after the initial event. The hematoma has a mass effect, potentially causing compression of the ventricular system and displacement of midline structures.

Intraparenchymal hematomas have several etiologies. Usually located at the level of the basal ganglia, the *hypertensive hematoma* can be large, extending into the ventricular system. In cases of *hemorrhagic infarcts,* the lesion appears as an ill-defined, hypodense area associated with a central, sometimes patchy hyperdense hemorrhagic component. They have a characteristic corticosubcortical distribution within the territory of one cerebral vessel, or are found in the basal ganglia area. Often the hemorrhagic component is represented by multiple small foci of hemorrhages, and less frequently by large hematomas.

Congophilic amyloid angiopathy is a common cause of intraparenchymal hemorrhages in the patient over 70. The hemorrhages are typically located in corticosubcortical position and may be multiple. They are often associated with chronic vascular changes of the periventricular white matter, lacunae, and diffuse cerebral atrophy.

Hematomas in tumors are usually contained by the tumor, which is often surrounded by edema. It is important that we emphasize the difference in appearance of tumoral versus hemorrhagic edema. With tumors, edema (vasogenic) spreads within the white matter to give a digitiform appearance. In contrast, edema secondary to an intraparenchymal hemorrhage appears, on an image slice, to surround the blood in a relatively smooth halo.

Intraparenchymal bleeding can be observed after rupture of a *vascular malformation* such as an arteriovenous malformation (AVM), or a venous or cavernous angioma. Usually, the hematoma hides the underlying lesion itself. AVMs are responsible for large intraparenchymal hematomas with severe mass effect. Venous angiomas usually bleed in the cerebellum, and rarely in the supratentorial compartment.

After complete reabsorption of the hematoma, a CT scan with infusion should be performed to assess the etiology of the bleeding, but angiography is usually the examination of choice. MRI allows the diagnosis of AVM and venous angioma (see below), but the feeding arteries of an AVM cannot be located precisely. These studies can be performed as the mass effect resolves, but the underlying pathology may still be obscured by the presence of the blood clot.

Signal intensities in MRI of intracerebral hematomas evolve in a complex way, as the products of hemoglobin degradation lead to very different water proton relaxation times. To demonstrate the importance of this point, we will outline the evolution of blood in a clot and the consequences for water proton relaxation times (for a 1.5T MR unit). In fresh blood, the hemoglobin is still present in the red blood cells (RBCs), predominantly as oxyhemoglobin. In this hyperacute phase (24 to 48 hours) of the hematoma, contrast is poor as the oxyhemoglobin does not change relaxation times of local tissue water. For this reason an early hematoma can be missed by MRI. Later in the acute phase (up to about 7 days), the hemoglobin deoxygenates. Intracellular deoxyhemoglobin in RBCs has little effect on signal in the T_1-weighted images, but it significantly shortens the water T_2-relaxation time, leading to a low intensity signal on the T_2-weighted image. From the acute to the subacute phase (1 to 4 weeks), the deoxyhemoglobin oxidizes, becoming first intracellular methemoglobin.

The intracellular methemoglobin leads to short T_1- and T_2-relaxation times for water protons and, consequently, a high intensity signal in T_1- and low intensity signal in T_2-weighted images. Eventually, the lysis of the red cells occurs and the methemoglobin becomes extracellular. Free methemoglobin (i.e., no longer in the RBCs) causes water protons to have a short T_1- and long T_2-relaxation time. Therefore, a late subacute hematoma has a high intensity signal both in the T_1- and T_2-weighted images. Starting from the end of the subacute phase and continuing into the chronic phase (past 1 month) of the hematoma, there is a progressive degradation of the free methemoglobin to hemosiderin and ferritin, beginning at the periphery of the hematoma and gradually extending toward its center. Because of the paramagnetic effect caused by the ferric iron, hemosiderin increases the T_1- and decreases the T_2-relaxation times of water protons, leading to a low intensity signal in both T_1- and T_2-weighted images.

Vascular Malformations

Three different types of vascular malformations can be detected with an infused CT scan of the head or MRI. *AVMs* are nests of vessels that appear hyperdense in the infused CT. Depending on the size and amount of flow through the AVM, the feeding arteries or draining veins may be seen. An area of focal atrophy is often associated with cortical AVMs. Flowing blood does not produce an MRI signal. Consequently, MRI displays the AVM as a nest of void signals (consistent with blood in the high flow vessels) both in T_1- and T_2-weighted images. Gliotic tissue, which may be visualized surrounding an AVM, produces a hyperintense signal in the proton density and T_2-weighted images.

Venous angiomas are formed from several medullary veins joined into a "caput medusa" that drains to a major transcerebral vein and eventually into the superficial (Fig. 3-7) or the deep venous system. Venous angiomas may be seen in either the supratentorial or infratentorial compartments. They appear similarly on MRI and CT but the signal is void.

Cavernous angiomas are partly calcified with ill-defined margins on CT, which can strongly enhance with infusion of intravenous contrast. They may bleed, usually causing small, well-circumscribed hematomas. CT, even with contrast injection, may not reveal the lesion (Fig. 3-8). On MRI, cavernous angiomas appear as well-defined lesions with mixed hypointense and hyperintense signals from blood in varying stages of degradation. MRI is the examination of choice because of its high sensitivity. Cavernous angiomas were much less known to the radiologist before the advent of MRI.

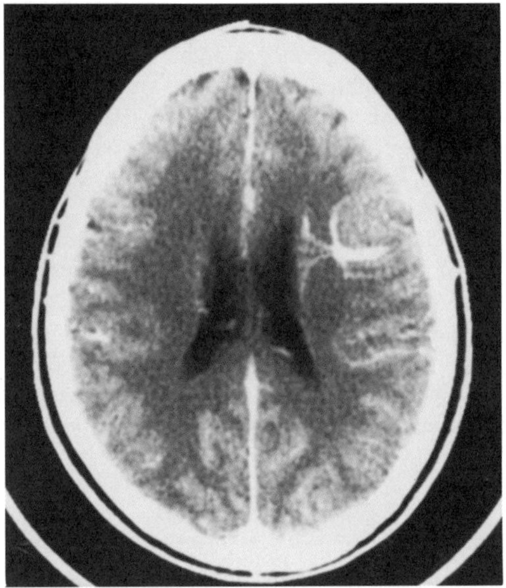

Fig. 3-7. CT scan of the head after infusion of intravenous contrast. A venous angioma is seen in the left frontal region. The so-called caput medusa formed by multiple subependymal veins is draining into a larger transcerebral vein directed toward the surface of the hemisphere.

In general, MRI is superior to CT for the evaluation and differential diagnosis of vascular malformations. However, in order to define the anatomy of an AVM (feeding arteries and draining veins) well enough to allow a therapeutic decision (e.g., between surgical, radiosurgical, or endovascular treatments) angiography is still needed.

Aneurysms usually appear as well-defined, round, hyperdense lesions along the course of the vessel in the infused CT scan (Figs. 3-9 and 3-10). If the lesion is large enough or the CT slice goes exactly through it, the aneurysm may be fully revealed. MRI will demonstrate the abnormal veins as a flow void.

Ischemic Lesions

Infarct

The appearance of an ischemic infarct of the brain on CT varies according to the time of the examination after infarction. Neuroradiologists classify infarcts as acute, subacute, or chronic. In the acute phase (first 24 hours)

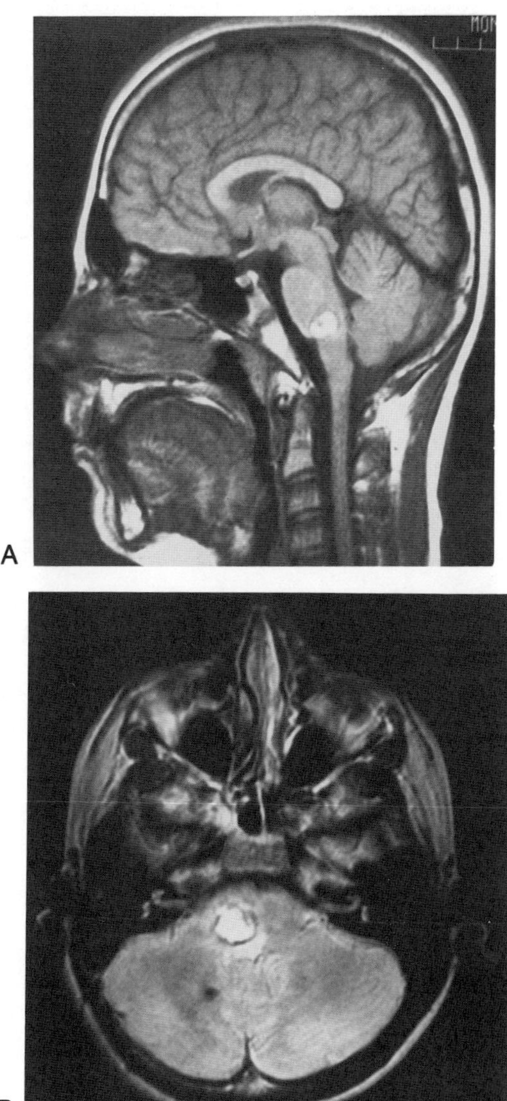

Fig. 3-8. MRI of the head from **(A)** T1-weighted (1.5 T, TR 400 msec, TE 30 msec) sagittal and **(B)** proton-density (TR 2000 msec, TE 30 msec) axial (right) sequences. A cavernous angioma in the right aspect of the pontomedullary junction is shown. Note that this lesion gives a high intensity signal with both pulse sequences. There is a rim of low intensity signal in the proton-density image from local hemosiderin deposition.

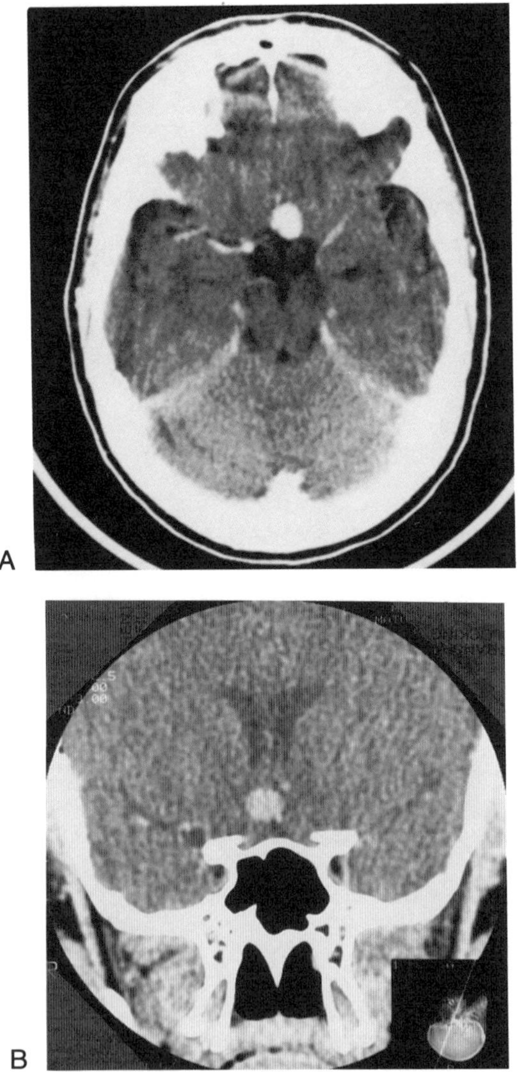

Fig. 3-9. CT scan of the head after infusion of intravenous contrast in **(A)** axial and **(B)** coronal planes. The well-circumscribed, hyperdense, round lesion seen in the anterior aspect of the suprasellar cistern was suspected to be an aneurysm of the anterior communicating artery. This was confirmed angiographically (see Fig. 3-10).

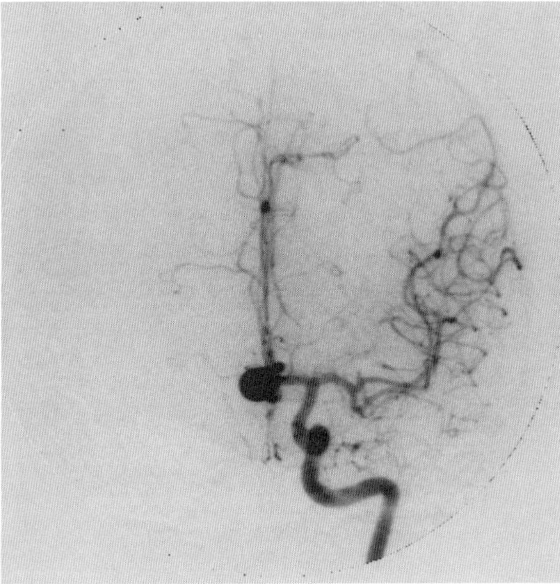

Fig. 3-10. Anteroposterior view from a left internal carotid angiographic study of the patient whose CT scan is shown in Fig. 3-9. The round vasular lesion filling in the arterial phase in communication with the anterior communicating artery confirms the diagnosis of an aneurysm, which was suspected from the CT scan.

little or no change occurs in the density of the infarcted tissue. There may be evidence of a mass effect with effacement of the subarachnoid spaces. In the subacute phase (2 to 7 days), the ischemic area starts to become relatively hypodense, and the mass effect increases, with obliteration of the subarachnoid spaces and compression of the homolateral lateral ventricle (Fig. 3-11). Of course, depending on the size of the lesion, the mass effect can be great enough to cause contralateral displacement of the midline structures. In the later subacute phase (5 to 7 days), the injection of contrast media may enhance the periphery of the ischemic area because of luxury perfusion phenomenon. In the chronic stage, the infarct appears as a well-defined hypodense area shaped according to the distribution of the vascular territory involved. Eventually (after months), loss of normal parenchyma will lead to an *ex vacuo* enlargement of the homolateral ventricle and of the adjacent subarachnoid spaces (Fig. 3-12).

MRI is more sensitive than is CT to edema associated with infarcts. It

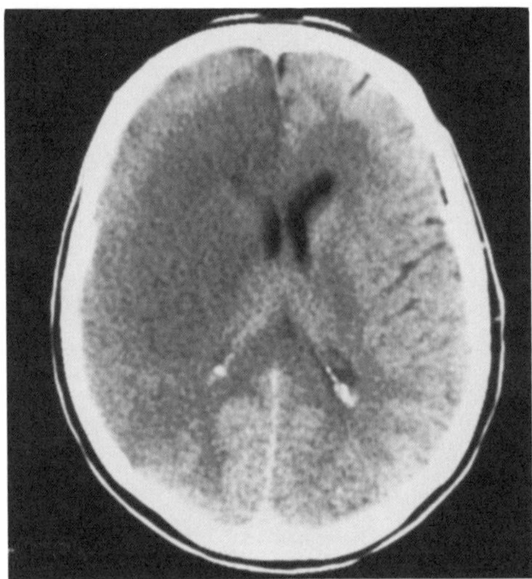

Fig. 3-11. Plain CT scan of the head. There is a diffuse hypodensity of the right hemisphere involving the frontal, temporal, and parietal lobes. Associated with this is a loss of the gray/white matter differentiation and some mass effect, with effacement of the subarachnoid spaces of the vertex and compression of the right lateral ventricle. These findings are consistent with a recent ischemic event in the territory of distribution of the right internal carotid artery.

can be particularily useful for defining early lesions in the posterior fossa and brainstem. Such lesions will appear isointense on T_1-weighted images, but are shown as hyperintense in T_2-weighted images. Chronic lesions will appear hypointense in T_1- and hyperintense in T_2-weighted images.

Lacunae

In the elderly patient, lacunae appear by CT as multiple small (under 1 to 2 cm diameter) hypodensities mainly in the basal ganglia. They are usually associated with diffuse corticosubcortical atrophy (Fig. 3-13). Whenever the periventricular white matter appear to be relatively uniformly hypodense (particularly around the frontal horns) the term *chronic vascular leukoencephalopathy* or *leukoariosis* is used to indicate probable diffuse vascular disease involving the perforator arteries (Binswanger's-type disease).

MRI is more sensitive than CT in demonstrating these lesions. On T_2-

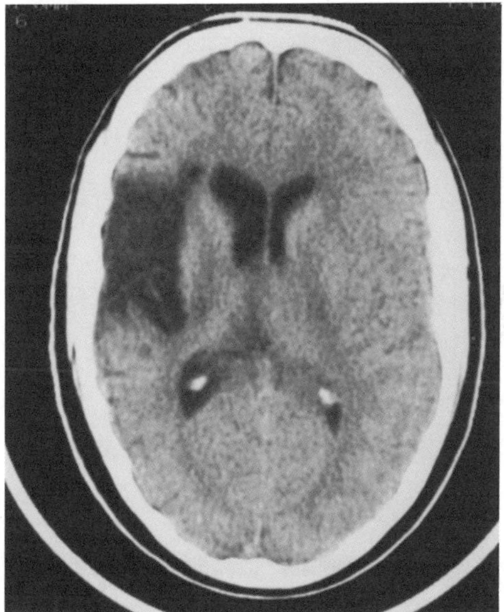

Fig. 3-12. Plain CT scan of the head. Chronic stage of an ischemic infarct of the right fronto-temporoinsular region. Ex vacuo enlargement of the right lateral ventricle is seen, a consequence of loss of brain parenchymal volume in the infarcted area.

weighted images they appear as areas of increased signal intensity, either focal (in lacunar disease) or periventricular and confluent (in leukoariosis). The same areas appear with hypointense signals on T_1-weighted images.

Subarachnoid Hemorrhages

A spontaneous subarachnoid hemorrhage is usually a dramatic event. The CT scan is the most useful initial examination to establish the diagnosis (Fig. 3-14). The blood within the subarachnoid space appears hyperdense. Blood (particularly from aneurysms of the anterior communicating artery) can dissect through the lamina terminalis and the third ventricle, resulting in flooding of the ventricles with blood. Acute hydrocephalus is a common but treatable complication. An early sign of hydrocephalus is bilateral enlargement of the temporal horn. Later diffuse ballooning of the ventricular system with compression of the sulci is seen.

Neurologic investigation is not complete until the etiology of the sub-

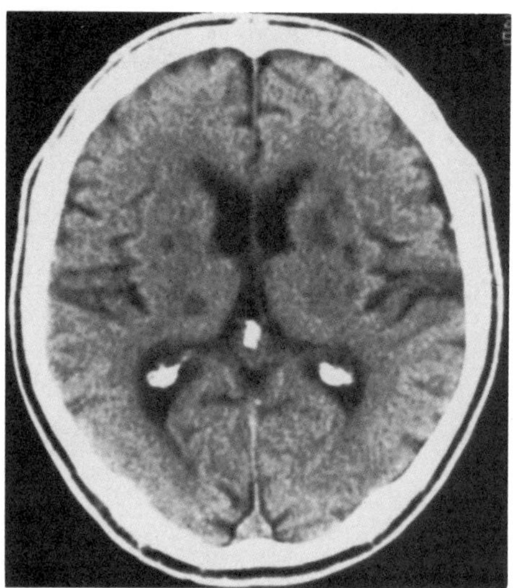

Fig. 3-13. Plain CT scan of the head. Lacunes are small hypodensities that are associated with long-standing hypertension and diabetes mellitis and are characteristically found in the basal ganglia, thalamus, pons, internal capsule, and corona radiata. In this patient, multiple lacunes are present in both basal ganglia and in the right thalamus. The ventricles are large and the subarachnoid spaces are prominent, consistent with moderate diffuse cortical atrophy.

arachnoid hemorrhage is known (if the patient survives the initial bleed). Detection of an aneurysm is not possible with a CT scan. Angiography is necessary if surgery is to be considered (Fig. 3–15).

Neoplastic Lesions

Intracranial tumors can be classified according to location, as either intra-axial or extra-axial.

Extra-axial Tumors

Meningiomas

Meningiomas appear as well-defined, hyperdense lesions in the infused CT scan. The image is often hyperdense in a plain CT as well, because of the presence of microcalcifications. They may also show macroscopic calcifications. Meningiomas are usually in close relationship with the inner

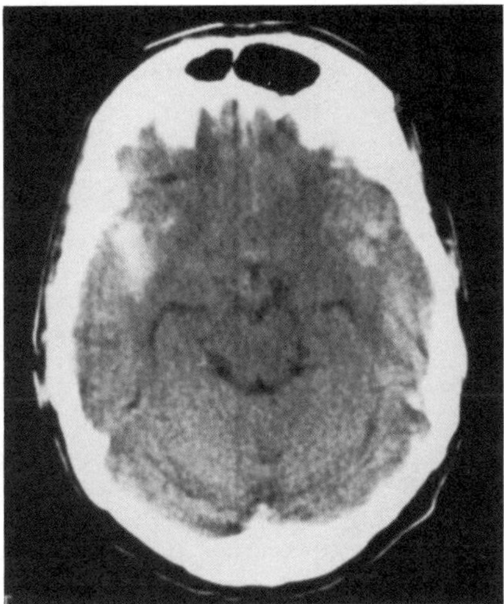

Fig. 3-14. Plain CT scan of the head. The hyperdensity seen in the interhemispheric and both sylvian fissures is from subarachnoid blood. The presence of the largest amount of blood in the right sylvian fissure suggests an aneurysm of the right middle cerebral artery, which was later confirmed by angiography (see Fig. 3-15).

table of the skull, falx cerebri, or tentorium cerebelli. The tumor is often surrounded by hypodensity consistent with edema, a consequence of tumor compression of the cerebral parenchyma. Posterior fossa meningiomas usually sit at the petroclival junction (Fig. 3-16) or close to the sigmoid sinus. Rarely, meningiomas may be intraventricular.

The angioblastic meningioma is particularly aggressive. Angioblastic meningiomas may show necrotic foci (hypodense areas) and usually enhance strongly.

Meningiomas are often easier to identify by CT than MRI because of the calcification visible on CT. On MRI meningiomas have a signal isointense to the normal parenchyma in T_1- and T_2-weighted images. However, in the intermediate echo they tend to increase their signal, becoming more intense.

Neurinomas

Neurinomas usually appear isodense or hypodense on the plain CT scan. After intravenous contrast infusion, the tumor usually enhances homogeneously, becoming hyperdense. Often small hypodense areas, consis-

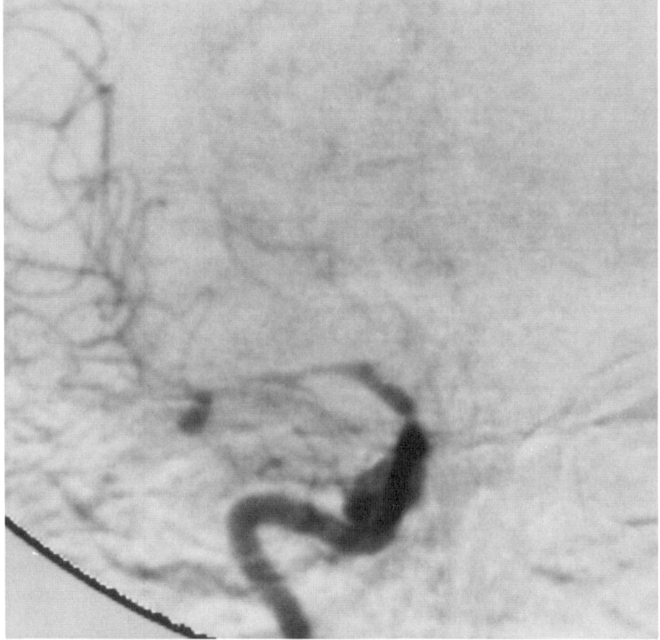

Fig. 3-15. Anteroposterior view from a right internal carotid interarterial angiographic study of the patient presenting with subarachnoid hemorrhage whose CT scan is shown as Fig. 3-14. A right middle cerebral artery aneurysm can be seen.

tent with necrosis, may be seen. The eighth cranial nerve is the most common location for neurinomas (Fig. 3-17). On MRI they are isointense in T_1- and hyperintense in T_2-weighted images. The injection of gadolinium DTPA as an MRI contrast agent can be extremely useful for showing small lesions that would otherwise be missed.

It is often difficult to distinguish between meningiomas and neurinomas in the cerebellopontine angle, but recognizing a few clues may be helpful. Neurinomas are usually centered at the level of the internal auditory canal, whereas meningiomas are usually located more anterior or more posterior to it. Usually neurinomas of the eighth cranial nerve cause an enlargement of the internal auditory canal that can be seen by CT with use of a bone window (Fig. 3-17). Finally, whereas neurinomas may form an acute angle with the posterior aspect of the petrous bone, meningiomas usually form an obtuse one.

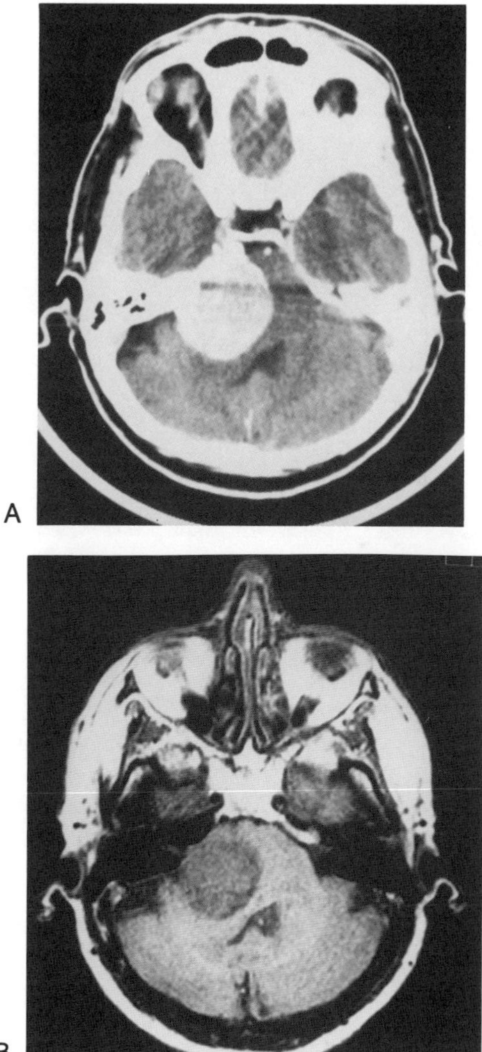

Fig. 3-16. CT scan of the head after **(A)** intravenous contrast infusion and **(B)** T_1-weighted MRI (1.5 T, TR 450 msec, TE 30 msec) from the same patient. A large petroclival meningioma causing compression of the fourth ventricle can be seen.

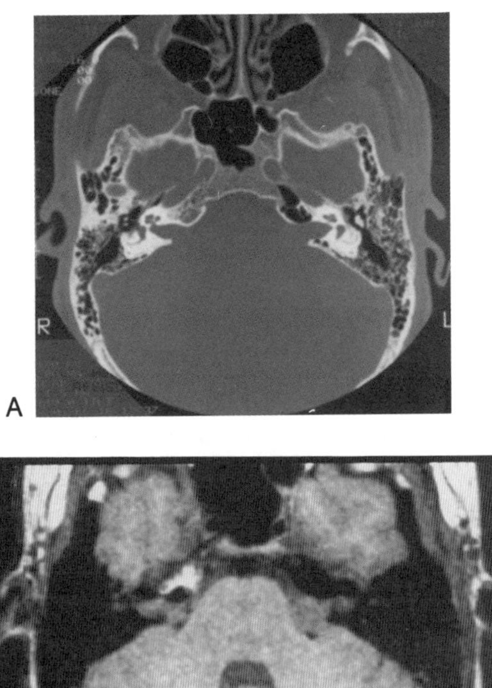

Fig. 3-17. **(A)** Plain CT scan of the head processed with bone "window" and **(B)** axial T_1-weighted MRI (1.5 T, TR 450 msec, TE 30 msec) of the same area. Bilateral intracanalicular neurinomas, causing enlargement of the internal auditory canals, are present in this patient. The CT image allows the visualization of enlargement and local bony destruction of the auditory canals near the tumors, a sign of chronic mass effect. MRI allows a better appreciation of the anatomic relationship between the tumors and adjacent soft tissue.

MRI is the examination of choice for evaluation of posterior fossa tumors because of the absence of bone artifacts. The differential diagnosis between meningioma and neurinoma is simplified since MRI allows direct evaluation of the eighth cranial nerve.

Other Extra-axial Tumors

Epidermoid Cysts. These lesions are often located in close relationship with the base of the skull in the middle or posterior cranial fossa. They are hypodense, rarely calcified, and do not enhance in the infused CT scan. If intraventricular (15 percent of cases) they are most commonly in the fourth ventricule.

Dermoid Cysts. These cysts are rarely intracranial (the most common location is in the spine). Located in the midline, they tend to be inhomogeneously hypodense and often have calcifications.

Teratomas. These tumors are most commonly located in the pineal region. They are inhomogeneous, largely hypodense lesions with multiple calcifications.

Chordomas. Chordomas are usually found in the posterior fossa in midline or paramedian positions in close relationship with the clivus. They are isodense and enhance slightly. They may erode the bone locally.

Craniopharyngiomas. These lesions are located in the sella region. They appear inhomogeneous with solid, hyperdense, and cystic portions. They may show calcifications.

Pituitary Adenomas. These tumors are divided into microadenomas and macroadenomas. Microadenomas (less than 10 mm in diameter) may be shown as hypodense areas within the homogeneously enhancing pituitary gland on an infused CT scan in the coronal plane, but are in fact seldom seen. Indirect signs, such as elevation of the superior border of the gland or contralateral displacement of the pituitary stalk, may be needed to make the diagnosis by CT. MRI is much more sensitive to microadenomas in the pituitary gland. The tumor appears hypointense in the T_1-weighted images. Evaluation of the cavernous sinus and internal carotid artery is possible during the same examination, eliminating the neurosurgeon's need to perform cerebral angiography to plan a transsphenoidal approach for microadenoma resection.

Macroadenomas. are visualized as well-defined, hyperdense lesions on the infused CT scan. They may cause destruction of the sella turcica and may involve the cavernous sinus. With suprasellar extension, they can compress the third ventricle. Subacute to chronic hemorrhages with macroadenomas are better detected by MRI than CT because in MRI, such blood presents a hyperintense signal in the T_1-weighted images while in CT it appears iso- or hypointense.

Intracerebral Tumors

Low-grade Astrocytomas. These (Fig. 3-18) are shown by CT as ill-defined, hypodense areas that do not enhance after contrast infusion. They may show calcifications and usually have little mass effect.

High-grade gliomas. More aggressive tumors such as *high-grade gliomas* (*glioblastomas*) (Fig. 3-19), are seen as areas of inhomogeneous density that enhance peripherally with hypodense, necrotic centers. They are surrounded by hypodensity consistent with edema and they cause severe mass effect.

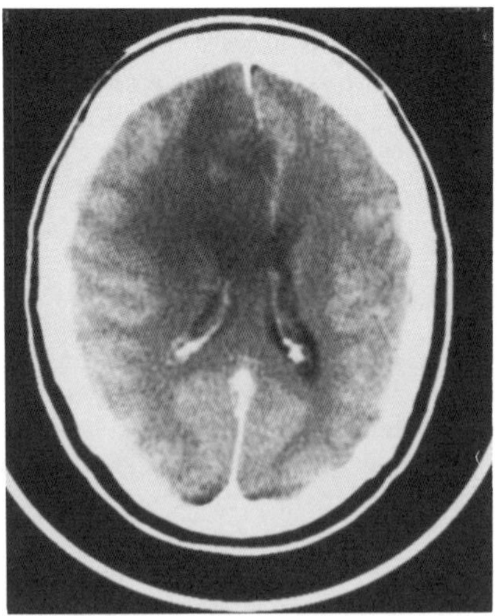

Fig. 3-18. CT scan of the head after infusion of intravenous contrast. A large, low grade astrocytoma in the right frontal region is illustrated. The tumor is compressing the right frontal horn and is probably beginning to infiltrate the genu of the corpus callosum.

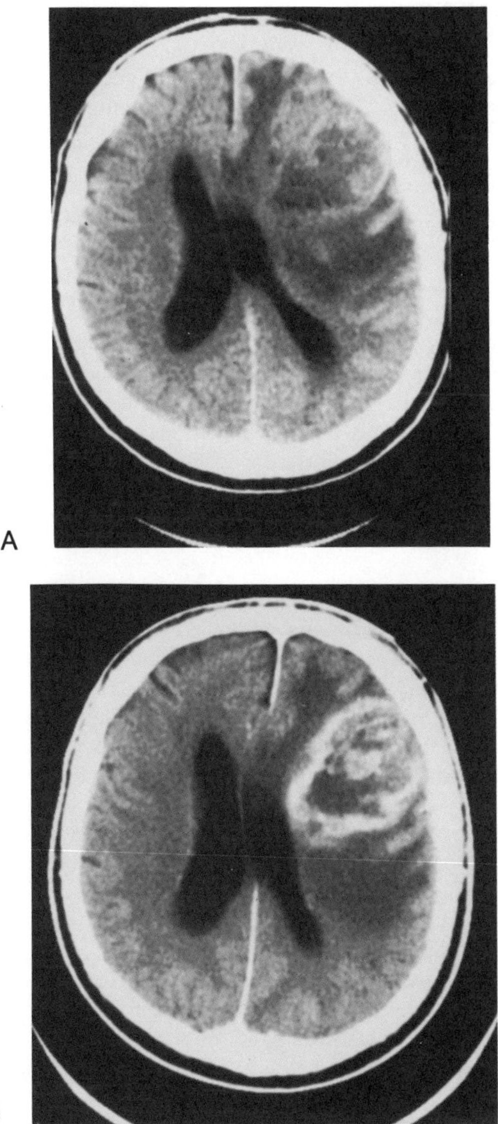

Fig. 3-19. **(A)** Plain CT scan of the head and **(B)** after infusion of intravenous contrast. A large glioblastoma is seen in the left frontal region. The infusion shows that the contrast-enhancing capsule has an irregular outline and that the tumor has a hypodense necrotic center; both are radiographic signs of an aggressive intracerebral malignancy. The tumor is surrounded by diffuse hypodensity consistent with edema. Also consistent with this is mass effect on the ventricular system and midline structures.

Butterfly glioma. This tumor (Fig. 3-20) is centrally located in the corpus callosum at the level of the splenium or genu and spreads bilaterally to involve both cerebral hemispheres.

Oligodendrogliomas. Oligodendrogliomas located in the frontal (Fig. 3-21) or occipital areas have an inhomogeneous density with multiple semilunar or nodular calcifications.

Lymphomas. These are commonly located periventricularly and usually strongly enhance.

Metastasis. Metastasis is the most common lesion of the posterior fossa in the adult and is usually characterized by dense enhancement and diffuse surrounding edema. The diagnosis of metastasis should be considered when multiple lesions are present.

Inflammatory Lesions

Abscesses

Classically an abscess appears as a well-defined, ring-enhancing lesion with a hypodense center and surrounding edema. Unfortunately, this characteristic picture may not always be recognized and the range of radiologic presentations of abscesses can be wide. In cysticercosis the ring-enhancing hypodense lesions are usually located at the corticosubcortical junction, and they may have a small calcification consistent with the dead cysticercus.

MRI is very sensitive in demonstrating intraparenchymal inflammatory lesions, particularly those in the brainstem. Its sensitivity is also especially helpful in cases (e.g., HIV-related encephalopathies) in which the differential diagnosis is between multifocal lesions and a diffuse encephalitis. Inflammatory lesions are usually isointense on T_1-weighted images, but appear hyperintense on T_2-weighted images. However, this appearance is nonspecific and does not identify specific inflammatory causes or distinguish between neoplastic and inflammatory lesions. An exception is cysticercosis; the cysticercus will appear as hyperintense within the cyst in T_1-weighted images.

Cerebritis

An area of focal cerebritis may appear inhomogeneously hypodense on plain CT, with irregular enhancement after infusion. Usually it is associated with mass effect and loss of white-gray matter differentiation.

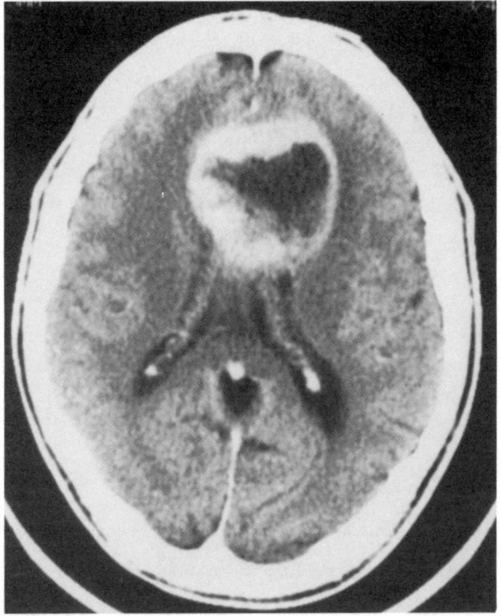

Fig. 3-20. CT scan of the head after infusion of intravenous contrast. An aggressive butterfly glioblastoma infiltrating the genu of the corpus callosum is illustrated. Note the large, hypodense, necrotic center.

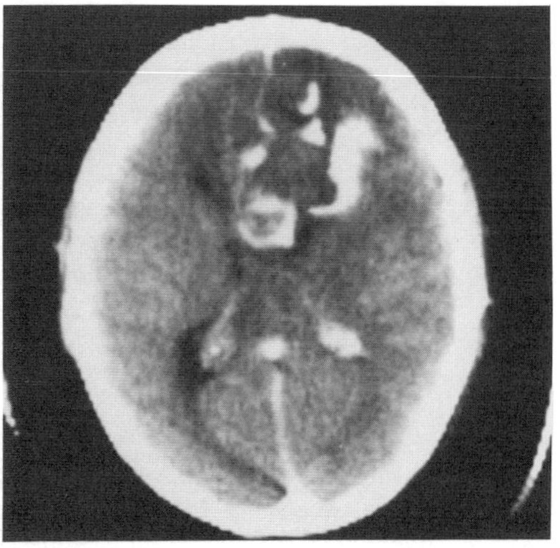

Fig. 3-21. CT scan of the head after infusion of intravenous contrast. Oligodendroglioma with multiple calcifications in the left frontal region. The tumor has already extended to involve the genu of the corpus callosum.

MRI has increased sensitivity for the edema associated with cerebritis and, in the case of herpes simplex encephalitis, allows better definition of contralateral spread. The better sensitivity allows improved assessment of the distribution and extent of lesions. The appearance is nonspecific (isointense on T_1- and hyperintense on T_2-weighted images), although evidence for microhemorrhages and a typical distribution (confined to the temporal lobes and limbic structures) of the edema considerably increase diagnostic certainty.

Meningitis

The plain CT scan may appear completely negative, but after infusion the meninges enhance dramatically. This hyperdensity is usually visualized in the posterior fossa, along both the notch of the tent of the cerebellum and the falx cerebri, and in the sylvian fissure.

Multiple Sclerosis

MRI is the technique of choice for the study of demyelinating disease in the CNS. Plaques appear on MRI as areas of hyperintense signal in the T_2-weighted images (Fig. 3-22). MRI has demonstrated that plaques can be located throughout the white matter and are often silent. Commonly, plaques in MS are found in and around the corpus callosum. Plaques can also be found in the brainstem and cerebellum. They need not be located only in the white matter; less commonly they are seen in the gray matter, particularly near the basal ganglia and thalami. However, these MRI changes are not specific to MS; a distribution of lesions with prominent involvement of the corpus callosum and both supratentorial and infratentorial plaques is more indicative of MS. The clinical presentation remains the major key to the differential diagnosis.

CT with double dose of contrast still remains a useful tool for demonstration of plaques when MRI is not available, but its sensitivity is far inferior. The acute demyelinating plaque appears hyperdense, whereas the chronic plaque appears hypodense on CT examination.

ANGIOGRAPHY

The role played by intra-arterial angiography has changed dramatically since the advent of CT and, more recently, MRI. Intra-arterial angiography is still mandatory for the complete evaluation of vascular malformations

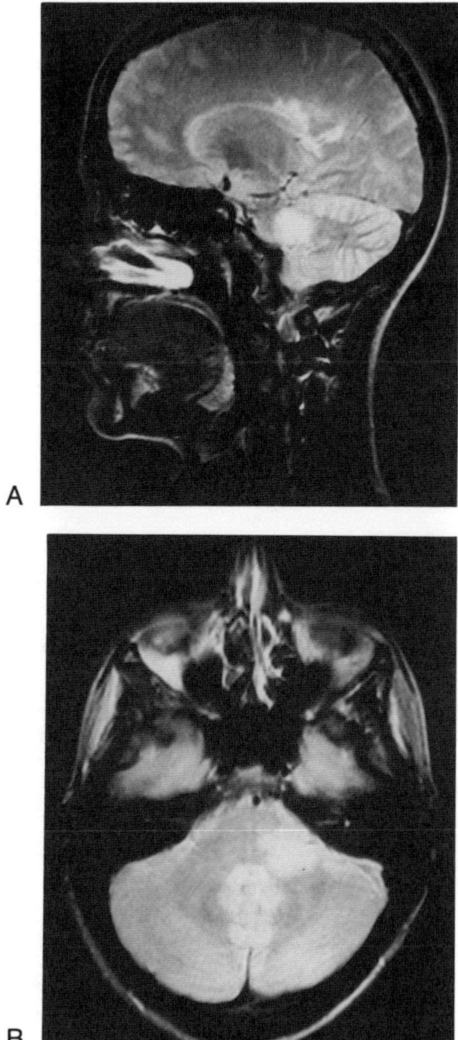

Fig. 3-22. T_2-weighted MRI (1.5 T, TR 2100 msec, TE 60 msec) of the head of a patient with MS. **(A)** The sagittal image shows prominent areas of hyperintense signal (plaques) in and adjacent to the posterior corpus callosum and in the anterior cerebellum. **(B)** The axial image from the posterior fossa further defines the large plaque in the left cerebellar hemisphere.

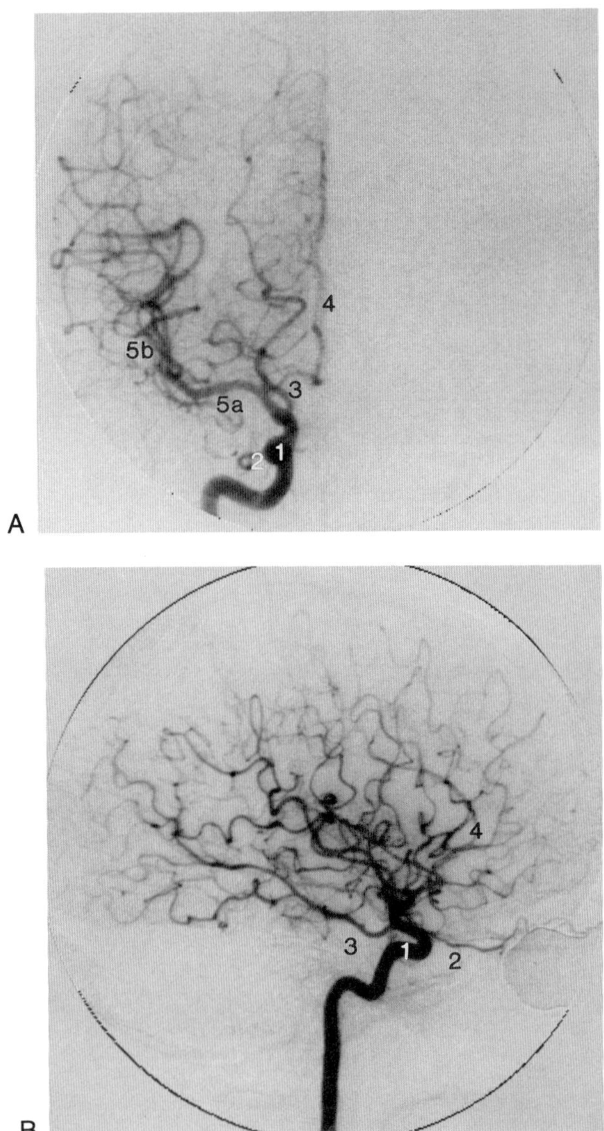

Fig. 3-23 (**A**) Anteroposterior and (**B**) lateral views from a normal study of the right internal carotid artery in the arterial phase after selective intra-arterial dye injection. 1, carotid siphon; 2, ophthalmic artery; 3, posterior cerebral artery; 4, anterior cerebral artery; 5, (a) middle cerebral artery M1 and (b) M2 portions.

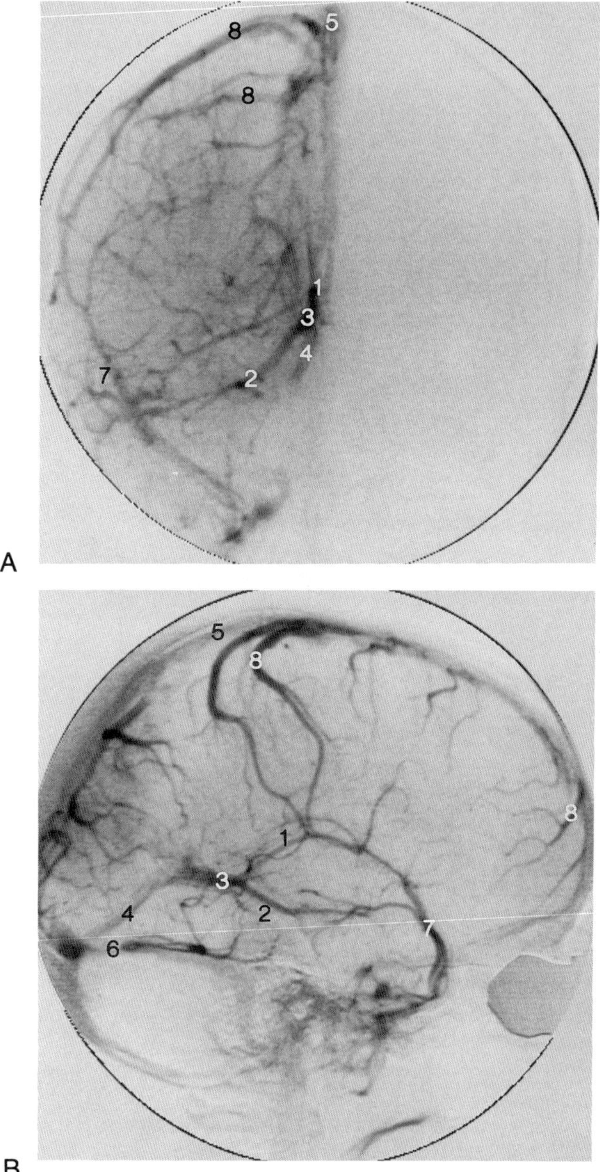

Fig. 3-24. **(A)** Anteroposterior and **(B)** lateral views from a normal study of the right internal carotid artery in the venous phase after selective intra-arterial dye injection. 1, internal cerebral vein; 2, basal vein of Rosenthal; 3, vein of Galen; 4, sinus rectus; 5, superior longitudinal sinus; 6, transverse sinus; 7, sphenoparietal sinus; 8, cortical veins.

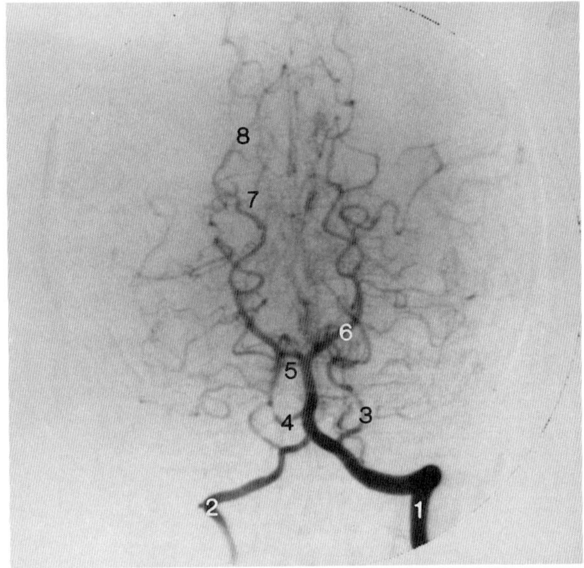

Fig. 3-25. (**A**) Anteroposterior (*Figure Continues.*)

(e.g., AVM, venous angiomas) and aneurysms. It remains essential for optimal definition of cerebrovascular disease and is usually an essential test for demonstration of CNS vasculitis (with the notable exception of temporal arteritis; see Ch. 8). Its role in evaluation of CNS neoplastic disease is variable and depends primarily on the needs of the neurosurgeon when biopsy or resection is being planned. Intra-arterial angiography can also be important in some cases in which the diagnosis is uncertain (e.g., abscess vs. neoplasm). Finally, angiography is essential for lesions (neoplastic or vascular) that may undergo an intravascular treatment (e.g., intra-arterial delivery of chemotherapy or embolization). In evaluation for any kind of embolization procedure, a complete angiographic study of the region of interest must be carried out. Images from normal anteroposterior and lateral angiograms are shown in Figures 3-23 to 3-26 with identification of key structures.

B

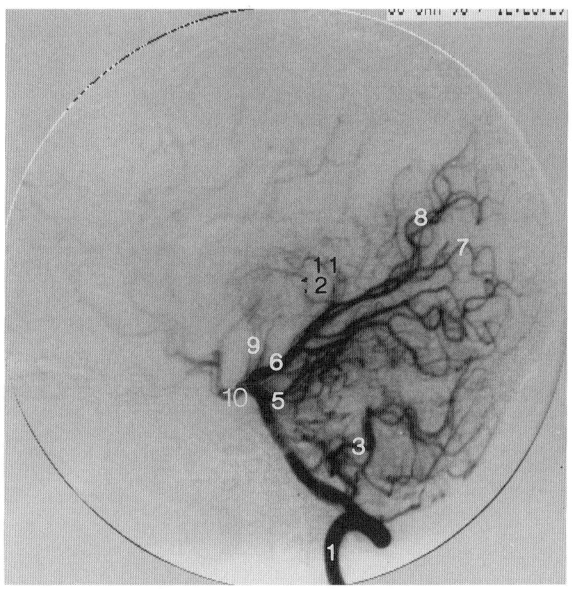

Fig. 3-25 *(Continued)*. and **(B)** lateral views from a normal study of the arterial phase of the left vertebral angiogram. 1, left vertebral artery; 2, right vertebral artery; 3, posteroinferior cerebellar artery (PICA); 4, anteroinferior cerebellar artery (AICA); 5, superior cerebellar artery; 6, posterior cerebral artery; 7, calcarine artery; 8, parieto-occipital artery; 9, thalamo-perforating arteries; 10, posterior communicating artery; 11, posterolateral choroidal artery; 12, posteromesial choroidal artery.

The risk-benefit ratio must be evaluated before performing angiography. It is important to appreciate that the likelihood of complications depends strongly on the technique used (direct puncture vs. femoral catheterization) and the experience of the physician. Femoral catheterization is usually the safest procedure. In experienced hands the risk of a transient neurologic deficit (i.e., resolving within 24 hours) should be less than 1 percent. The risk of a permanent deficit is 0.1 percent or less.

Three types of complications can occur with angiography: local, distal, or related to the contrast medium. Local complications resulting directly from the femoral puncture and catheter manipulations include hematoma at the puncture site, dissection of the artery, and formation of an arteriovenous fistula. These complications are usually easily controlled, al-

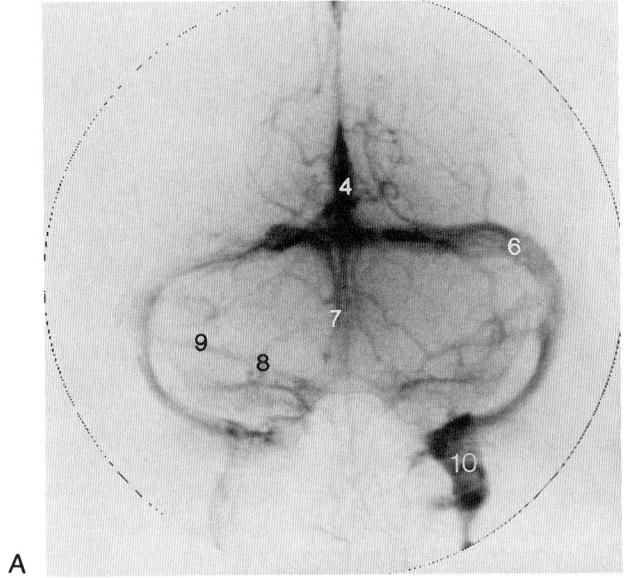

Fig. 3-26. (A) Anteroposterior (*Figure Continues.*)

though (e.g., in the case of an arteriovenous fistula) the intervention of a general surgeon may be required. Patients must be watched carefully for signs of local hematomas after angiography, as considerable blood may be deep in the femoral region before the mass effect of the hemotoma is readily appreciated.

Distal complications are those caused by the tip of the guide wire or catheter. Dissection of vessels, dislodgment of arteriosclerotic plaques, or accidental injection of a blood clot formed during the catheter manipulation are the most common. All of these complications can lead to strokes.

The risks associated with use of contrast medium are largely independent of the radiologist's skill. Most patients feel an uncomfortable hot flush with dye injections. The most serious complications arise with allergic reactions, although these are usually not as severe as those that can be seen with intravenous injections. Patients with histories of allergic reactions to other substances (e.g., seafood) are at higher risk. The use of low-osmolality and non-ionic contrast media has been demonstrated to

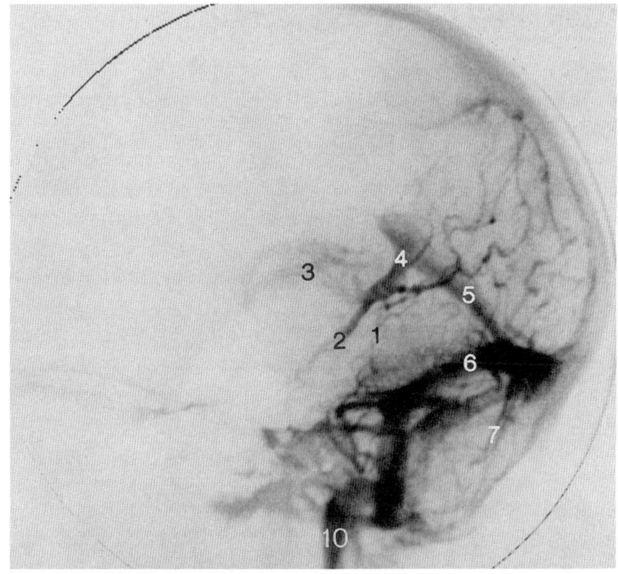

Fig. 3-26 (*Continued*). and (**B**) lateral views from a normal study of the venous phase of the left vertebral angiogram. 1, precentral cerebellar vein; 2, basal vein of Rosenthal; 3, internal cerebral vein; 4, vein of Galen; 5, sinus rectus; 6, lateral sinus; 7, inferior vermian vein; 8, petrosal vein; 9, superior petrosal sinus; 10, jugular vein.

reduce the complication rate. If there is a break in the integrity of the blood-brain barrier (e.g., around an infarct), local toxicity of the contrast medium may lead to a transient neurologic deficit. The use of smaller amounts of dye (as allowed by the digital subtraction imaging techniques) and low-osmolality contrast media have reduced the incidence of this complication.

MR angiography has an exciting potential, which is only beginning to unfold. Currently its application is limited to the study of large aneurysms, and of vessels found in the neck and the base of the brain. The quality of these images is similar to that of images from intravenous digital subtraction angiography, and usually demand corroboration by intra-arterial angiography when significant pathology is suspected. The resolution is still too poor for evaluation of medium to small vessel disease.

MYELOGRAPHY

Just as for angiography, indications for myelography have changed since the advent of spinal CT and MRI.

When the patient presents with a myelopathy and an intradural lesion is suspected (either intramedullary or extramedullary), MRI with gadolinium-DTPA for contrast enhancement is the examination of choice. If MRI is not available, myelography followed by CT has reasonable sensitivity for such lesions and can define their relationship with the spinal cord.

On the other hand, when the patient presents with a radiculopathy and an extradural lesion is suspected, the approach varies in relationship to the level of the suspected lesion. In cases of cervical or thoracic radiculopathies (including cervical spondylosis), the examination of choice is myelography followed by local CT. This combination allows a thorough evaluation of the dural tube and its contents and, at the same time, of the surrounding bony canal. If the problem is located at the lumbar level, the initial examination should be a plain CT scan at the levels of suspected disc disease. In cases in which the patient presents with multiple levels of pathology, or the spinal canal is known to be narrow from plain films of the spine, myelography and CT postmyelography may represent the optimal study. MRI is not completely satisfactory for the study of nontumoral extradural lesions (e.g., disc disease, degenerative disease with bony changes), because the evaluation of the bone is poor and thus inadequate for preoperative neurosurgical assessment.

Abnormalities (both congenital malformations and acquired lesions) of the craniocervical junction are best evaluated by MRI because this technique allows simultaneous visualization of the bony canal and its contents. The T_1-weighted images in the sagittal plane allow the best anatomic definition (See Fig. 3-3). T_2-weighted images highlight the CSF space as in a myelogram, allowing graphic demonstration of extradural compression.

READINGS

Brant-Zawadzki M, Norman D: (eds): Magnetic Resonance Imaging of the Central Nervous System. Raven Press, New York, 1987

Daniels DL, Haughton VM, and Naidich TP: Cranial and Spinal Magnetic Resonance Imaging: An Atlas and Guide. Raven Press, New York, 1987

Enzman DR, DeLaPaz RL, Rubin JB: Magnetic Resonance of the Spine. CV Mosby, St Louis, 1990

Latchaw RE (ed): Computed Tomography of the Head, Neck and Spine. Year Book Medical Publishers, Chicago, 1985

Lee SH, Rao K: Cranial Computed Tomography and MRI. 2nd Ed. McGraw-Hill, New York, 1987

Osborn AG: Introduction to Cerebral Angiography. Harper & Row, Hagerstown, MD, 1980

Pomeranz SJ: Craniospinal Magnetic Resonance Imaging. WB Saunders, Philadelphia, 1989

Shapiro R: Myelography. 4th Ed. Year Book Medical Publishers, Chicago, 1984

ELECTROPHYSIOLOGIC TESTS OF PERIPHERAL NERVES, MUSCLE FUNCTION, AND CENTRAL SENSORY PATHWAYS

4

ANATOMY

Cord, Roots, and Mixed Spinal Nerves

Rootlets leave the spinal cord anterolaterally and enter posterolaterally within the subarachnoid space where they join together to form roots (Fig. 4-1). When they reach the intervertebral foramina, the roots join to form the mixed spinal nerves, which then exit the protective bony spinal column. About one-third of the fibers are myelinated. Their myelin is formed by Schwann cells.

Mixed spinal nerves (loosely called "roots") divide into the anterior and posterior primary rami almost immediately after they leave the intervertebral foramina. The anterior primary rami innervate the bulk of the trunk and the limbs. The posterior primary rami innervate myotomes of the paraspinous muscles and dermatomes adjacent to the spine. Root and mixed spinal nerve lesions can interrupt fibers in the posterior primary rami, whereas they will be spared damage with more distal lesions in nerve plexuses or peripheral nerves.

Preganglionic sympathetic autonomic fibers exit in the mixed spinal nerves (Fig. 4-2). Between T1 and L4, white rami composed of preganglionic fibers leave the spinal nerve to enter the paraspinal sympathetic ganglia at each level. Postganglionic fibers rejoin the spinal nerve via the gray rami located more proximally. More distal damage in nerve plexuses

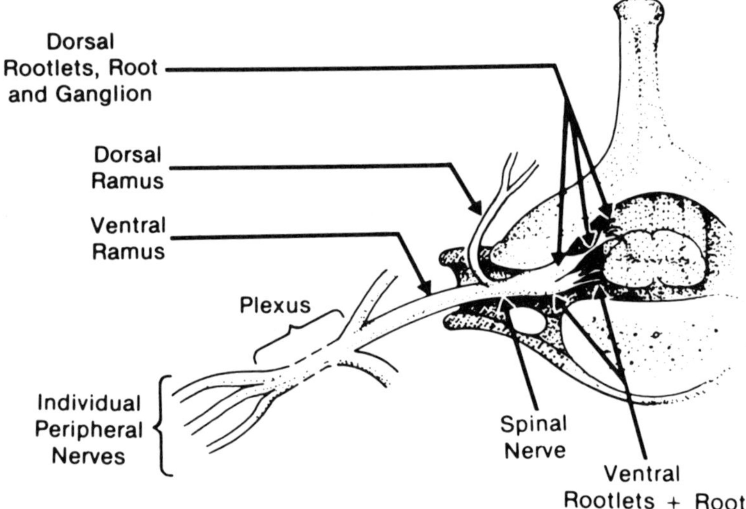

Fig. 4-1. General organization of the somatic peripheral nervous system. (From Stewart, 1987, with permission.)

or peripheral nerves can interrupt postganglionic sympathetic fibers and result in sympathetic denervation of the affected segments.

Cell bodies for motor neurons in the mixed peripheral nerves are found in the ipsilateral anterior horn of the spinal cord. Cell bodies of the bipolar sensory nerve cells are found in the dorsal root ganglia (located just distal to the openings of the intervertebral foramina), from which axonal processes are directed proximally toward the dorsal columns of the spinal cord and distally into the mixed spinal nerve.

To understand the pathophysiology of myelopathies and radiculopathies it is important to appreciate the relation between the spinal cord, the spinal nerve roots, and the bony structures of the spine (Fig. 4-3). The vertebral canal accommodates the spinal cord and is formed by the posterior surface of the vertebral bodies and intervertebral discs ventrally, the pedicles laterally, and the vertebral arches dorsally. The intervertebral foramina through which a mixed spinal nerve exits is limited anteriorly by the edge of the vertebral body and the lateral portion of the intervertebral disc, posteriorly by the facets, superiorly by the pedicle of the uppermost vertebra, and inferiorly by that of the lower vertebra. The foramina are nar-

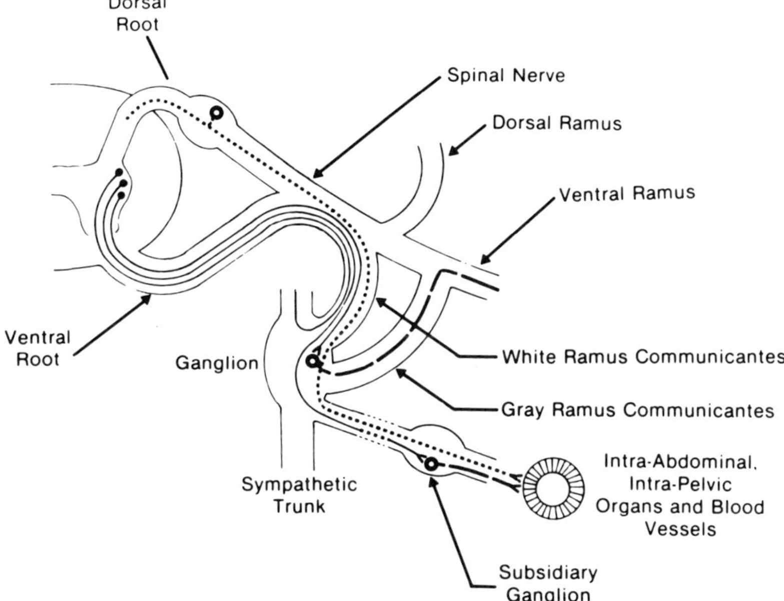

Fig. 4-2. The course of peripheral sympathetic nerve fibers. Solid lines, preganglionic fibers; stippled lines, postganglionic fibers; short stippled lines, sympathetic afferent fibers. (From Stewart, 1987, with permission.)

rowed usually by encroachment anteriorly or posteriorly. Disc prolapse and local extrusions or sequestration of nucleus pulposus are frequent causes of anterior compression. Osteophytes formed around the facets may compress posteriorly.

In the cervical spine (C1 to C7) roots exit via foramina above the vertebral body of the same number, with C8 exiting between C7 and T1. Thus, a C5 to C6 disc protrusion will generally result in a C6 radiculopathy. Thoracic, lumbar, and sacral roots exit below the associated vertebral body (e.g., the L5 root exits between the L5 and S1 vertebral bodies). In the lumbosacral region, the roots are more laterally situated and stretched under the pedicle of the vertebral body of the same number. Thus, disc protrusions usually compress the root exiting from the next most caudal foramina, which is somewhat more medially located (e.g., an L5 to S1 disc protrusion generally compresses the S1 root with only a very lateral protrusion compressing the L5 root). Below the level at which the spinal

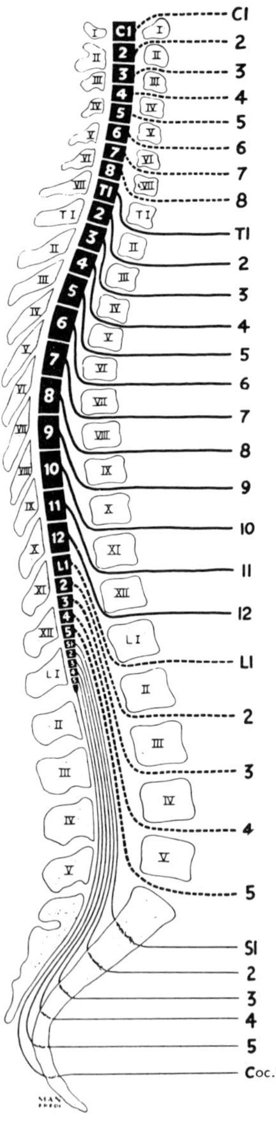

Fig. 4-3. Relationship of spinal segments and roots to the vertebral bodies and spinous processes. (From Haymaker et al., 1953, with persmission.)

cord ends (approximately L2) the nerve roots to all lower segments travel together in the vertebral canal (as the cauda equina) to the appropriate foramina. Medial compressions of the canal here, therefore, can produce polyradiculopathies. The more caudal nerve roots lie toward the center of the cauda equina.

The Motor Unit

The motor unit is defined as including the anterior horn cell, its axon, and the muscle fibers innervated by its terminal branches. The number of muscle fibers innervated by a single anterior horn cell varies tremendously: in the orbicularis oris a motor unit may contain only 5 to 10 fibers, whereas in the powerful gastrocnemius muscles large motor units may include many hundreds of fibers. A muscle is composed of multiple motor units derived from a brainstem motor nucleus or anterior horn cells from one to a few adjacent spinal segments. Although each anterior horn cell innervates many muscle fibers, each muscle fiber has a single neuromuscular junction innervated by only a single fascicle. Fibers from different motor units are interspersed in the body of the muscle.

Terminal fascicles to different fibers of the same motor unit are of slightly different lengths. This fact, plus the fact that the terminal branches are not fully myelinated, results in a small variation in the time at which signals for acetylcholine release arrive at the presynaptic terminal. The time required for acetylcholine to trigger a muscle action potential is also variable and is normally the major source of the small differences (a few tens of microseconds) in depolarization times for different muscle fibers. The time is minimized in normal muscle by release of considerably more acetylcholine than is needed to depolarize the motor endplate enough to reach the threshold for triggering a propagated action potential. This excess establishes a safety factor for neuromuscular transmission. An early sign of diseases of the neuromuscular junction that impair release of acetylcholine or the response of the motor endplate is an increased variability of the delays in motor endplate potential generation between different fibers.

Motor units in a muscle are recruited in strict order from smallest to largest with progressively more powerful movements. The activation frequency of neurons rises with greater recruitment. Control of the process is complex and occurs at many levels. Recruitment of fibers in a muscle can be decreased by loss or dysfunction of anterior horn cells or their axons, as well as by upper motor neuron dysfunction.

The Somatosensory System

The organization of the somatosensory system is less well understood than that of the motor system. Primary sensory stimuli generate changes in sensory nerve membrane potentials, often through modality-specific receptors. The nature of a sensation is determined by the durations, amplitudes, and frequencies of these changes; the variety of afferent nerves stimulated and their specific types; and their central processing. Sensory afferents are carried in the mixed peripheral nerves. Afferents from pacinian corpuscles, annulospiral endings, Golgi tendon organs, and joint capsule receptors are transmitted in rapidly conducting, large, myelinated fibers (class Ia, Ib sensory axons) with central projections that travel primarily in the dorsal columns. Secondary afferents travel in the medial lemniscus, decussating in the upper medulla and pons, to synapses in the contralateral ventral posterolateral thalamus. Tertiary projections continue to the contralateral sensory cortex. Pain and temperature sensation involves predominantly small diameter fibers that follow spinothalamic and other less well-defined central pathways.

NERVE CONDUCTION STUDIES

Sensory Nerve Action Potentials and Conduction Velocity Measurements

Normal nerve conduction velocities depend on the specific nerve, the section studied, the age of the patient, and environmental factors such as limb temperature. Measured velocities, therefore, can vary somewhat with the technique used to obtain them. Each laboratory develops its own standards.

Sensory nerve conduction velocities can be measured orthodromically or antidromically. Selective distal stimulation of sensory nerve fibers with recording more proximally over the appropriate mixed nerve fiber is known as orthodromic stimulation because the physiologic direction of impulse conduction is being followed. The orthodromically recorded superficial sensory nerve action potential (SNAP) amplitude is smaller (10 to 20 μV) and more variable in amplitude than with antidromic stimulation. The ratio of SNAP to random electrical noise can be increased by computer averaging of signals from repeated stimulations. The changing waveforms from random noise do not reinforce with repetition linked to the stimulation pulse, unlike the sensory action potential elicited synchronously with stimulation.

Let us consider measurement of a median nerve sensory nerve conduction velocity (SNCV) in order to illustrate the principles of measurement. Stimulating electrodes are placed superficially over the distal sensory branches of the median nerve in the index finger and recording electrodes are placed over the median nerve at the wrist. This allows measurement of the orthodromically recorded distal median SNCV:

$$\text{SNCV} = \text{D/T (m/sec)}$$

where D is the distance between the two electrodes and T is the delay between the stimulus pulse at the index finger and the *onset* of the recorded action potential at the wrist. Calculation of the SNCV from the onset of the action potential selectively determines the conduction velocity of the fastest conducting fibers.

Needle recording electrodes may be placed along the course of the nerve to increase the recorded potential amplitude. However, as they record from a more restricted field than do superficial skin electrodes, velocities measured with needle electrodes may be different from those measured with superficial electrodes.

In antidromic sensory nerve conduction studies, both motor and sensory fibers are stimulated *proximally* in the nerve and the SNAP is recorded from a superficial electrode placed over distal branches (e.g., using a ring electrode on the fifth finger for ulnar nerve studies) (Fig. 4-4). The relative positions of the recording electrode and the nerve can be reproduced more consistently with antidromic stimulation, decreasing the variation in amplitude between different measurements. Supramaximal nerve stimulation is used to minimize differences in the degrees of nerve activation arising from variable location the stimulating electrode with respect to the nerve. A disadvantage of antidromic stimulation is that muscle contraction (motor nerves are also excited by the stimulus) can introduce large-movement artifacts. Amplitudes measured antidromically are not directly comparable with those made orthodromically.

It is generally important to consider only the lower limits of the normal range for nerve conduction velocities (2 standard deviations below the mean). In the upper extremities the lower limits of normal sensory nerve conduction velocities are around 45 m/sec. Velocities are somewhat slower in the distal lower extremities where the lower limit of normal is around 35 m/sec.

In general, sensory nerve conduction studies are well tolerated by patients. The stimulation currents are large enough to give a strong electrical

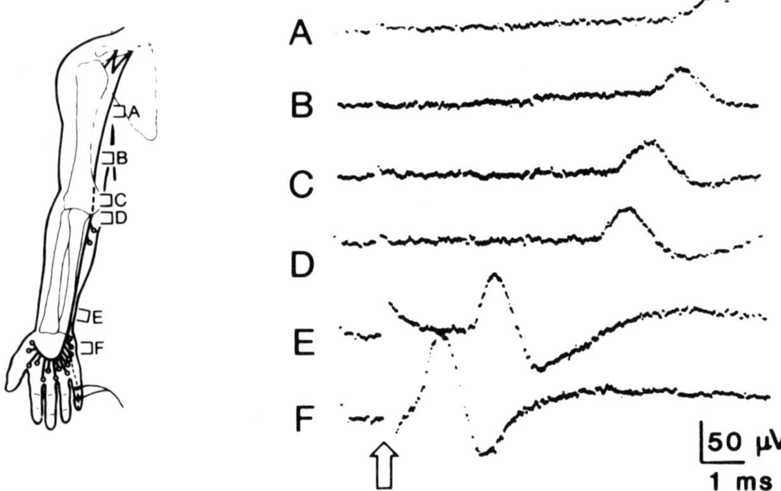

Fig. 4-4. (A–F) Diagram showing sites for stimulation of the ulnar nerve with recording of antidromically conducted sensory fiber impulses over the fifth digit using ring electrodes. To the right are the recorded potentials. Note the progressive increase in latency as the stimulating electrode is moved more proximally. (From Kimura, 1983, with permission.)

tingling along the course of the nerve. Antidromic stimulation leads to a brief contraction of the muscles innervated by the motor fibers and thus is more uncomfortable. Stimulation is frequently surprising and often mildly unpleasant, but not painful.

Useful nerves for routine study include the distal radial nerve and the mixed median and ulnar nerves in the upper extremities. In the lower extremities, the sural and peroneal nerves are commonly studied.

Compound Motor Action Potentials

Three parameters are important in the electrophysiologic characterization of motor nerve function: the compound motor action potential (CMAP or M wave) amplitude, the conduction velocity, and the distal motor latency. The amplitude of the M wave depends on the bulk of the muscle from which the recording is made and the number of motor units activated. It is diminished in an atrophic muscle, for example. A typical M wave has a biphasic or triphasic shape. Positive potentials are conventionally represented by downward deflections. The usual duration is about 10 to 15 msec. M waves have much higher amplitude (1 to 6 mV) than do sensory nerve action potentials (10 to 100 μV). In the former, synchronous firing of many motor units amplifies the propagated nerve action potential.

Motor nerve conduction velocity (MNCV) is measured using a recording electrode placed over the motor point (which is usually at the middle of the muscle belly) (Fig. 4-5). The voltage is measured with respect to a second electrode potential at the insertion site of the muscle. To perform the measurement, supramaximal stimulation current must first be determined. The latency between stimulation of the nerve and recording of the CMAP is recorded (L_1), using an oscilloscope triggered by the stimulus pulse. The stimulating electrode is then moved more proximally along the motor nerve by a measured distance (D), stimulation is repeated, and a second latency recorded (L_2). The MNCV over the portion of the nerve between the two stimulation sites is then calculated as:

$$\text{MNCV} = \frac{D}{L_2 - L_1} \text{ m/sec}$$

It is important to appreciate that because latencies L_1 and L_2 are measured from the *onset* of the recorded action potential, just as for SNCVs, the measured MNCV represents that for conduction in the fastest conducting fibers only.

The latency to the CMAP with most distal stimulation at a standard site is known as the distal motor latency for that nerve. One cannot calculate a conduction velocity over this segment because it includes contributions from the relatively slow conduction along the terminal unmyelinated portions of the nerve and the much slower *chemical* transmission across the neuromuscular junction. However, it can be somewhat useful to probe conduction velocities along the terminal stretch of the motor nerve. For example, in carpal tunnel syndrome the median nerve conduction velocity between the wrist and above the elbow is likely to be normal, whereas the distal latency measured from stimulation the wrist with recording over the abductor pollicis brevis is prolonged.

MNCVs in the upper extremities lower than about 45 m/sec are probably abnormal. Distal motor latencies for median nerves (measured with stimulation at the wrist) greater than 4.5 msec are abnormal. In the lower extremities, the lower limit of normal is (just as for sensory nerve conduction velocities) slower, 40 m/sec.

Motor nerve conduction studies are somewhat more uncomfortable for the patient than are sensory nerve conduction studies, because an invol-

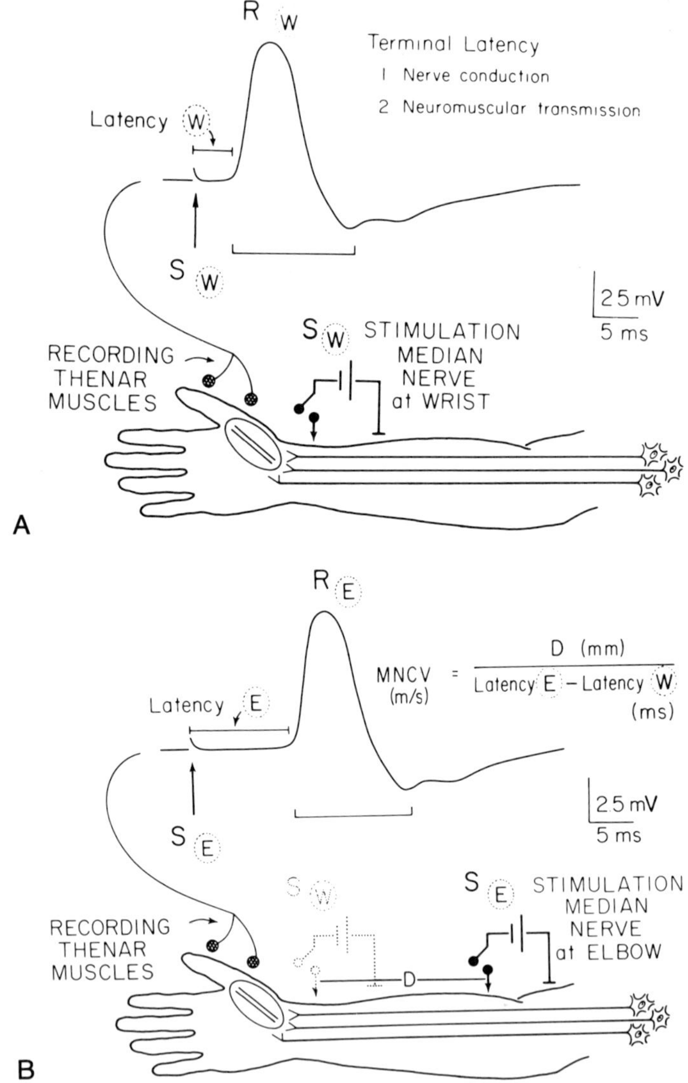

Fig. 4-5. **(A)** Diagram of the CMAP recorded from the thenar eminence after stimulation of the median nerve at the wrist (5w). The terminal latency (latency W) includes time for nerve conduction of the impulse from the stimulation site to the muscle (including transmission along the distal unmyelinated fascicles of the motor nerve) as well as the delay for neuromuscular transmission. **(B)** Results of stimulation more proximally at the elbow. The median nerve conduction velocity over the distance (D) from elbow to wrist can be calculated from the difference in latencies after stimulation at the two sites as shown. (From Kimura, 1983, with permission.)

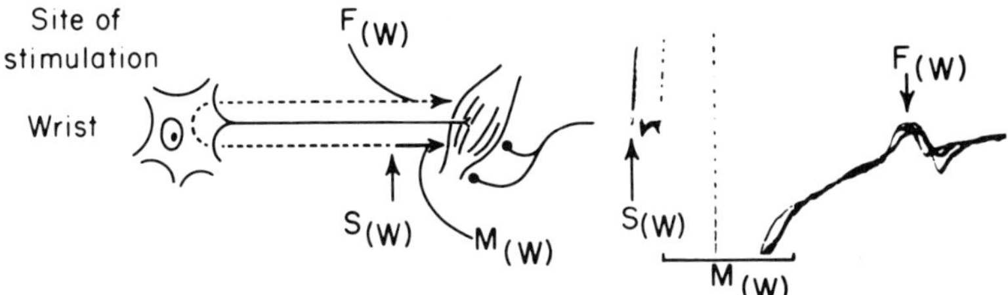

Fig. 4-6. Stimulation of a motor nerve produces an orthodromic impulse (solid arrow), which gives rise to the M wave. Antidromic impulses return from the anterior horn cell to give rise to a much smaller, longer latency, F wave response. To the right is illustrated an expanded tracing demonstrating superposition of three successive F waves. Note that the latency after stimulation (Sw) is greater than for the M wave (Mw), the amplitude is smaller (on this scale the M wave cannot even be accommodated), and the morphology is variable. (From Kimura, 1983, with permission.)

untary contraction is elicited in the stimulated muscle; however, studies of single nerves are usually performed rapidly. Easily studied motor nerves useful in screening for the presence of a polyneuropathy include the median and ulnar nerves in the upper and the posterior tibial and peroneal nerves in the lower extremities. It must be recalled that median, ulnar, and peroneal nerves are entrapable. Other nerves can also be studied and are often helpful in the diagnosis of focal neuropathies.

Late Responses

Late responses are lower amplitude potentials with latencies (several tens of msec) much longer than the M wave (about 10 msec or less) that arise in response to antidromic (distal to proximal) conduction of the depolarizing wave. They can be useful in defining more proximal pathology of motor neurons. There are three commonly measured types of late responses: the F wave, the H reflex, and the blink reflex.

F Wave

The amplitude of the F wave is about 5 percent that of the M wave. It has a variable, often polymorphic (i.e., the signal crosses the baseline more than four times) waveform (Fig. 4-6). It is generated at the anterior horn cell with antidromic stimulation. No synapses are crossed. The variable morphology results from activation of different subsets of the group of anterior horn cells whose axons contribute to the nerve stimulated. Its latency is sensitive to focal slowing anywhere along its path (including at the level of the root). Prolonged latencies or unobtainable F waves are often the only abnormalities in early or mild Guillain-Barré syndrome. They may be absent with radiculopathies; but, as most muscles are innervated by roots from multiple segments, the F wave latency is not a very sensitive index of root dysfunction. Also, interpretation of results can be difficult, as F waves are occasionally unobtainable even in normal subjects.

H Reflex

The H reflex most commonly recorded is an electrophysiologic equivalent of the ankle jerk. It is obtained by submaximal electrical stimulation of the posterior tibial nerve in the popliteal fossa performed while recording a CMAP over the soleus muscle. Submaximal stimulation excites afferents from soleus muscle stretch receptors, which trigger bisynaptic or polysynaptic activation of anterior horn cells belonging to motor units in that muscle. The amplitude is increased by facilitation maneuvers (e.g., tightly closing the fists or the jaw) and upper motor neuron lesions. It is decreased or unelicitable with dysfunction of either afferent or efferent branches of this reflex are by neuropathies or radiculopathies.

Blink Reflex

The blink reflex is the bilateral involuntary contraction of the orbicularis oris muscles after a glabellar tap or electrical stimulation of either supraorbital nerve. There are three distinct phases of muscle response: an early ipsilateral contraction, followed by a late ipsilateral contraction and a contralateral consensual response. Afferent and efferent limbs of the reflex together test the fifth and seventh cranial nerves and an extensive territory in the mid pons and upper medulla.

The early ipsilateral contraction of the orbicularis oculi is a monosynaptic reflex. The afferent limb is the fifth cranial nerve (the supraorbital nerve is a branch of cranial nerve V_1). In the brainstem, there is a putative excitatory interneuron running between the mid and lower pons to the ipsilateral seventh cranial nerve nucleus. The efferent limb is then the seventh cranial nerve. Latencies are about 10 msec. The late ipsilateral contraction arises from an ipsilateral *polysynaptic* pathway in the lower pons and upper medulla involving the spinal nucleus of cranial nerve V. Latencies may be as long as 40 msec. The consensual response arises from another polysynaptic pathway with projection to the contralateral seventh cranial nerve nucleus. The latency is similar to that of the ipsilateral late response.

Latency measurements are simply and rapidly performed. Superficial recording electrodes are placed over the orbicularis oculi muscles below the eye with ground electrodes placed lateral to the outer canthi of both eyes. A superficial stimulating electrode placed over the supraorbital nerve on one side delivers a supramaximal stimulus. The stimulus should trigger oscilloscope sweeps on two channels, one for the output of recording electrodes from each eye.

Unilateral lesions of the afferent limb (cranial nerve V) lead to prolonged latencies for all responses after stimulation of that side (Fig. 4-7). Lesions of the ipsilateral efferent limb (cranial nerve VII) will prolong both early and ipsilateral late responses, whereas the contralateral response latency will be normal. Mild dysfunction may be reflected in significant side-to-side variations in the usual latencies (i.e., differences greater than approximately 2 msec for the early and 8 to 10 msec for the late responses). With intrinsic brainstem lesions, ipsilateral responses are delayed by lesions of the main sensory nucleus of cranial nerve V and late responses by more caudal lesions involving the spinal nucleus of cranial nerve V. Contralateral responses will be affected by dysfunction of interneurons in the contralateral motor nucleus of cranial nerve VII.

In cases where damage to the efferent limb on one side is suspected, a side-to-side comparison of the orbicularis oculi CMAP amplitudes with direct stimulation of the facial nerves may help to localize the lesion. A difference in amplitude of greater than 50 percent suggests distal axonal loss or demyelination. These two possibilities can be distinguished by electromyography (EMG). The absence of asymmetry with facial nerve stimulation suggests more proximal conduction block in the seventh cranial nerve or its nucleus.

Repetitive Stimulation

Acetylcholine is released from an active pool of presynaptic vesicles at the neuromuscular junction with depolarization of a motor nerve. This pool turns over with each discharge as new vesicles from a much larger reserve reservoir enter the active pool. The amount of acetylcholine released is determined by the instantaneous cytosolic free Ca^{2+} concentration in the presynaptic terminal. In normal muscle, considerably more acetylcholine is released with each discharge-induced Ca^{2+} transient than is necessary for postsynaptic threshold depolarization at the motor endplate. Intracellular free Ca^{2+} concentration decays toward normal resting levels after each depolarization as Ca^{2+} is resequestered.

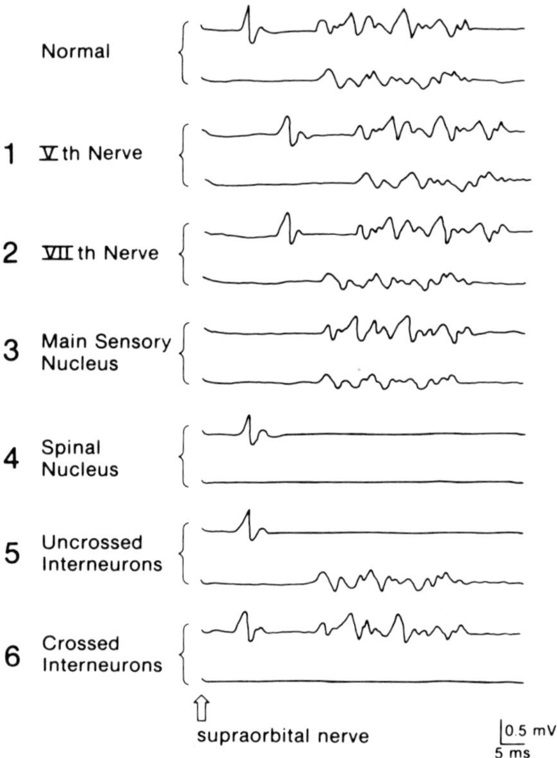

Fig. 4-7. The upper tracing shows a normal blink response recorded from electrodes placed ipsilaterally (top) and contralaterally (bottom) to the stimulation. Note the early (R_1) ipsilateral and late (R_2) ipsilateral and contralateral responses. The latter are of longer duration. The basic patterns of abnormality are shown: (1) all responses are delayed with dysfunction of the afferent arc (ipsilateral cranial nerve V); (2) ipsilateral responses are delayed with dysfunction of the ipsilateral afferent arc (ipsilateral cranial nerve VII); (3) dysfunction of the ipsilateral main sensory nucleus can selectively affect the early (R_1) responses; (4) dysfunction of the ipsilateral spinal tract and nucleus of cranial nerve V or medullary interneurons to the facial nuclei bilaterally will affect both late responses (R_2); (5 and 6) unilateral dysfunction of medullary interneurons between the spinal nucleus and the facial nuclei can affect either late response selectively. (From Kimura, 1983, with permission.)

Repetitive stimulation at 3 Hz is rapid enough to deplete the active acetylcholine vesicle pool slightly. Such slow repetitive stimulation releases fewer quanta of acetylcholine after each of the first few stimuli. Normally enough should still be released to activate the entire motor unit in muscle because of the large safety factor in neuromuscular transmission (i.e., the amount of acetylcholine released per discharge in excess of that needed to produce threshold depolarization). Thus, with 3 Hz stimulation, a normal individual shows at most only a minimal (<5 percent) decrement in the CMAP amplitude.

Stimulation at 20 to 30 Hz (or voluntary maximal contraction) is rapid enough to prevent full normalization of intracellular free Ca^{2+} concentration between depolarizations, allowing a new, increased steady state level to be achieved. However, in normal muscle, rapid stimulation usually produces no further change in the CMAP amplitude. Although more acetylcholine is released per contraction, it does not cause an increased CMAP amplitude, as the depolarization threshold for each of the fibers in the normal motor unit has already been surpassed; however, as we will discuss later, this is not always true with disorders of the neuromuscular junction.

PATHOLOGY OF NERVE LESIONS AND INTERPRETATION OF ABNORMAL NERVE CONDUCTION STUDIES

Axonal Degeneration

Polyneuropathies may result from demyelination or axonal degeneration. Those resulting from the latter are characterized by functional and pathologic changes more prominent distally than proximally. Toxic, metabolic, and some hereditary polyneuropathies often develop in this manner.

Amplitudes of SNAPs and CMAPs are reduced with advanced axonal degenerating processes. However, significant clinical signs may be present with SNAP or CMAP amplitudes still in the normal range. Nerve conduction velocities are slowed proportionally to the loss of the large myelinated fibers. Therefore, slowing may occur only late and is not a sensitive index for axon damage. When present, slowing is usually more prominent distally than proximally. The neuropathic process may selectively involve motor or sensory nerves. EMG is an important adjunct in evaluation and will be discussed later.

Segmental Demyelination

Myelin increases the effective resistance across the axon membrane and, in conjunction with specializations of ion-channel distribution, allows for rapid saltatory conduction. Loss of myelin will slow conduction velocity, often dramatically. Loss from several adjacent segments may block conduction altogether. Conduction block is probably the most important mechanism of early clinical deficits in acquired demyelinating neuropathies. Demyelinating disease may give rise to a classically neuropathic progression of deficits worsening distally to proximally. However, this gradient is not always seen, and there may be a pattern of predominantly proximal or asymmetric dysfunction.

Differential involvement of fibers in a mixed nerve and blocking of conduction in some can lead to dispersion of action potentials. A normal SNAP duration is less than 4 msec. The SNAP is significantly dispersed when there is more than 8 msec between the initial and terminal deflections. Inherited demyelinating diseases often show the most profound slowing of conduction velocity, but have relatively much less dispersion than *acquired* demyelinating diseases. The CMAP should also be evaluated for increased dispersion when acquired demyelinating disease is suspected.

Neuronopathies and Ganglionopathies

In contrast to neuropathies due to primary axonal degeneration, neuronal cell death secondarily accompanied by axonal degeneration can be caused by some metabolic, toxic, infectious, and heritable processes. The processes are frequently relatively selective for either anterior horn cells (neuronopathies, e.g., amyotrophic lateral sclerosis, [ALS]) or dorsal root ganglion cells (ganglionopathies, e.g., herpes zoster). In general, nerve conduction studies are not very sensitive indices of disease in these conditions. There is decreased amplitude and slowing proportional to the loss of large fibers. Consideration of the clinical presentation, any selectivity of damage to sensory or motor nerves, and EMG studies are useful in distinguishing these disorders from the primary axonal degenerating neuropathies.

Neuromuscular Junction Disorders

Disorders of the neuromuscular transmission may originate presynaptically or postsynaptically. Myasthenia gravis is associated with an impaired response to acetylcholine due to a decrease in acetylcholine receptors at the postsynaptic motor endplate. In the Lambert-Eaton syndrome and botulism, acetylcholine release is impaired presynaptically. Both processes reduce the likelihood that the threshold for propagated depolarization will be reached at the motor endplates with each presynaptic discharge.

The number of quanta of acetylcholine released with each depolarization will initially decrease with slow repetitive stimulation (3 Hz). This may result in a progressive decrease in the CMAP for the first 3 to 4 stimuli in patients with myasthenia gravis. A decrement of greater than 10 percent is considered significant. Mobilization of Ca^{2+} tends to partially repair this decrement after subsequent stimuli. A brief period of voluntary tetanic contraction will also repair a decrement.

In Lambert-Eaton syndrome, rather than merely repairing a decremental response, increased release of acetylcholine induced by such a short period of exercise may result in dramatic increases (>100 percent) in the CMAP amplitude.

ELECTROMYOGRAPHY

Standard Electromyography

EMG is performed by insertion of a needle electrode into a muscle to record local potentials produced by depolarization of muscle fibers. Studies are performed both with voluntary activation and at rest. EMG studies are an important complement to nerve conduction studies in investigation of dysfunction of motor nerves and the only electrophysiologic approach to diagnosis of myopathies. EMG is more unpleasant for the patient than nerve conduction studies, as needle insertion is somewhat painful. A complete study demands cooperation from the patient.

The standard EMG recording needle is a concentric, coaxial electrode. The inner recording electrode has a 0.2 mm diameter with an outer needle diameter of 0.3 mm. Recall that individual muscle fibers have a diameters only betwen 0.025 and 0.050 mm. The pickup area includes a volume with a diameter of about 1 mm around the electrode tip. Thus recordings represent composite signals from many nearby fibers, usually from several motor units with even modest contractions.

With care and a small, constant amount of muscle recruitment by the patient, potentials from single motor units may be isolated. The normal waveform is triphasic. Potentially pathologic polyphasic waves are defined as those crossing the baseline four or more times. The morphology varies with the position of the electrode relative to the motor unit, due to the

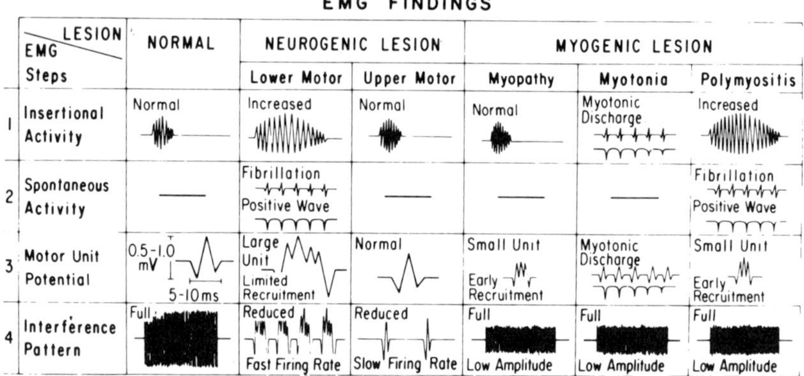

Fig. 4-8. Idealized illustrations of EMG findings in normal and diseased muscle during the four essential observation periods for a standard examination: during initial insertion, after insertion with the muscle at rest, with minimal voluntary contraction activating only a few motor units, and will full voluntary recruitment (interference pattern). Abnormalities in each of the stages of the examination define characteristic patterns of disease. Fibrillation potentials and positive sharp waves are manifestations of the same phenomenon of spontaneous excitability of individual muscle fibres. Myotonia is a much more regularly varying and sutained phenomenon secondary to specific defects of muscle membrane ion fluxes. (From Kimura, 1983, with permission.)

selective loss of higher frequency components of the potential as it travels through intervening muscle and connective tissue. This effect causes more distant units to have a broad, slowly rising shape. Accurate analysis, therefore, demands placement of the electrode near fibers of interest.

Experienced electromyographers rely heavily on the audio output of the recording amplifier in addition to the visual display. Distant units have a low-pitched, muted sound that changes to a crisp pop as the motor units are approached more closely.

Polyphasic units seen after reinnervation lead to a motor unit in which fibers depolarize at slightly different times (Fig. 4-8). The pathologic significance of polyphasic potentials is determined by their relative numbers and their stability. Normal muscle may have 10 to 15 percent polyphasic potentials, perhaps even up to 20 percent, as does tibialis anterior, where a minor degree of chronic denervation is expected even in normal subjects. Chronic changes lead to polyphasic potentials with stable morphology. Ongoing denervation may yield unstable polyphasic potentials in which the amplitudes and latencies of different components of the waveform are continuously changing. These are usually pathologic.

Motor unit potential amplitudes increase with the diameters of the muscle fibers and the size of the motor unit. They are normally small (0.25 mV) in the orbicular oris. Potential amplitudes from larger muscles vary between 1 and 4 mV. Potentials greater than about 6 mV are giant and should be considered pathologic. These imply an abnormally large distribution of terminal axons of the motor unit and are a consequence of loss of axons of adjacent motor units, followed by reinnervation of the denervated muscle fibers by new terminal branches of the surviving axons.

With minimal voluntary effort, smaller motor units discharge at relatively low frequencies. As effort increases, more and larger units are activated and the frequency of discharges rises. Full recruitment should give rise to a full interference pattern composed of overlapping potentials of different sizes from all of the simultaneously activated motor units in the muscle.

The duration of the motor unit action potential reflects differences in times for transmission of depolarization down the terminal fascicles of each motor fiber, delay at the neuromuscular junctions, and conduction along the muscle fibers. Larger muscle fibers and motor units have longer potential durations. The mean motor unit potential duration is around 10 to 15 msec, depending on the muscle and the age of the patient.

When normal muscle is at rest there are no recordable potentials. In pathologic conditions (usually after denervation, but also with some myopathic processes involving secondary denervation), fibrillation potentials and positive sharp waves may be seen (Fig. 4-8). Fibrillation potentials are spontaneous action potentials generated by irritable motor fibers. They are recognized as low-amplitude negative potentials. Positive sharp waves are larger, of shorter duration, and have opposite polarity. Spontaneous activity can be elicited by movement of the electrode or percussion of the muscle belly. Fibrillation potentials and positive sharp waves are abrupt in onset and discharge at a regular rate. They must be distinguished from voluntary recruitment, which yields motor unit potentials with amplitudes and frequencies that vary with time.

Myotonic discharges are rapid trains of repetitive high-frequency depolarizations (said to have the sound of a dive bomber) elicited after either spontaneous or voluntary excitation of a motor fiber; they are always pathologic.

Single-Fiber EMG

Single-fiber EMG has proved particularly useful for investigation of the neuromuscular junction. The single-fiber EMG recording needle is smaller than the standard EMG needle and is sensitive to a volume that is only a few muscle fiber diameters wide. The action potential from a single fiber within a motor unit may be identified with the single fiber electrode. The amplitude and morphology of the potential depend critically on the precise position of the electrode with respect to the muscle fiber. Stabilizing potentials to allow measurements to be made requires skill on the part of the examiner and considerable cooperation from the patient.

In normal limb muscles, most random insertions of a single-fiber recording needle allow recording of only a single potential from a given motor unit at one time, because fibers in a given motor unit are usually separated from each other by muscle fibers from different motor units. However, it is possible to find areas where potentials from two or more fibers in a single motor unit may be recorded. Such potentials are simultaneously displayed when the oscilloscope is triggered from the onset of the first potential. Quantification of the proportion of sites from which two or more fibers in the same unit are recorded relative to those in which only single units are seen gives a measure of *fiber density* in the motor unit.

The relative times of activation of two potentials in the same motor unit, expressed as the mean consecutive difference (MCD), is normally between 20 and 50 μmsec. The MCD (a quantitative measure usually referred to as jitter) arises mostly from differences in the transmission delays across the terminal axons and neuromuscular junctions for the two fibers. The upper limit of normal for jitter is age- and muscle group-dependent.

Occasionally, the second discharge may fail to appear. This phenomenon is called blocking. Although both increased jitter and blocking can be seen in normal older individuals, they usually suggest disease involving the neuromuscular junction (either primarily or secondarily).

PATHOLOGIC NERVE AND MUSCLE CHANGES AND THE INTERPRETATION OF ABNORMAL EMG STUDIES

Nerve Disease

The earliest change in the EMG after denervation is reduced recruitment in muscles of the affected myotome(s). Even with maximal effort a full interference pattern may not be seen on the oscilloscope; the audio output gives an anemic popping sound in which individual potentials are easily recognized rather than the roar of full recruitment. Within 7 to 14 days after acute denervation, spontaneous activity at rest (fibrillations and positive sharp waves) may be observed as the needle is moved (Fig. 4-8).

Axons of affected neurons may also be hyperexcitable and spontaneously discharge, producing activation of entire motor units, which is seen as the larger fasciculation potentials by EMG. As the disease becomes more chronic, new neuromuscular junctions may be formed on denervated fibers after sprouting of new terminal branches from preserved axons. Conduction is relatively slowed along new fascicles causing CMAPs to become polyphasic and possibly large (6 to 10 mV). The potentials may also be unstable with intermittent blocking along the new fascicles.

These abnormalities are found with a broad range of etiologies. Diagnosis of a radiculopathy is based on recognizing the patterns in which these characteristic changes occur. A radiculopathy is characterized by changes confined to the distribution of a specific myotome. In contrast, changes confined to the distributions of innervation of single nerves or portions of a nerve plexus are seen with focal neuropathies or plexopathies, respectively. Asymmetric involvement of myotomes throughout the body is a feature of motor neuron disease. Selective involvement of those supplying the most distal (or, more rarely, most proximal) limbs characterizes some of the inherited motor neuronopathies. Diffuse changes affecting sites in proportion to axonal length are seen with polyneuropathies.

Neuromuscular Junction Disorders

Disorders of neuromuscular transmission may show typical decremental (myasthenia gravis) or incremental (Lambert-Eaton syndrome) responses with repetitive stimulation as described earlier. The morphologies of the motor units are normal and spontaneous activity is generally not seen. Single-fiber EMG is significantly more sensitive to changes associated with myasthenia gravis than are other electrophysiologic tests. The decreased probability of neuromuscular transmission after the motor nerve depolarization is reflected in increased jitter and blocking in single-fiber studies of involved muscles. There is a useful difference between the jitter seen with myasthenia gravis and that in the Lambert-Eaton syndrome. In the former, the jitter should increase after exercise; in the latter it should decrease. Often changes can be seen in subclinically involved muscles.

Muscle Disease

Myopathies decrease the maximal contractile force that can be generated by motor units. Thus, a larger number of units must be recruited to complete a given movement. This hyper-recruitment is characterized by an interference pattern that is full, despite less than full muscle power (Fig. 4-8). However, unless this is dramatic, hyper-recruitment may be difficult to recognize without computer quantitation. Myopathies frequently lead to increased variability in fiber size with atrophy of some fibers, compensatory hypertrophy in others, and regeneration. Conduction can be slower along smaller fibers. Focal necrosis can lead to fiber splitting and formation of new neuromuscular junctions. Such changes can give rise to polyphasic motor unit potentials and spontaneous activity at rest. Fiber atrophy reduces the volume of individual fibers and there is a decrease in volume of the motor unit as fibers on the edges of the motor unit are lost. These changes lower the mean motor unit potential duration. Abnormally increased jitter may be found with single-fiber studies if there is fiber splitting.

SOMATOSENSORY EVOKED POTENTIALS

Peripheral sensory nerve studies test function of the distal axons of the bipolar sensory ganglion cells. Study of somatosensory evoked potentials (SEPs) gives information about the proximal axons and the postsynaptic central sensory pathways of the dorsal column-medial lemniscal system. They are useful only when it has been established that the peripheral nerve function is intact.

The measurements are usually not difficult and involve minimal discomfort to the patient. A peripheral sensory nerve is electrically stimulated by discrete square wave (0.2 to 2 msec duration) applied superficially at a rate of 3 to 5 Hz. Common stimulation sites include the radial or median nerves at the wrist, the common peroneal nerve at the knee, and the posterior tibial nerve at the ankle. Cutaneous stimulation localized to a specific dermatome rather than to a nerve may also be used, but this procedure is technically more difficult as the signal is of lower amplitude and more dispersed.

Potentials generated in the CNS after stimulation are best detected at specific sites. The sites are said to be near potential generators, but precisely what these are is unclear. They may be synapses in ganglia or merely related to local changes in volume conduction properties. Although some texts identify them with some anatomic precision, results are less likely to be misinterpreted if it is clearly recognized that their real nature and exact locations are uncertain. It has been found empirically that useful potentials can be recorded after upper limb stimulation from Erb's point, over the second or seventh cervical vertebrae, and over the parietal cortex of the contralateral side. The latter electrode is placed 40 percent of the way along an imaginary line connecting the vertex of the skull and tragus of the contralateral ear. A midfrontal electrode acts as ground. When the lower limb is stimulated, recordings are made from electrodes placed over L1, C2 or C7, and the vertex.

Evoked potentials are small, with amplitudes of only about 10 μV, which is of the same order as the random electrical noise. Averaging of the signal (usually 512 to 1,024 transients are needed) increases the signal-to-noise ratio as described earlier in discussion of SNAP measurement. Potentials recorded at each site have characteristic waveforms and latencies. Abnormal waveforms alone may be interpreted as evidence for pathology, especially if there is a clear and reproducible side-to-side difference. Major differences in amplitude between the two sides may sometimes be significant, although amplitudes are not usually diagnostically useful.

The major diagnostic information is obtained by measuring absolute and interpeak latencies. Block or dispersion of the afferent volley at one level may prolong latencies of potentials from all of the more proximal generators or prevent them from being recorded. For example, prolongation of the Erb's point latency after stimulation of the median nerve at the wrist suggests a lesion at the level of the brachial plexus or more distally. Peripheral nerve conduction studies can rule out dysfunction of the median nerve itself. Study of late responses can help in evaluation of conduction through the brachial plexus. Prolongation of Erb's point to C2 or C7 interpeak latency occurs with a lesion in the spinal cord. More rostral abnormalities in the central nervous system can prolong the cervical to cortical latency. Stimulation of the lower extremity allows the lumbar (or sacral) plexus to be investigated.

The dorsal column-medial lemniscal system subserving the lower and upper extremities are anatomically distinct. Thus prolongation of the L1-cortex latency with a normal cervical-cortex latency need not necessarily imply localization of a lesion in the posterior columns of the cord between cervical and lumbar levels.

The technique may be used to help diagnose plexopathies, but is otherwise poorly suited to evaluation or peripheral nerve lesions. It may help identify nerve root avulsion. A normal Erb's point (N9) latency with an absent or prolonged cervical (N13) latency can distinguish an avulsion of the spinal root proximal to the ganglion from a more distal injury. A major application in the past has been in defining subclinical myelopathies for the diagnosis of multiple sclerosis. In definite MS without myelopathic signs, about 50 percent of patients will show an abnormality. The sensitivity is greater with symptoms localizing for a lesion in the spinal cord. It can be used to develop evidence of a further, clinically occult lesion when attempting to establish the presence of multifocal disease in suspected MS (although, as discussed elsewhere, MRI is much more sensitive). Similarly, other myelopathies, syrinxes, metabolic disorders (e.g., subacute combined deficiency), or degenerative disease (e.g., Friedreich's ataxia) affecting the posterior columns can lead to increased latencies and dispersion of the somatosensory evoked potentials. However, as noted previously, it is critical to ascertain that the peripheral nerves are relatively intact before ascribing any changes to posterior column lesions.

Lesions in the deep white matter of the brain may also lead to prolonged cortical latencies. In such cases, sensory evoked potential studies might be used in an attempt to localize the lesion responsible for sensory loss in a limb to either the brain or spinal cord.

STRATEGIES IN EVALUATION

Focal Neuropathies

Radiculopathies

Diagnosis of a radiculopathy involves recognition of motor and sensory deficits in the distribution of a single mixed spinal nerve or root. EMG is the most useful electrodiagnostic test as it can define degrees of denervation not apparent on clinical examination or equivocal because of pain. Often the question arises of whether spontaneous activity has resulted from recent or old lesions. As denervated fibers atrophy, the amplitude of the spontaneous potentials decreases. Thus large spontaneous potentials suggest a more recent lesion.

The SNAPs are normal with radiculopathies, but may be reduced with more peripheral lesions (e.g., plexopathy). Motor nerve conduction studies usually provide little additional information. The CMAP will decrease with significant large fiber axonal loss but spontaneous activity on EMG is a more sensitive index of denervation. Late responses (H response, F wave) are often absent, but because all the motor nerve axons in the mixed nerve contribute to them, they may be normal if damage is confined to just a fraction of the fascicles of the nerve.

A further point should be made about the electromyographic distinction of a motor neuron disease (e.g., ALS) from a polyradiculopathy. The usual very widespread nature of changes in motor neuron disease is often the best clue. Unequivocal involvement of muscle of the face and/or three limbs makes the diagnosis of a motor neuron disease more likely (*in the absence of a neuropathy*). Giant potentials (6 to 10 mV) are characteristic of the chronic denervation/reinnervation of motor neuron disease, but are not specific.

Plexopathies

A plexopathy is distinguished from a radiculopathy by abnormalities in a limb that involve multiple myotomes and include the territories of more than one peripheral nerve in a distribution consistent with a lesion or lesions in a nerve plexus. The electrophysiologic changes depend on the nature of the pathology. Demyelination alone may lead to decreased recruitment in affected muscles only. Axonal degeneration will lead to denervation. However, in plexopathies, the paraspinous muscles, whose nerve supply branches dorsally, proximal to the origin of the plexus, should be normal (the notable well-recognized exception being a diabetic plexopathy in which paraspinous muscle changes may be seen).

Because a plexus lesion is by definition distal to the sensory ganglion, the sensory nerve action potentials in affected nerves may be reduced. Changes occur first at about 5 to 6 days after an acute lesion and reach their maximum after 9 to 10 days. CMAPs show similar changes.

Focal Peripheral Neuropathies

In focal neuropathies, changes are confined to the distribution of a single peripheral nerve (or nerves). Conduction studies may show a focal decrease in conduction velocity (defined by comparing velocities measured over several adjacent lengths of the nerve). More severe lesions may give rise to blocking, which will decrease the CMAP or SNAP amplitude measured with conduction across the site of damage. If axonal degeneration has occurred, CMAPs and SNAPs remote from the site of the lesion will also be decreased.

The EMG of distal muscles may show decreased recruitment, but will otherwise be normal. With more severe damage, the EMG may show denervation changes in muscles within the field of innervation of the damaged nerve.

Polyneuropathies

Polyneuropathies may be classified by electrodiagnostic studies as either axonal or demyelinating, a distinction of great importance in establishing etiology. Axonal neuropathies involving the large motor and sensory fibers are characterized by (1) decreased SNAP and CMAP amplitudes; (2) sensory and motor nerve conduction velocities decreased proportional to the loss of large diameter myelinated axons; and (3) decreased recruitment, spontaneous activity, and, if chronic, polyphasic potentials with EMG studies of affected muscles. The common, painful, small fiber distal neuropathies may show none of these changes despite clear pathologic evidence of axonal degeneration because of the relative insensitivity of these electrophysiologic tests to dysfunction of the small diameter, slowly conducting fibers in the mixed nerves.

The characteristic finding in a demyelinating neuropathy is slowing of the nerve conduction velocities or, in milder cases, only prolongation of late-response latencies. As discussed earlier, inherited demyelinating diseases show dramatic slowing (20 to 30 m/sec) with minimal dispersion, whereas acquired demyelinating diseases usually show increased dispersion even with modest slowing. In pure demyelinating neuropathies, the EMG shows only decreased recruitment. Severe cases may lead to secondary axonal degeneration and denervation changes in muscle.

Myopathies

EMG is the most important electrodiagnostic test in investigation of myopathies. Nerve conduction studies are useful only to better rule our neuropathic processes. The EMG may show abnormal motor unit morphology with stable or unstable polyphasic potentials and even spontaneous activity at rest in processes accompanied by fiber necrosis. Measurement of motor unit potential durations normalized for age and the muscle group studied may show decreases. Myotonic dystrophies, myotonia congenita, and paramyotonia are associated with myotonic discharges. Myopathies classically show hyperrecruitment.

Myasthenic Syndromes

Routine nerve conduction studies should be normal in myasthenic syndromes. Usually the standard EMG studies are also normal, although blocking can sometimes be seen even with a routine examination. More sensitive tests for diagnosis involve repetitive nerve stimulation tests and single fiber EMG measurements of jitter as described earlier.

READINGS

Brown WF, Bolton CF (eds): Clinical Electromyography. Butterworths, Boston, 1987

Buchthal F: Electromyography in the evaluation of muscle disease. p. 573. In Aminoff MJ (ed): Neurologic Clinics. Vol. 3. No. 3. WB Saunders, Philadelphia, 1985

Buchthal F: Electrophysiologic abnormalities in metabolic myopathies and neuropathies. Acta Neurol Scand 46:suppl. 43, 129, 1970

Chiappa KA, Ropper AH: Evoked potentials in clinical medicine. New Engl J Med 306:1140, 1205, 1982

Cornblath DR, Mellits ED, Griffin JW, et al: Motor conduction studies in Guillain-Barré Syndrome: description and prognostic value. Ann Neurol 23:354, 1988

Eisen A: Electrodiagnosis of Radiculopathies. p. 495. In Aminoff MJ (ed): Neurologic Clinics. Vol. 3. No. 3. WB Saunders, Philadephia, 1985

Gillmore R (ed.): Evoked potentials. Neurologic Clinics. Vol. 6. No. 4. WB Saunders, Philadelphia, 1988

Haymaker W, Woodhall B: Peripheral Nerve Injuries. WB Saunders, Philadelphia, 1953

Kimura J: Electrodiagnosis in Diseases of Nerve and Muscle: Principles and Practice. FA Davis, Philadelphia, 1983

Kimura J: Principles and pitfalls of nerve conduction studies. Ann Neurol 16:415, 1984

Shahani BT, Young RR: Clinical electromyography, p. 6-1. In Joynt RJ (ed): Clinical Neurology. Vol. 1. JB Lippincott, Philadelphia, 1985

Stalberg E, Sanders DB: Electrophysiological tests of neuromuscular transmission. p. 88. In Stalberg E, Young RR (eds): Clinical Neurophysiology. Butterworths (Publishers), Sevenoaks, Kent, England, 1981

Stalberg E, Trontelj JV: Single Fibre Electromyography. Mirvalle Press, Old Woking, Surrey, England, 1979

Stewart JD: Focal Peripheral Neuropathies. Elsevier Science Publishing, New York, 1987

EVOKED POTENTIALS IN THE EVALUATION OF VISUAL AND AUDITORY PATHWAYS

5

Andrew N. Wilner

As described earlier, an evoked potential results from the electrical activity of the central nervous system in response to an external stimulus. For routine neurology three types of evoked potential tests are generally available. These are:

Visual evoked response (or potential) (VER, VEP)

Brainstem auditory evoked response (BAER, BAEP)

Somatosensory evoked response (SEP, SER, SSEP)

The last type was discussed in Chapter 4.

Evoked potential tests verify the functional integrity of visual (VER), auditory (BAER), or somatosensory (SEP) pathways using a well-defined sensory stimulus to elicit a specific neurophysiologic response, just as a tap on the knee demonstrates the integrity of the local spinal reflex arc. For example, to obtain a VER, a repetitive stimulus such as a shifting checkerboard pattern is used to activate retinal receptors, which initiate conduction of a signal to neurons of the occipital cortex. The cortical neurophysiologic response is seen as a change in the electrical field detected by a scalp electrode. In assessing *dynamic* physiologic responses, therefore, evoked potentials differ from imaging studies such as magnetic resonance imaging (MRI) and computed tomography (CT), which provide only anatomic views of the CNS.

The nature of the stimulus must vary with the sensory system evaluated.

For the visual system it is a changing pattern of light, for the auditory system it is clicks, and for the somatosensory system it is generally direct electrical stimulation of a nerve. More recently, stimulation of deeper structures in the CNS using a magnetic stimulator has become possible.

A response is said to be near field or far field, depending on the relative distance of the electrode detecting the evoked response from the source of the electrical potential changes. In the case of the VER, the recording electrode is relatively close to the signal generators, which are cortical neurons in visual area 17 (association areas 18 and 19 may also contribute). This is a near field response. In contrast, BAEPs originate relatively far from the recording electrodes, producing a far field response. All evoked responses have a very small amplitude, on the order of 0.1 to 20 μV. Because the amplitude of a response decreases as the square of the distance from the source of the signal to the receiving electrode, amplitudes of far field evoked responses are smaller than those of near field responses.

Neither type of response is sufficient to be discerned after a single stimulus. To observe evoked responses above the background of brain electrical activity (the EEG normally has an amplitude of 20 to 60 μV), one must use computer averaging of responses after repetitive stimulation. For a VER approximately 128 repetitions are needed, for a SER between 256 and 512, and for a far field BAER as many as 2,048 repetitions. The waveforms are recorded electronically for each trial. As the evoked response always occurs at the same time after each stimulus, it reinforces with each repetition, whereas the EEG signal waveforms, which are not timelocked to the stimulus, will progressively cancel. Averaging augments the signal-to-noise ratio as the square root of the number of responses in the average. Thus, in order to double the size of the signal obtained with 128 responses, 512 responses must be performed.

Electronic malfunctions, excessive patient movement, poor electrode contact, or lack of patient cooperation (for VERs and SEPs) can degrade the signal-to-noise ratio.

VISUAL EVOKED RESPONSES

A schematic description of the stimulus-receptor response sequence for the VER appears in Figure 5-1. The patient views a checkerboard screen that reverses its patterns with a frequency of 1 to 2 Hz. In this way, repeated contrast stimuli are provided without changing the total luminance of the checkerboard. One eye at a time is tested. Electrodes record from OZ and CZ of the standard 10–20 EEG electrode classification system (see Ch. 5). The first evoked potential occurs from the retina (and

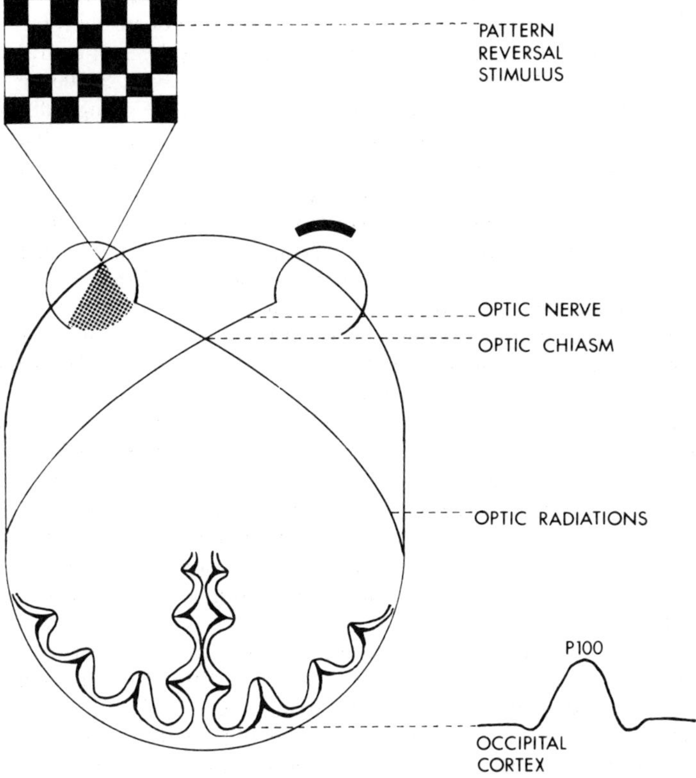

Fig. 5-1. Diagram illustrating the stimulus-receptor response of a VEP. With one eye covered, the patient views a checkerboard stimulus, which produces a retinal response. The signal then travels through the optic nerve, optic chiasm, and optic radiations to the occipital cortex, which produces the P100 wave (Redrawn by Yerulshalmi from Spehlmann, 1985, with permission.)

can be separately recorded as the electroretinogram, a useful measure of retinal ganglion function), but this is not often recorded for standard VERs. The response to the visual stimulus then traverses the optic nerve, chiasm, and optic radiations to arrive at the occipital cortex where the synchronized depolarization of the regularly arrayed neurons produces the measured evoked potential response. The most reproducible wave is called the P100 response, because the positive peak of this wave occurs with a latency of about 100 msec from the time of the stimulus.

A delayed or morphologically abnormal wave can occur with a lesion anywhere in the visual pathway. The problem may be non-neurologic, such as a severe refractive error (acuity poorer than about 20/200) or corneal opacities. These can be ruled out before the test. Neurologic diseases altering the VER may affect the retina, optic nerve, chiasm, radiations, or the visual cortex. However, in most cases, disease in the optic nerve or chiasm is responsible for abnormalities in the VER.

When interpreting VER results, an attempt is made to localize the lesion to the prechiasmal, chiasmal, or retrochiasmal regions. From the anatomy of the visual pathways (Fig. 5-1), it can be appreciated that a unilateral abnormality indicates a lesion anterior to the chiasm.

Bilateral abnormalities are more difficult to localize. The most reliable abnormality is a prolongation of the latency. Side-to-side differences in amplitude may also be used, if they are large.

VERs are very sensitive to optic neuritis or atrophy or compressive lesions of the optic nerve. Because of the wide anatomic distribution of the optic radiations, a lesion must be very large in this area to significantly affect the VER. Similar considerations apply to diseases involving the retina or cortex. Note that a patient may be blind because of extensive damage to the visual association areas, yet have a normal VER because the evoked potential generator neurons in the primary visual cortex have been spared.

When an abnormality is detected, correlation with the patients's history and physical examination is essential. A word with the technician may also be required to ensure that cooperation or technical difficulties were not responsible for an abnormal waveform. Unlike with BAERs or SERs, the patient must cooperate by staring at the screen when using the pattern reversal checkerboard stimulus. If the patient cannot (or will not) fixate, a strobe light flash stimulus can be used, reducing the need for cooperation. However, changing the nature of the stimulus somewhat changes the response. Latencies obtained with strobe light and shifting checkerboard stimuli are not directly comparable.

Common indications for ordering VERs include the following.

1. Suspected optic or retrobulbar neuritis

2. Location of a second lesion to help establish a diagnosis of MS (e.g., it may be useful to order VERs in a young person with transverse myelitis to establish the presence of more widespread demyelinating disease)
3. Evaluation of hysterical blindness (note the caution above)
4. Postoperative follow-up of a patient after resection of a compressive tumor of the optic nerve or chiasm
5. Monitoring response to treatment of a pituitary tumor compressing the chiasm.

BRAINSTEM AUDITORY EVOKED RESPONSES

BAERs assess the functional integrity of pathways from the peripheral eighth nerve through the medulla, pons, and midbrain. Repetitive (1,024 to 2,048) rarefaction clicks of 50 to 100 μsec duration are given with a frequency of 10 Hz via headphones to one ear at 60 to 70 dB above the hearing threshold. A masking noise excludes participation by the contralateral ear. Recording electrodes are placed over the mastoid bone and at the skull vertex. As with all evoked responses, the precise way in which the measurement is performed can influence the evoked potential waveforms and perhaps even latencies. Thus all stimulus parameters, such as a click rarefaction polarity, frequency, and intensity, must be standardized.

The classic BAER waveform contains seven peaks that occur in the first 10 msec after stimulation (Fig. 5-2). By convention, these are labeled with Roman numerals. Although the exact signal generator(s) for each peak remains controversial, a generally accepted guide for localization is the following.

I—Eighth nerve

II—Cochlear nucleus (medulla)

III—Superior olive (pons)

IV—Lateral lemniscus (pons)

V—Inferior colliculus (midbrain)

VI—Medial geniculate (thalamus)

VII—Auditory radiations (thalamocortical)

For evaluation of the brainstem auditory pathways, wave I must be

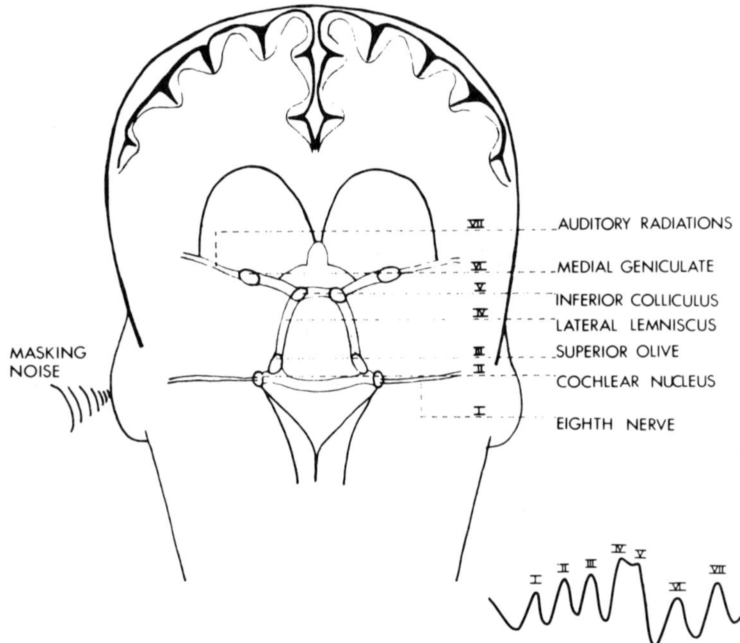

Fig. 5-2. The approximate anatomic correlate of each of the seven short latency brainstem auditory evoked responses recorded after a transient auditory stimulus. The first recorded wave is generated primarily from the distal portion of the eighth cranial nerve. As the signal continues through the brainstem, peaks are generated at the cochlear nucleus (II), superior olive (III), lateral lemniscus (IV), inferior colliculus (V), medial geniculate (VI), and auditory radiations (VII). The inset in the lower right corner illustrates the morphology of the evoked potential (Redrawn by Yerushalmi from Gilmore, 1988, with permission.)

present, indicating successful stimulation of the acoustic nerve. If waves I, III, and V occur at the appropriate latencies, with minimal side-to-side variation, and with wave V at least 50 percent of the amplitude of wave I, the study may be considered normal. Waves II and IV may be absent as a normal variant. For routine testing, waves VI and VII have proved too variable to be useful. In an abnormal study, if wave I is present, a lesion can be electrophysiologically localized in the brainstem to an area just distal to the anatomic area to the generator of the last recognizable waveform. For example, a pontine lesion affecting the left lateral lemniscus may lead to a BAER with stimulation of the left ear that has normal waveforms and latencies for waves I to III, but no later identifiable peaks. Less severe dysfunction may be reflected in delays in peak latencies. The central conduction time (calculated as the difference between the latencies of waves V and I) assesses conduction along the intra-axial brainstem auditory pathway. This is the most important and reliable measurement and should not exceed 4.75 msec. Side-to-side differences in the central conduction time should not be greater than about 0.4 msec. Reproducible, unilateral abnormalities in wave amplitudes alone may also suggest brainstem lesions, but are less reliable.

BAERs may be abnormal in many conditions. Acoustic neuromas, posterior fossa meningiomas, pontine gliomas, and ischemic lesions may also be detected and localized with the BAER. Demyelination from multiple sclerosis will prolong central conduction times and may lead to loss or decreased amplitude of later waves (e.g., wave V). Other diseases of white matter (e.g., adrenoleukodystrophy) or neuronal degenerative processes (e.g., Friedreich's ataxia) may produce similar abnormalities.

Common indications for ordering BAERs include the following.

1. To obtain evidence for a second lesion in suspected multiple sclerosis
2. To evaluate compressive or infiltrative lesions of the posterior fossa
3. To evaluate dysfunction secondary to brainstem ischemia
4. To evaluate hearing in infants and other uncooperative patients
5. To screen for acoustic neuromas in high-risk patients
6. To perform an ancillary study in the evaluation of coma or the diagnosis of brain death.

INTRAOPERATIVE MONITORING

The most widespread application of evoked potentials in intraoperative monitoring has been the use of SEPs (see Ch. 4) during scoliosis or other spinal surgery. One of the potential pitfalls of SEP monitoring in spinal surgery is that only posterior columns, which are supplied by the posterior spinal arteries, are evaluated. Consequently, it is theoretically possible to damage the anterior two-thirds of the cord without a significant change in the SEPs. Combined use of SEPs and a magnetic stimulator for excitation of the lateral columns may potentially overcome this limitation by allowing simultaneous assessment of the posterior columns and the corticospinal tracts.

SEPs have also been used to monitor cortical function in procedures potentially leading to ischemia in the cerebral hemispheres such as carotid endarterectomy, repair of carotid circulation aneurysms, or coronary artery bypass surgery. The SEP is not as sensitive to ischemia as is the EEG and, therefore, may be more specific for clinically significant impending ischemic damage. BAER measurements may also be useful in the operating room. For example, Radtke (1989) has reported that BAER monitoring reduced morbidity related to damage to cranial nerve VIII in a series of patients undergoing local microvascular decompressive surgery.

READINGS

Aminoff M (ed): Electrodiagnosis. Neurologic Clinics. Vol. 3. No. 5. WB Saunders, Philadelphia, 1985

Deiber M, Ibanez V, Bastuji H, et al: Changes of middle latency auditory evoked potentials during natural sleep in humans. Neurology 39:806, 1989

Gilmore R (ed): Evoked Potentials. Neurologic Clinics. Vol. 6. No. 4. WB Saunders, Philadelphia, 1988

Niedermeyer E, Lopes da Silva F: Electroencephalography. 2nd Ed. Urban & Schwarzenberg, Baltimore, 1987

Radtke R, Erwin CW, Wilkins RH: Intraoperative brainstem auditory evoked potentials: significant decrease in post-operative morbidity. Neurology 39:187, 1989

Seyal M, Sandhi LS, Mack YP: Spinal segmental somatosensory evoked potentials in lumbosacral radiculopathies. Neurology 39:801, 1989

Spehlmann R: Evoked Potential Primer: Visual, Auditory, and Somatosensory Potentials in Clinical Diagnosis. Butterworths, Boston, 1985

THE ELECTROENCEPHALOGRAM 6

Norman K. So

This chapter is intended to introduce the basic principles of EEG and serves as a user's guide for clinicians treating adult patients. Texts useful for learning EEG interpretation are cited at the end of the chapter. The guidelines of the International Federation of Societies for Electroencephalography and Clinical Neurophysiology on terminology are recommended.

PHYSIOLOGIC BASIS OF THE ELECTROENCEPHALOGRAM

The EEG is a measure of the extracellular field potentials of the brain. By convention, the EEG refers to brain activity recorded by electrodes placed on the scalp, which reflects electrical activity of large neuronal aggregates.

With deep intracerebral electrodes, large potentials (200 to 1000μV) are recorded. EEG potentials at the scalp surface are considerably smaller (20 to 200μV). This is related not only to the falloff in potential, which occurs in proportion to the square of the distance from the source, but also to boundaries, created by the intervening CSF, tissues, and skull, which attenuate the signal. The factor of attenuation between cortex and scalp ranges from a ratio of 2:1 to 50:1. Attenuation is greater for higher frequencies and for activities in which synchronous activity involves only a small area of the cortex. Consequently, any EEG signal as seen on the scalp reflects summated activity over several square centimeters of cortex. Detection is also related to the orientation of the electrode to the generator. A generator deep in a sulcus and oriented perpendicularly to the surface may be undetectable by standard scalp electrodes.

Potential Sources

Changes in electrical potential are related to current flow. In nervous tissue, current flow is caused by ionic fluxes. These fluxes result from either synaptic transmission, which generates graded postsynaptic potentials, or all-or-none action potentials. Summated postsynaptic potentials (not the action potential) in cortical gray matter are the sources of EEG activity. Correlation of electrophysiologic and histologic studies indicates that the vertically oriented pyramidal cells, with their long apical dendrites, are the most important generators of the cortical EEG.

Rhythm Generation

Given that the EEG reflects electrical activity in neuronal aggregates, the characteristic rhythmic waveforms can only arise if individual neurons are synchronized in their activities. Intense but unsynchronized neuronal activity, as occurs during arousal and sometimes at the onset of seizures, actually causes an attenuation or flattening of the EEG. Modeling experiments show that signals resembling EEG can result from interactions within local neuronal networks alone. Direct recordings in animals and humans have revealed rhythmic EEG activity in both the cortex and thalamus, leading to the proposal of a thalamocortical loop. Within the thalamus, excitation and reciprocal inhibition in local neuronal networks or groups of neurons in the different thalamic nuclei have long been favored as a mechanism for the generation of rhythmic activity such as the alpha rhythm. Thalamic neurons may also exhibit intrinsic oscillatory behavior. The exact mechanisms for the generation of specific EEG activities remain uncertain.

RECORDING THE ELECTROENCEPHALOGRAM

The standard EEG is a noninvasive procedure using electrodes applied to the scalp surface. EEG signals can also be recorded by needle electrodes inserted into the scalp or soft tissues of the head, by intracranial electrodes placed subdurally or epidurally over the brain surface (electrocorticogram), or by depth electrodes in the brain substance.

Electrodes

Conventional electrodes are usually small cups made of chlorided silver, tin, or other metals. After the scalp under the electrode site is cleaned, the electrode is applied and secured with collodion adhesive. Electrode jelly is then injected through a hole in the dome of the electrode. When properly and securely applied, the electrodes are very sturdy and can provide excellent recordings for many hours. The use of adhesive electrode paste and pressure contact electrodes can also give satisfactory recordings, but only for short durations, since they tend to dry out. Needle electrodes can also give good quality EEGs, but there is no indication for their use in a routine setting. Insertion is painful and electrodes cannot always be securely anchored. There is also the risk of spreading diseases transmissible in body fluids.

Protection of staff and patients demands attention to the last point. The referring physician should alert the EEG laboratory about diseases potentially transmissible by contamination of body fluids, especially hepatitis B, human immunodeficiency virus (HIV) infection (acquired immune deficiency syndrome [AIDS]), and Creutzfeldt-Jakob disease. This regimen allows laboratory personnel to take appropriate precautions and to disinfect, sterilize (by steam autoclaving), or dispose of contaminated materials.

Electrode Positions

Twenty-one standard electrodes are placed according to the International 10-20 system (Fig. 6-1). This system is based on direct measurement of the head, with electrodes placed proportionately at 10- or 20-percent intervals along measured meridians. Electrode positions, therefore, are correlated with the underlying cerebral anatomy. Additional electrodes are placed to act as ground or reference electrodes or sometimes to monitor extracerebral electrical activity (e.g., ECG, potentials generated by eye movement, surface electromyelogram [EMG]).

The Electroencephalograph

The pins of the electrodes are inserted into a headbox and then connected to the EEG machine (Fig. 6-2). The most important and characteristic feature of the EEG machine is the differential amplifier in each channel. Each amplifier compares the difference in signal between two inputs and rejects any potentials that are common to them with respect to the ground or the reference electrode. The pattern of electrodes linked to the inputs of channels is given by the montage selector on the EEG machine. The EEG signal is further filtered and amplified. The final output amplifiers drive moving coil galvanometers that are attached to pens, and in some machines to ink jets, to provide a paper record. In the printout, vertical displacement of the EEG signal is proportional to potential magnitude (in

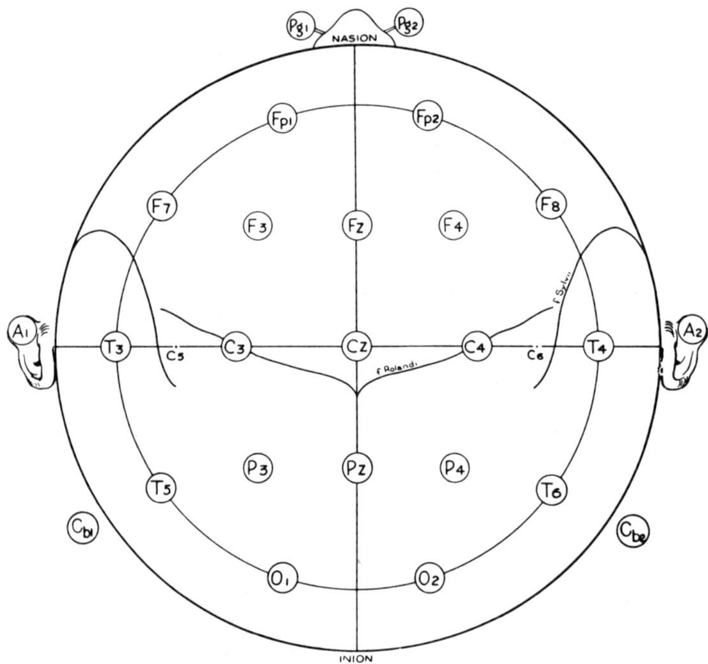

Fig. 6-1. Standard electrode positions of the International 10-20 system. (From Jasper, 1958, with permission.)

μV), and the horizontal time base is determined by the speed of the running paper.

Conventional Display of the Electroencephalogram

Polarity Convention

The output from each channel is a differential signal (input 1–input 2) of the two original inputs. By convention, when the potential in input 1 is negative relative to input 2 (whether because input 1 has a negative or input 2 a positive signal or both), the potential difference is represented by an upward deflection (Fig. 6-3). In the reverse situation (when input 2 is negative relative to input 1) a downward deflection results.

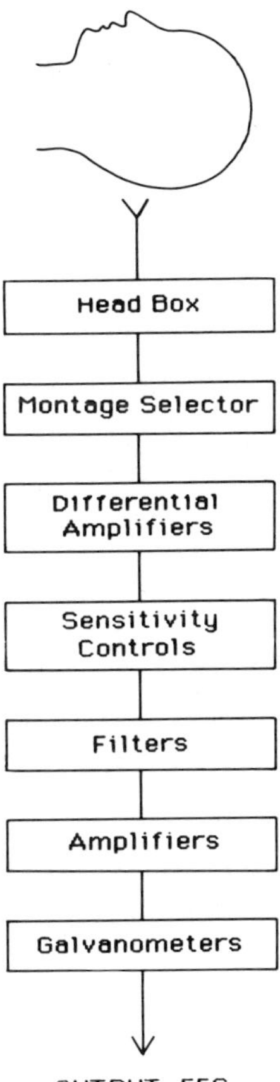

Fig. 6-2. Schematic diagram of the major functions in an EEG machine.

Derivations and Montages

Modern EEG machines have at least 16 sometimes 21 channels. Older instruments and some portable units may be limited to eight channels. The manner in which electrodes are connected to the channels is called the derivation. The selection and specific sequence of electrodes for all channels in use constitute the montage. In principle, the ability to identify and localize EEG abnormalities increases with the number of channels. It also

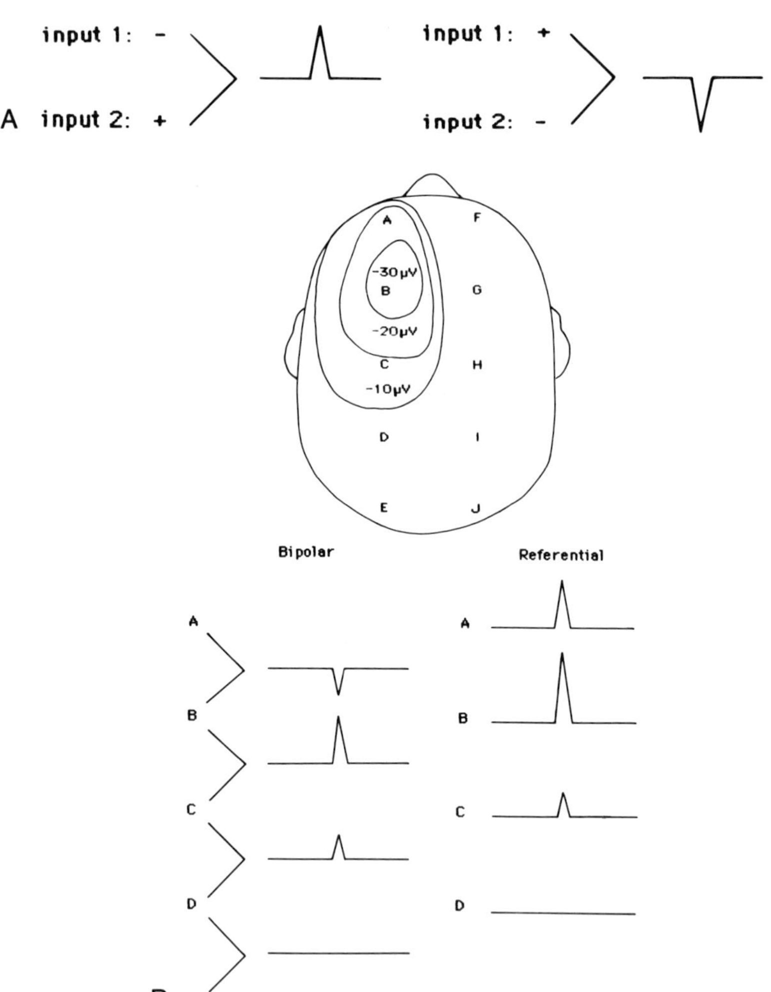

Fig. 6-3. **(A)** Polarity convention in EEG: an upward deflection results whenever input 1 is negative relative to input 2. A downward deflection occurs when input 1 is positive relative to input 2. **(B)** Bipolar and referential derivations and their display in the EEG (see text).

depends on the judicious choice of montage(s) to optimally display the area(s) and activities of interest.

There are two basic types of derivations (Fig. 6-3). In a bipolar derivation, pairs of electrodes are connected to each channel for comparison. In practice, consecutive electrodes along a linear chain are connected to successive channels. This bipolar arrangement plots a map of potential gradients between one electrode site and another. The point of potential maximum when localized to one electrode along a chain will cause pen deflections in opposite directions in the two adjacent channels connected to that electrode, giving rise to a phase reversal.

In a referential derivation (also called a monopolar derivation), the potentials from different electrodes (input 1 of each channel) are all compared with a common reference point (input 2). With all channels sharing the same baseline, the referential montage is like a map measuring the magnitude of the potential field at each electrode relative to the baseline provided by the reference. The point of potential maximum in a monopolar derivation is found in the channel measuring the largest deflection.

Standard Recording Conditions

The EEG changes with the patient's physiologic state. EEG abnormalities may be apparent only in specific states. Thus even a routine EEG should include recording during hyperventilation and photic stimulation.

Hyperventilation for 3 to 5 minutes often causes varying degrees of generalized rhythmic slowing in normal individuals, the topography, frequency, and voltage of which depends on age, effort, and the blood glucose level. Hyperventilation frequently activates generalized epileptiform abnormalities and precipitates absence seizures. It can also increase the incidence of localized epileptiform discharges, magnify slow wave abnormalities, and occasionally precipitate partial seizures. Photic stimulation uses a strobe light usually placed 30 cm in front of the subject's eyes, flashing at rates varying from 1 to 50 Hz. Its main role is to elicit epileptiform abnormalities in subjects with epilepsy. An abnormal photoparoxysmal response and high voltage occipital spikes should be distinguished clearly from nonspecific spiky or slow activities and the photomyogenic response (see *Epileptiform Abnormalities*). The photic driving response may be absent or show some asymmetry in the normal population.

A sleep study is often invaluable. There is a characteristic progression of EEG patterns through the different stages of non-REM (NREM) and REM sleep. Daytime sleep studies in the EEG laboratory usually only record the earlier stages of NREM sleep. For this purpose, pharmacologically induced sleep using an oral hypnotic (e.g., a short-acting barbiturate or chloral hydrate) is as satisfactory as natural sleep. Extended overnight sleep studies that simultaneously monitor the EEG and extracerebral variables, such as eye movements, EMG, respiration and oxygen saturation, can be performed in a specialized sleep laboratory. The sleep EEG provides information on the organization of sleep activity and can increase the chance of detection or reveal new abnormalities, particularly epileptiform discharges.

A routine recording in an awake, relaxed patient takes approximately 30 minutes after initial preparation. Sweating because of poor ventilation, tremor, and movements in an anxious or restless, confused patient can all create artifacts that obscure the tracing and confound interpretation.

PRINCIPAL NORMAL AND ABNORMAL ELECTROENCEPHALOGRAPHIC ACTIVITIES

The central features in analysis of the EEG concern the wave forms, their distribution, and the context in which they occur. This section introduces terminology used to describe waveforms and patterns. Abnormalities found in different pathologic states will be described later (see *Clinical Applications and Limitations of the EEG*).

There is considerable interobserver variability even among experts in EEG analysis. Given a wide choice of nonstandardized jargon and terminology, traditions of practice in each EEG laboratory, and personal idiosyncrasies, it is small wonder that clinicians sometimes have trouble deciphering oracular pronouncements and doubt the reliability of EEGs. Overdiagnosis is often a greater offender than underdiagnosis, and it has taken many decades to dispel the myths attached to patterns now regarded as clinically insignificant. Particularly in the investigation of a patient for a possible seizure disorder, such terms as *paroxysmal irritative focus, potentially epileptiform,* or *possibly epileptogenic* when used without explanation are confusing and misleading. When met with these uncertainties, the clinician should seek every opportunity to discuss them with the electroencephalographer.

Normal Activities

Features of some of the most commonly encountered normal patterns in wakefulness and in sleep of adults are listed in Table 6-1 (Fig. 6-4). The terms alpha, beta, theta, and delta activity are not only used to describe certain normal background activities but also nonspecifically to denote

Table 6-1. Normal EEG Activities in Adults Awake and Asleep

Activity	Frequency (Hz)	Amplitude	Topography	State
Alpha (α)	8–13	20–60 μV	Usually occipital maximum	Relaxed wakefulness with eyes closed
Beta (β)	>13	10–20 μV	Frontocentral	Wakefulness, drowsiness, NREM1&2, REM
Theta (θ)	4–8	Variable	1. Frontocentral, temporal 2. Diffuse	1. Minimal awake 2. Drowsiness, NREM
Delta (δ)	<4	Variable	1. Occasional posterior[a] 2. Diffuse	1. Awake 2. Drowsiness, NREM
Mu (μ)	8–10	20–60 μV	Central	Awake, suppressed by volitional movement
Vertex waves (V waves)	Usually sporadic	Variable	Central vertex	NREM1 onward
Spindles	10–14	20–50 μV	Frontocentral	NREM2 onward
K complexes	Sporadic	Variable	Frontocentral	NREM2 onward
Positive occipital sharp transients of sleep (POSTS)	Sporadic or short trains	Variable	Occipital	NREM1 onward

[a] Posterior slow waves of youth.

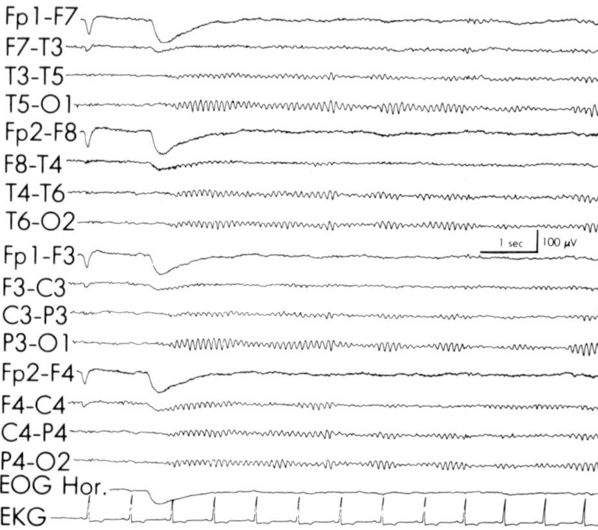

Fig. 6-4. Normal awake EEG in an adult with eyes closed. Well-regulated, sinusoidal 10 Hz alpha rhythm is seen over the posterior head regions.

frequency bands, either normal or abnormal. The ongoing activity (whether normal or abnormal) from which other distinct rhythms or waveforms emerge is referred to as the background activity.

Spiky or sharp phenomena often appear to be very dramatic, yet can be of no clinical significance. Above all, remember that not all spikes fit, just as not all sharp objects are dangerous. A broad range of phenomena are clearly not diagnostic of and are not associated with epilepsy (Table 6-2). Indeed, they have not been shown to indicate any definite clinical abnormality. Spiky or sharp waveforms can also occur as the result of a haphazard co-incidence of waveforms of different frequencies. They can arise in NREM sleep (e.g., vertex waves, K complexes, positive occipital sharp transients of sleep (POSTS]) and during hyperventilation or photic stimulation.

Abnormal Activities

Abnormalities in the EEG are signified by the appearance of abnormal waveforms, the disappearance of normal background activities, or alterations in the distribution of normal background activities. The different

Table 6-2. Spiky or Sharp Phenomena of No Clinical Significance

Phenomena	Features	Topography	State	Usual Age
14 and 6 Hz positive spikes	Low voltage, positive polarity, short bursts	Posterior temporal[a]	Drowsiness, light NREM sleep	Children, adolescents, young adults
6 Hz spike and wave (phantom spike and wave)	Low voltage spikes, short bursts	Bilateral frontal or occipital	Waking, drowsiness, light NREM sleep	Adolescents, young adults
Rhythmic temporal theta burst of drowsiness (psychomotor variant)	4–7 Hz, notched waves, sometimes in long trains	Midtemporal[a]	Drowsiness, light NREM sleep	Adolescents, young adults
Benign small sharp spikes (BSSS, BETS)	Low voltage, short duration, biphasic, sporadic	Shifting bilateral, widespread frontotemporal	Drowsiness, NREM sleep	Adults
Wicket spikes	Sporadic or in short trains	Temporal[a]	Waking, drowsiness, light NREM sleep	Adults
Subclinical rhythmic EEG discharge of adults (SREDA)	4–7 Hz, in long trains	Parieto-occipital[a]	Waking, drowsiness	>50 years

[a] Bilateral, occasionally unilateral.

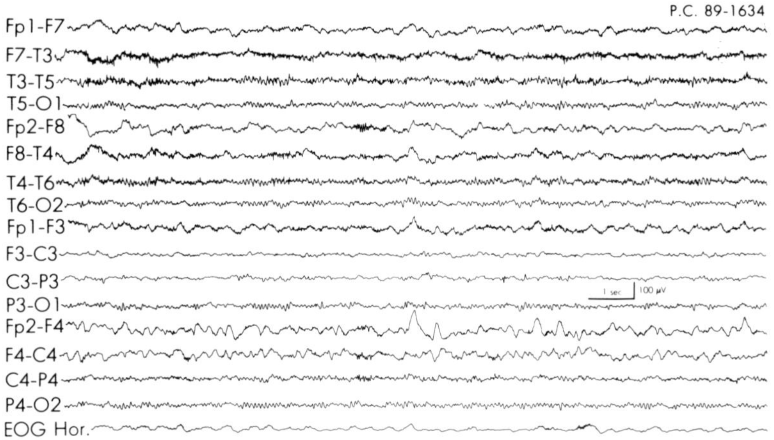

Fig. 6-5. Localized polymorphic slow activity over the right frontal region, with extension to the left. The patient has a right frontal glioma and presented with left arm weakness.

abnormalities often occur together in the same EEG or may follow one another in the course of evolution of the EEG.

Slow Wave Abnormalities

There are two main types of slow wave abnormalities. Bilateral intermittent slow activity (also called intermittent rhythmic delta activity or IRDA) is characterized by intermittent (1 to several seconds) bursts of bilateral, more or less regular, 1.5 to 4 Hz delta waves, which are usually roughly symmetric over the two hemispheres. In adults the activity is commonly of maximal voltage over frontal regions. The pathophysiologic correlate is usually a diffuse disturbance involving cortical and subcortical structures, as in toxic-metabolic encephalopathies. Deep midline lesions in the diencephalon and midbrain are an *occasional* causative factor.

Polymorphic slow activity (also called polymorphic delta activity [PDA]) consists of delta and sometimes theta activity, irregular both in frequency and morphology, occurring intermittently or continuously. Although frequently localized, it can be diffuse or generalized. It is correlated with dysfunction in white matter and may be related to deafferentation of the overlying cortex. Localized polymorphic slow activity (Fig. 6-5) suggests the possibility of a localized lesion involving the white matter (e.g.,

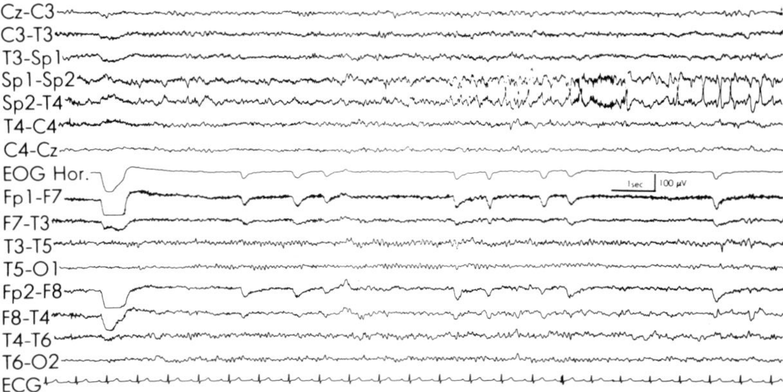

Fig. 6-6. Frequent epileptiform spike discharges localized to the right sphenoidal (Sp2) electrode, recording from the right basal (mesial) temporal region. The patient suffered from medically intractable complex partial seizures, later treated by a right anterior temporal resection.

tumor, hematoma), but can also occur in the postictal state and in patients with migraine. Localized intermittent rhythmic slow activity is a variant distinguishable by its rhythmicity and intermittency. It is most commonly seen as an interictal disturbance in the epilepsies. In partial epilepsy, it frequently arises from the same area as epileptiform discharges. In idiopathic generalized epilepsies, it seems to be a genetic trait, manifest as rhythmic posterior delta activity or parietal theta rhythms. The underlying pathophysiologic disturbance of this latter variant is unknown.

Epileptiform Abnormalities

Interictal epileptiform discharges (Fig. 6-6) are called spikes if they are less than 70 msec and sharp waves if they last between 70 and 200 msec, and are often associated with slow waves. While interictal epileptiform abnormalities alone are not diagnostic of epilepsy, they are strongly associated with it. Spikes and sharp waves are caused by synchronized electrical discharges in a population of neurons. The intracellular electrophysiologic counterpart is the paroxysmal depolarizing shift and is associated with early burst firing of action potentials (Fig. 6-7). The slow wave that follows appears to represent inhibitory postsynaptic potential-mediated hyperpolarization and inhibition.

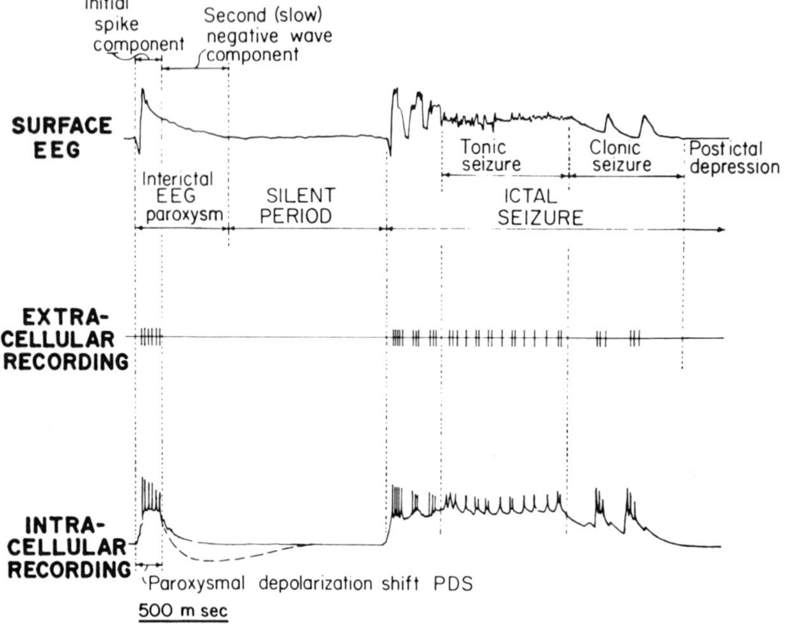

Fig. 6-7. Relationship between paroxysmal depolarizing shift (PDS) recorded by intracellular electrode, and EEG field potential (see text). (From Ayala et al., 1973, with permission.)

Ictal EEG activity clearly establishes the diagnosis of a seizure disorder, but the ictal EEG pattern is quite variable and should always be correlated with clinical phenomena. The EEG may exhibit localized, lateralized or generalized voltage attenuation, rhythmic spikes, sharp waves, spike and wave complexes, or other activity ranging from delta to very fast beta (40 to 60 Hz) frequency bands. These changes can occur singly or in any combination or may show a sequence of evolution in the course of the same seizure. Frequently, muscle and movement artifacts obscure much or all of the tracing. Postictally, slow waves of varying distribution and severity are frequently found.

The photoparoxysmal (photoconvulsive) response is characterized by the development of bilateral spike or multiple spike and wave discharges, which are not time-locked to the rate of stimulation. They are usually generalized, but may predominate over frontal or occipital regions. Self-sustained discharges may outlast the stimulus by some hundreds of milliseconds or longer. A response having these characteristics is correlated with the presence of epilepsy, usually idiopathic generalized epilepsy. The response is frequently accompanied by symptoms and signs of visual discomfort, headache, impaired consciousness (absence), myoclonic jerks of the eyelids or extremities (or both); and may culminate in a generalized tonic-clonic convulsion. It can occur transiently in patients without a seizure disorder after drug withdrawal or in toxic-metabolic states.

Photic stimulation may elicit high voltage spikes over the occipital regions time-locked to the flashes. They represent large amplitude visual evoked potentials, have a weaker association with epilepsy, and are most dramatic in neuronal ceroid lipofuscinosis.

These abnormal photic responses should be distinguished from the photomyogenic response, nonspecific spiky driving responses, and from slow wave activities during photic stimulation, none of which are correlated with epilepsy. The photomyogenic response consists of muscle potentials with spiky morphology that are maximal over the frontal regions. It may be accompanied by eyelid fluttering and jerking of the facial muscles. The response is more likely seen in tense subjects or after alcohol or sedative withdrawal.

Repetitive or Periodic Patterns

Repetitive or periodic patterns are characterized by clear intervals between successive paroxysmal elements. Background activity is usually severely disturbed. When the interval of repetition is regular with only slight variability, the term periodic can be used. In all these patterns, the patient's state of responsiveness is likely to be impaired. Some are associated with myoclonic jerks and other abnormal movements. As a rule, they should not be considered ictal discharges, although it is sometimes difficult to separate them from patterns seen in status epilepticus. There is no satisfactory neurophysiologic explanation of the mechanisms for periodic phenomena in EEG. Pathologically, the associated diseases all tend to involve large regions or the brain diffusely.

The burst suppression pattern consists of bursts of generalized high voltage mixed frequency waveforms, usually with admixed spikes and sharp waves of variable duration, alternating with regular periods of generalized voltage suppression. The latter last from 1 to several seconds, with no intervening normal background activity. The patient is invariably comatose and may experience myoclonic jerks. The burst suppression pattern indicates a severe generalized disturbance of cerebral activity but

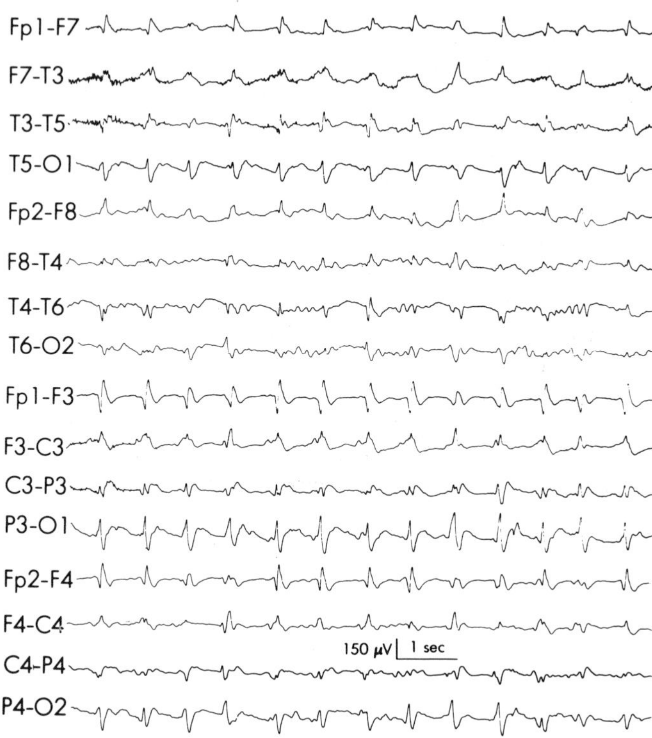

Fig. 6-8. Generalized, periodic sharp waves, and loss of normal background activities in a patient with Creutzfeldt-Jakob disease.

can also occur transiently in anesthesia, drug overdose, and postictal states.

Periodic spikes or sharp waves describe a pattern of repeated spikes or sharp waves of biphasic or multiphasic morphology, usually at a rate of between 0.5 to 2 Hz. The discharges are generalized and bilaterally synchronous, but can be asymmetric. This finding in a patient with a rapidly dementing illness and myoclonic jerks supports the diagnosis of Creutzfeldt-Jakob disease (Fig. 6-8). Indicative of a severe encephalopathy, the pattern can occur after anoxic cerebral damage, as after cardiac arrest, and in toxic-metabolic states (uremia, dialysis dementia, lithium toxicity, tricyclic antidepressant overdose).

Runs or trains of broad, triphasic waves, at 1.5 to 3 Hz, that are bilateral or generalized with bifrontal maxima, usually indicate a moderate to se-

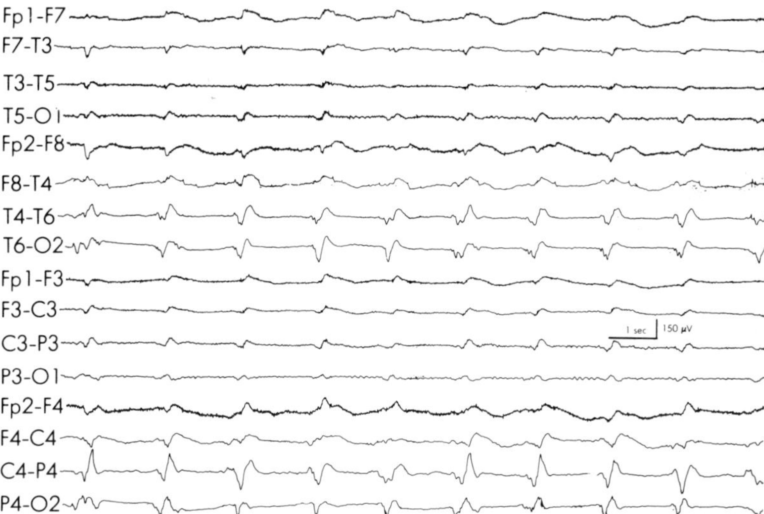

Fig. 6-9. PLEDs arising from right posterior head region and severe generalized depression of normal background activities. Patient underwent resection of a right temporal glioblastoma 1 month previously, then developed focal motor seizures of the left body.

vere metabolic encephalopathy. The pattern is nonspecific in etiology. Hepatic and renal failure are the most common causes.

The pattern of bilateral or generalized high voltage, repetitive complexes with multiphasic sharp and slow wave components from 0.5 to 2 seconds in duration, recurring every 4 to 15 seconds or longer, has a high specificity for subacute sclerosing panencephalitis (SSPE). Jerks, spasms, or sudden loss of tone may accompany the periodic complexes in SSPE.

Localized or lateralized sharp or slow wave complexes of 0.2 to 1 seconds in duration, usually recurring every 1 to 5 seconds (Fig. 6-9), are known as periodic lateralized epileptiform discharges (PLEDs). They may also be bihemispheric (BIPLEDs). The pattern is nonspecific, but is most commonly seen as a result of an acute localized cerebral injury, such as can occur with acute cerebral infarction, brain tumor, focal encephalitis, or subdural hematoma. BIPLEDs are usually seen with more widespread insults such as cerebral anoxia or CNS infections. In an acutely febrile and confused patient, the presence of PLEDs or BIPLEDs on the EEG strongly raises the suspicion of herpes encephalitis or other focal CNS

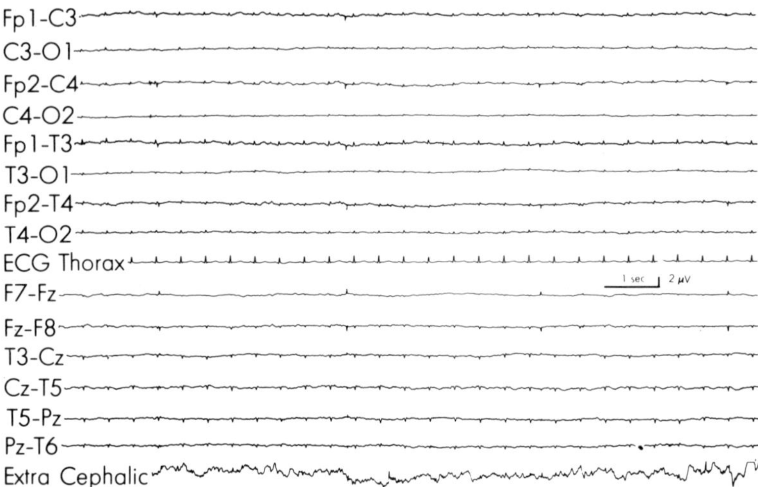

Fig. 6-10. Electrocerebral inactivity in a patient who was clinically brain dead after cardiac arrest. Note the use of wide interelectrode distances and the high amplification for gain. Aside from ECG artifact, no cerebral activity over 2 μV was present. Ambient noise monitored by the extracephalic lead exceeded that level.

infections. Because of the underlying etiologies, PLEDs are often found in patients who are obtunded and have repeated partial seizures, but should not be regarded as an ictal EEG pattern. Depending on the nature, reversibility, and severity of the insult, PLEDs, seizures, and obtundation often improve spontaneously over a period of days to weeks. PLEDs sometimes also occur in epilepsy of focal origin and in migraine.

Disappearance of Cerebral Activity

Localized loss of cerebral activity indicates focal damage or loss of function of the underlying cerebral gray matter. When reversible causes have been excluded (e.g., barbiturate overdose), generalized disappearance of EEG activity is consistent with loss of brain function. When this is accompanied by neurologic findings of unresponsive coma, apnea, and areflexia, it indicates brain death (see *Stupor, Coma, and Brain Death*). Such electrocerebral inactivity (Fig. 6-10) should be carefully distinguished from the so-called low voltage record found in 5 to 10 percent of normal subjects, in anxious individuals, and in patients with Huntington's disease. Localized attenuation of background activities may also result

Table 6-3. Approximate Correlation Between EEG and Pathological Abnormalities

Lesion or Dysfunction	EEG Abnormalities
Localized	
Localized cortical gray matter	Voltage attenuation, loss of EEG activity, epileptiform abnormalities
Localized subcortical white matter	Polymorphic slow activity
Localized subcortical gray matter	Sometimes unilateral or bilateral intermittent slow activity
Generalized	
Diffuse cortical gray matter	Voltage attenuation, loss of EEG activity, epileptiform abnormalities
Diffuse subcortical white matter	Polymorphic slow activity
Diffuse cortical and subcortical	Bilateral intermittent slow activity, periodic patters, epileptiform abnormalities

when there is increased impedance to current flow in the tissues between the brain and scalp surface, as may occur with a subdural hematoma.

CLINICAL APPLICATIONS AND LIMITATIONS OF THE ELECTROENCEPHALOGRAM

Overview of Information Provided

The clinician should appreciate four basic points when considering use of the EEG:

1. EEG findings are not specific for etiology. However, EEG findings in the appropriate clinical context can suggest or confirm a diagnosis (e.g., Creutzfeldt-Jakob disease, SSPE, complex partial status).
2. Although there is an approximate correlation between EEG and pathologic abnormalities (Table 6-3), the neurophysiologic basis for the different abnormalities in EEG remain imperfectly understood and unknown in many instances.
3. The EEG cannot compare with modern imaging techniques such as CT or MRI for the detection or localization of lesions, although the EEG frequently detects localized abnormalities in epilepsy that are not revealed by imaging tests. Computerized quantitative EEG anal-

ysis and display may increase the ability to detect subtle changes in the EEG. It should be remembered that EEG abnormalities are not generated by the lesion itself, which is electrically silent, but by affected yet viable nerve tissue in the vicinity. This fact sometimes accounts for the apparently false localization of structural lesions by EEG.

4. EEG changes in disorders causing diffuse cerebral disturbance, as in the encephalopathies, or those resulting in stupor and coma tend to parallel the clinical course (see Table 6-5).

The remainder of this section describes EEG abnormalities found in different pathologic states.

Epilepsy

The diagnosis of epilepsy and seizures is clinical, but the EEG can reveal confirmatory electrophysiologic evidence of epileptic excitability. Ictal EEG activity with altered behavior or convulsions is proof of an epileptic seizure.

Significance of Interictal Epileptiform Abnormalities

The significance of epileptiform abnormalities is not always clear. Epileptiform discharges occur in about 2 percent or less of normal adults and children. Closer questioning may reveal a past history or a family history of epilepsy. In a nonepileptic hospital population, the incidence of epileptiform discharges is somewhat higher (2 to 4 percent) and related to other evidence of cerebral dysfunction. These discharges cannot be considered entirely incidental or without significance because approximately 10 percent of these patients may subsequently develop seizures.

The location and morphology of the discharges modifies the association with clinical epilepsy. Anterior and basal temporal spikes are strongly correlated (90 percent) with temporal lobe epilepsy.

Correlations with Epileptic Syndromes

Idiopathic (Primary) Generalized Epilepsies

The hallmark of the primary generalized epilepsy is the presence of generalized, bilaterally synchronous epileptiform discharges with normal or only minimally abnormal background activity. Intermittent trains of biocipital 2 to 3 Hz rhythmic slow activity or runs of 4 to 7 Hz biparietal theta rhythms are not rare. In absence epilepsy, the discharges are typi-

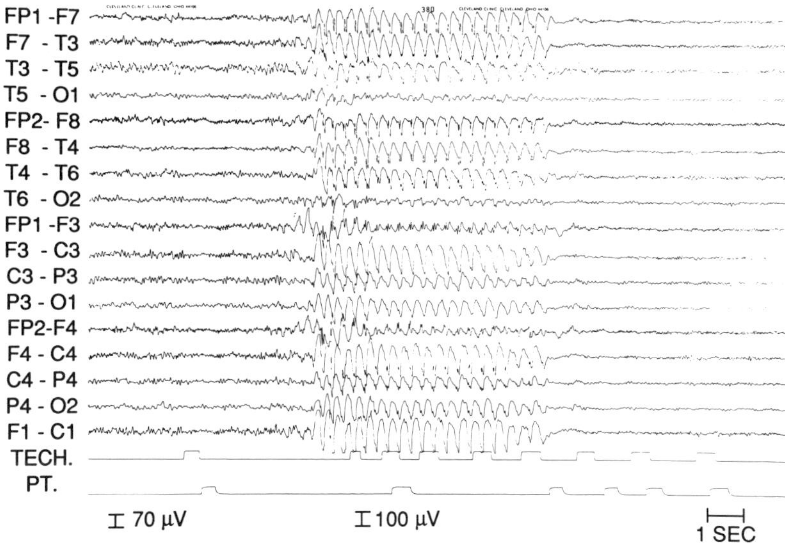

Fig. 6-11. Generalized 3 Hz spike and wave complexes with clinical absence seizure. Note the impaired ability of the patient to deliver clicks closely following those made by the technologist.

cally well-formed, symmetric, 3 Hz (range 2.5 to 4 Hzs) spike and wave complexes (Fig. 6-11) that are readily precipitated by hyperventilation. Trains of discharges, when longer than 3 seconds, are frequently obvious as clinical absence. Conditions with prominent myoclonus, as in juvenile myoclonic epilepsy, tend to show multiple spike and wave complexes or faster discharge rates around 6 Hz or both. Irregular spike or multiple spike and wave complexes occur more frequently in epilepsy with generalized tonic-clonic seizures. Discharges increase but become more irregular and fragmented in NREM sleep. Photoparoxysmal responses and clinical photosensitivity are not uncommon, particularly in absence and juvenile myoclonic epilepsy.

The onset of a grand mal generalized tonic-clonic seizure is marked by generalized voltage attenuation and low voltage fast activity. This later develops into a generalized approximately 10 Hz-discharge, in the form of repetitive spikes or sharp waves (epileptic recruiting rhythm) during the tonic phase of the seizure. Coincident with the clonic phase, the EEG shows generalized multiple spike and wave complexes.

Symptomatic (Secondary) Generalized Epilepsies

The EEG patterns are much more variable among the secondary generalized epilepsies in keeping with the wide spectrum of etiologies. Interictal background activity is abnormal with excessive slowing. Interictal epileptiform discharges consist of irregular spikes, multiple spikes, or sharp and slow waves. Although variable between 1 and 4 Hz, the epileptiform discharge frequency is usually around 2 to 2.5 Hz (slow spike and wave). The discharges are usually generalized, but frequently show asymmetric features. Localized or multifocal discharges may also occur. Generalized multiple spike and wave complexes are associated with disorders with prominent myoclonus.

Ictal EEG changes are equally variable. Generalized rhythmic fast (10 to 20 Hz) spikes or sharp activity can accompany tonic seizures. Some seizures show no apparent EEG change.

Idiopathic Localization-related Epilepsies (Benign Partial Epilepsies of Childhood)

Idiopathic localization-related epilepsies are age-related and occur in childhood, usually between the ages of 4 and 15 years. Background activity should be normal. The epileptiform discharges are typically high voltage, biphasic spikes or sharp waves that have slightly blunted peaks and a low voltage after going slow wave. They arise (in order of frequency) over the centrotemporal (rolandic), occipital, parietal, and frontal regions, depending on the exact type of epilepsy.

Symptomatic Localization-related Epilepsies (Partial Epilepsies)

Interictal abnormalities include localized epileptiform discharges, localized intermittent rhythmic or more continuous polymorphic slow activity, and disturbances of background activity. The location, spatial extent, and type of abnormalities are determined by the location and size of the epileptogenic zone and the underlying pathologic process. Bilateral independent discharges over homologous regions occur in 20 to 30 percent of patients with temporal lobe epilepsy, and bifrontal synchronous discharges can occur in frontal lobe epilepsy. Bihemispheric independent discharges can occur, even in patients with a well-defined unilateral pathology who become seizure free after localized surgical resection. Multifocal discharges (three or more foci involving both hemispheres) usually indicate multiple or extensive regions of abnormality.

The ictal EEG pattern can take many forms (Fig. 6-12). The earliest changes can be subtle; for example, a mild localized voltage attenuation,

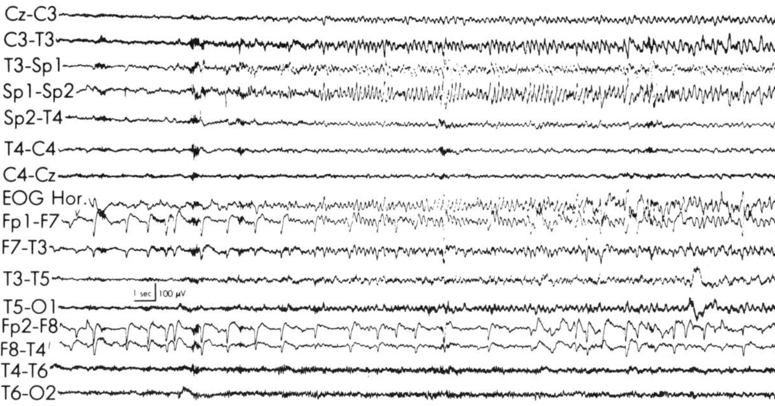

Fig. 6-12. Localized EEG ictal onset over the left temporal region, in the form of rhythmic 6 Hz sharp activity.

or cessation of ongoing epileptiform discharges. Low amplitude rhythmic fast activity, rhythmic spikes, sharp waves, or sinusoidal activity may then emerge. The seizure discharge typically shows sequential evolution over time in morphology, frequency (acceleration or deceleration), amplitude, and topography (spread to other regions). However, the extracranial EEG may be obscured by artifact, or the generator at the epileptogenic zone may be too small or too deeply buried in mesial or deep sulci to be detectable on the scalp surface. In these circumstances, the EEG may be unrevealing or only demonstrate ictal activity after it spread diffusely, creating the false impression of a seizure generalized from onset. As many as 70 to 80 percent of simple partial seizures (including temporal lobe auras) may show no EEG change during recordings by extracranial electrodes. Complex partial seizures are usually accompanied by ictal EEG changes, owing to frequent bilateral spread of the seizure discharge. However, only about 50 to 60 percent of temporal lobe seizures and probably no more than a third of frontal lobe seizures show clear ictal localization or lateralization at onset on the extracranial EEG. Partial seizures that become secondarily generalized (seizure spread leading to generalized convulsions with loss of consciousness) always show generalized ictal EEG changes at that stage unless the cortical electrical activity is obscured by artifacts. Intracranial EEG recording is sometimes necessary in order to identify the epileptogenic zone before planning for surgical treatment of epilepsy.

Factors Influencing the Detection of Epileptiform Abnormalities

From a technical point of view, the yield of detection of interictal epileptiform abnormalities is related to (1) the duration of sampling; (2) the state of recording and activation procedures; and (3) the number and position of electrodes and the choice of montages. Biologic factors also influence the likelihood of detection; the yield is higher (1) in children, (2) in patients with generalized epilepsies, and (3) when the recording is performed within 1 week of a clinical seizure. Deeply situated epileptic generators may be undetectable at the scalp surface.

The longer a patient is monitored, the more likely it becomes that an EEG abnormality will be found. A first routine EEG has approximately a 55 percent chance of detecting interictal epileptiform abnormalities in patients with epilepsy. The yield increases upward to 90 percent after three to four EEGs with sleep, but about 8 percent of patients fail to show epileptiform discharges despite repeated EEG follow-up for 1 year. Prolonged monitoring for 24 hours or more detects discharges in about 40 percent of patients who had a previously normal routine record.

The physiologic state is also important. Monitoring frequently demonstrates marked fluctuations in discharge rates and patterns throughout the day and night. Discharge rates tend to show a circadian pattern with increases during sleep and cyclic changes with the NREM-REM cycle. Both localized and generalized discharges are activated during NREM sleep. Localized discharges often show spread in spatial extent and may appear as independent contralateral foci. Generalized discharges often become fragmented and irregular.

Prolonged sleep deprivation can precipitate seizures and tends to activate epileptiform discharges. However, 24 hours of sleep deprivation is hard to enforce. Partial sleep deprivation (no more than 4 hours of overnight sleep) is much easier to accomplish and is useful to ensure an adequate spontaneous sleep study. The role of hyperventilation and photic stimulation in the activation of epileptiform abnormalities has already been discussed.

Anticonvulsant drug withdrawal can precipitate seizures and is only justified when there is a clear clinical need to record seizures. Nonspecific paroxysmal and generalized spike and wave discharges may occur in the postwithdrawal period. Thus anticonvulsant withdrawal is not recommended for enhancing detection of interictal discharges in routine recordings. Intravenous methohexitol or pentobarbital at low doses induces light narcosis and nonspecific fast activities and increases spiking rates. Seizure induction by drugs (e.g., pentylenetetrazole) is not recommended, as the resultant seizures and ictal EEG can be unreliable and misleading.

Special or additional extracranial electrodes and the appropriate selection of montages can increase the detection of abnormalities over certain brain regions. Nasopharyngeal electrodes in the upper nasopharynx are prone to artifacts and can be uncomfortable. Generally they are not superior to scalp electrodes for detection of abnormal discharges arising from the temporal lobes. Anterior temporal (T_1, T_2) or similar electrodes (e.g., D_9, D_{10}) are simply applied as extra scalp electrodes to record from temporal areas not covered by standard electrodes of the 10-20 system. In temporal lobe epilepsy, the maximal potentials and highest incidence of discharges are frequently found with these electrodes. The sphenoidal electrode is a fine flexible wire that is introduced with a needle to rest below the greater wing of the sphenoid near the foramen ovale. In temporal lobe epilepsy, a small but significant number of patients show only discharges with sphenoidal electrode recordings. The basal position of this electrodes allows identification of discharges from the anterior basal portion of the temporal lobe. Supraorbital electrodes placed on the supraorbital ridge sometimes improve the detection of frontopolar and orbitofrontal discharges.

Recommendations for Initial Electroencephalogram Series in Suspected Epilepsy

The first routine recording should include hyperventilation and photic stimulation. If this recording proves negative, a spontaneous sleep recording or one with pharmacologically induced sleep is performed. If this recording is also negative, one with partial or complete 24-hour sleep deprivation is recommended. The three recordings have an 80 to 90 percent probability of detecting epileptiform abnormalities in patients with epilepsy. When no EEG confirmation is available and the clinical diagnosis or management remains in doubt, long-term monitoring with electroclinical correlation of attacks may be indicated.

Electroencephalography in the Management of Epilepsy

Advantages

The EEG can help clarify the nature of behavioral and subjective disturbances when there is doubt as to whether they are epileptic in origin. Interictal epileptiform abnormalities may or may not coexist. The ideal goal is to obtain electroclinical correlation of the actual attacks and usually entails long-term video-EEG monitoring. This can be supplemented when indicated by the use of special electrodes and the recording of extracerebral physiologic variables such as the ECG, EMG, and respiration.

If the diagnosis of epilepsy has been established, the EEG may allow precise classification of the seizure disorder and the epileptic syndrome. It can help in distinguishing between seizure types, such as prolonged absences from brief complex partial seizures, or generalized seizures with asymmetric manifestations from partial seizures that become secondarily generalized. Classification may improve clinical management by allowing choice of the appropriate pharmacotherapy or sometimes a decision for surgical treatment. It may also provide prognosis of the seizure disorder. Prolonged video-EEG monitoring is usually required for this purpose.

In other cases, EEG monitoring can be used to assess seizure frequency. Patients and witnesses cannot always accurately identify all seizures. This information may be useful to evaluate the therapeutic response to medications. Practically, assessment of seizure frequency is limited to patients with frequent absence, tonic, atonic, and myoclonic seizures. Documentation can be obtained by ambulatory cassette EEG or video-EEG monitoring. Patients with other seizure types usually do not experience them frequently enough to make EEG monitoring of seizure frequency worthwhile. The efficacy of antiepileptic drugs can also sometimes be assessed by quantification of interictal discharge rates in certain syndromes. The generalized discharges in absence epilepsy and the photoparoxysmal response in photosensitive patients have been shown to be suppressed by effective anticonvulsant drug treatment and correlated with seizure control. This can be documented by repeated trials of photic stimulation and by ambulatory or video-EEG, depending on the problem. In the partial epilepsies, there is no convincing evidence that interictal discharge rates are correlated with drug efficacy and seizure control.

When surgical treatment of epilepsy is considered, EEG investigation is indispensable for the localization, lateralization, and assessment of the extent of the epileptogenic zone, as well as for understanding how it relates to the clinical seizure disorder. Adequate investigation requires prolonged video-EEG monitoring, often with special extracranial and sometimes intracranial electrodes for assessment of interictal and ictal abnormalities.

The EEG probably plays only a secondary role (in relation to the primary one of precise diagnosis and classification of the epileptic disorder) when assessing the prognosis for seizure recurrence after an isolated seizure, the probability of seizure remission while on treatment, and the risk of relapse after anticonvulsant withdrawal. The risks of seizure recurrence and relapse appear increased in children when interictal epileptiform abnormalities are present. Generalized discharges seem to pose a greater risk for recurrence compared with other discharges. The presence or absence of epileptiform discharges does not appear to be predictive of the risk for late post-traumatic seizures after head injury.

Misconceptions

Misconceptions regarding the use of EEG in epilepsy include the following.

1. A negative interictal EEG excludes epilepsy. Absence of interictal discharges should *never* be interpreted as evidence against a diagnosis of epilepsy. As already discussed, detection of interictal epileptiform discharges is subject to technical factors in sampling and to biologic factors in the patient. The diagnosis of epilepsy should remain clinical.
2. Interictal spikes indicate epilepsy. The clinical interpretation depends on the context. In a patient with suspected epilepsy on clinical grounds, epileptiform discharges in the EEG can be regarded as confirmatory evidence. But when found in an otherwise healthy subject during screening, the risk for development of seizures is probably only minimally raised above that of the whole population.
3. A negative ictal EEG indicates nonepileptic seizures (pseudoseizures). Aside from the fact that the ictal EEG is often obscured by artifacts, it often shows no definite change in simple partial seizures and sometimes even in brief complex partial seizures. Seizures of frontal lobe origin can manifest with complex axial and bilateral motor signs with no detectable changes on the scalp EEG. On the other hand, a normal EEG during bilateral convulsions with loss of consciousness is incompatible with an epileptic event. Absence of ictal EEG changes, therefore, must be interpreted in the light of clinical seizure behavior.

Focal Cerebral Dysfunction

EEG findings in cerebral infarction, hemorrhage, tumor, and focal infection are nonspecific. Detection and localization of abnormalities are modified by the size, location, and temporal evolution of the underlying process and depend on techniques of recording and analysis. Lesions of small size, deep location, or slow growth (e.g., lacunar infarcts, demyelinating plaques, meningiomas) often show no detectable EEG abnormalities. Lesions overlying the cortical surface such as a subdural hematoma may cause asymmetric attenuation of the voltage of background activity. Lesions directly involving cortical gray matter (e.g., Sturge-Weber disease) or cortical infarctions cause alteration or loss of normal EEG activities and may be associated with epileptiform abnormalities. Lesions involving subcortical white matter, such as gliomas or hematomas, cause localized polymorphic slow activity. Deep subcortical diencephalic and posterior fossa lesions tend to produce widespread slow wave disturbances that are sometimes bilaterally synchronous and rhythmic.

Large lesions can sometimes produce periodic lateralized epileptiform discharges (PLEDs). Lesions causing general clinical deterioration from factors such as mass effect are associated with greater alteration of background activity, unreactive polymorphic slow activity, and sometimes bilateral intermittent slow activity. The degree of EEG slowing, however, does not appear to correlate with the presence of cerebral edema. The temporal profile of EEG changes follows that of the particular pathologic process. The disturbances sometimes seen in uncomplicated migraine and small cerebral infarcts are often fully reversible. Progressive lesions such as tumors, on the other hand, cause progressive deterioration in EEG patterns.

Central Nervous System Infections

Creutzfeldt-Jakob disease and subacute sclerosing panencephalitis (SSPE) are the two infectious conditions that stand apart because EEG findings are relatively specific (see *Repetitive or Periodic Patterns*). In most cases of meningitis and encephalitis, the EEG shows a diffuse disturbance of background activity and polymorphic or bilateral intermittent slow wave abnormalities of varying degrees. The severity of the disturbances is usually greater in encephalitis than in meningitis and is related to the extent of cerebral involvement, the rate of disease progression, and secondary complications, such as hypoxia, metabolic derangements, and sepsis. Focal or localized predominance of slow wave abnormalities occurs with abscesses and certain focal encephalitides, particularly in herpes simplex encephalitis. Sometimes the localized abnormalities take the form of PLEDs.

In herpes simplex encephalitis, PLEDs are usually seen 2 to 5 days after the onset of illness and may be unilateral or bilateral. The EEG can provide the earliest evidence for localized brain involvement in herpes encephalitis with greater sensitivity even than CT. Epileptiform abnormalities may arise in patients with encephalitis and frequently develop as chronic sequelae of brain abscesses.

The EEG pattern does not always parallel the clinical state. Slow wave abnormalities indicating subclinical CNS dysfunction can be seen in uncomplicated measles, mumps, rubella, and varicella infections without other evidence for CNS involvement. EEG abnormalities may persist for days to weeks after clinical recovery.

Dementia

Except for its value in the diagnosis of Creutzfeldt-Jakob disease and SSPE, the EEG does not provide specific findings in individual dementing illnesses. The EEG remains clinically useful as a simple test to screen for potentially treatable disorders such as toxic-metabolic encephalopathies, localized cerebral dysfunction, and nonconvulsive status epilepticus.

EEG evaluation of adults with suspected dementia must be based on solid knowledge of age-related changes seen in healthy subjects. Slowing of background activity and its rate of decline often falls beyond the normal range in patients with Alzheimer's disease. Although the posterior background frequency often falls to 5 to 7/sec, it may overlap with the normal alpha frequency range (8 to 13/sec), at least in early disease. Unfortunately, this is the situation in which EEG findings would be most helpful. Mild but progressive slowing may be best appreciated by serial quantitative EEG analysis. In more severe stages of Alzheimer's disease, increased delta slowing becomes apparent. Clinical deterioration appears to be faster in those who show more severe EEG slowing early on. The EEG is frequently normal in Pick's disease. In Huntington's disease, a low voltage (<10 μV) pattern has been reported.

Altered Behavior, Confusion, and Psychosis

The main role of the EEG in states of altered behavior, confusion, and psychosis is to screen for possible cerebral dysfunction as a cause of these conditions, rather than as a specific investigative tool in psychiatric illnesses. In absence and complex partial status epilepticus, behavioral disturbances can range from relatively subtle personality change and cognitive impairment to hallucinations, agitation, confusion, and stupor. Seizures of frontal lobe origin may appear so bizarre as to invite ridicule as hysterical attacks. To determine whether episodic psychological and behavioral disturbances represent seizures, more intensive EEG investigations, as previously outlined, may be needed.

Toxic and Metabolic Encephalopathies

The EEG is invariably abnormal in toxic-metabolic encephalopathies (Table 6-4). In milder stages, there is diffuse slowing, the degree of which tends to parallel the clinical course. In later, more severe stages, new patterns may emerge, such as triphasic waves, periodic sharp waves, and monotonous patterns (e.g., as in alpha coma, described later) (Table 6-5).

Table 6-4. Common EEG Patterns in Toxic and Metabolic Encephalopathies

EEG Patterns	Etiologies
Diffuse slowing of background activity; Bilateral intermittent slow activity; Diffuse polymorphic slow activity	All etiologies
Excess activity	Barbiturate and benzodiazepine toxicity
Prolonged theta activity	Phencyclidine toxicity
Triphasic waves	Hepatic failure, uremia, anoxia, hypoglycemia, hyperosmality
Periodic spikes or sharp waves	Anoxia, uremia, dialysis dementia, lithium and tricyclic antidepressant toxicity
Monotonous alpha activity; Burst suppression pattern	Anoxia, severe CNS depressant drug toxicity

In hepatic failure and in Reye syndrome, EEG grading scales have been used to help provide an index of disease progression and prognosis.

Stupor, Coma, and Brain Death

The EEG sometimes helps yield information on the underlying causes of the comatose state. Localized abnormalities point to the possibility of a

Table 6-5. Relative Severity of EEG Patterns in Coma

Severity		EEG Pattern (Does Not Imply Serial Evolution)
Least ↓	With spontaneous variability and reactivity	Predominance of normal activities
		Slowing with preservation of some normal activities
		Bilateral intermittent slow activity
		Sleeplike patterns (e.g., spindle coma)
		Continuous polymorphic slow activity
		Triphasic waves
Worst	Without variability or reactivity	Periodic spikes or sharp waves
		Episodic voltage attenuation
		Monotonous alpha activity (i.e., alpha coma)
		Burst suppression pattern
		Scattered low voltage ($<20\ \mu V$) delta activity
Brain death		Electrocerebral inactivity (ECI)

supratentorial mass lesion. Toxic-metabolic and anoxic encephalopathies and diffuse encephalitis tend to cause widespread diffuse abnormalities. Persistent rhythmic epileptiform abnormalities indicate unrecognized status epilepticus. Infratentorial lesions are difficult to diagnose on EEG.

The monotonous alpha frequency activity sometimes found in coma is also called *alpha coma*, but does not constitute a specific etiologic entity. Monotonous, unreactive alpha activity with a reversed anterior distribution is most commonly seen after circulatory or respiratory arrest and severe drug overdoses. Monotonous but partially reactive posterior alpha activity is sometimes seen in brainstem infarcts. Reactive, normally distributed alpha activity in an otherwise unresponsive patient raises the possibility that the unresponsiveness is not so much due to coma as to either a locked-in state or psychogenic unresponsiveness. Trains of rhythmic 10 to 12/sec activity resembling sleep spindles are found in some stuporous or comatose patients and has been labeled the *spindle coma* pattern. It is without etiologic specificity and represents partial preservation of organized sleep activity.

The greater role of the EEG in coma is to provide an assessment of the severity of cerebral dysfunction (Table 6-5). Serial EEGs are more informative than a single record, as they allow follow-up of the evolution of the illness. Broadly speaking, preservation of any recognizable EEG activity from patterns of normal wakefulness or sleep is better than when they are absent. Spontaneous variability, sleep-wake changes, and reactivity to external stimuli suggest a better prognosis than when no variability or reactivity exists. In contrast, the presence of an invariant pattern of any form generally carries a poorer prognosis. With increasing global dysfunction, the EEG may show increasing voltage suppression, continuously or in bursts, and eventually loss of all activity.

Electrocerebral inactivity (ECI) (Fig. 6-10) is operationally defined as "no EEG activity over 2 μV when recording from scalp electrode pairs 10 or more cm apart with interelectrode impedance under 10,000 ohms, but over 100 ohms" (American EEG Society). Recording conditions are demanding and often technically difficult to achieve in an intensive care unit. ECI confirms total brain death, provided the clinical criteria of irreversibility, unresponsive coma, apnea, and brainstem areflexia are met. A minority of patients display some residual EEG activity incompatible with the criteria of ECI, despite clinically established brain death. The United Kingdom Code for the Diagnosis of Brain Death (1976) does not recommend EEG as a necessary confirmatory test. The United States Guidelines for the Determination of Death (President's Commission 1981) recommend the EEG as a confirmatory test, but stop short of making its use explicit and mandatory.

SPECIAL ELECTROENCEPHALOGRAM RECORDINGS

Several modern technical developments have extended the scope of clinical EEG. Ambulatory cassette monitoring uses a compact portable unit to record four or eight channels of EEG for up to 24 hours onto conventional cassette tapes for subsequent analysis. It has the advantage of allowing extended EEG sampling under relatively normal living conditions. Limitations include a restricted number of channels and vulnerability to a wide range of artifacts from environmental causes and from patient activity. Its main application is in the extended sampling of interictal and some ictal epileptiform EEG abnormalities in patients with known or suspected epilepsy. Video-EEG monitoring allows simultaneous recording of the EEG and a video image of the patient's behavior. It is the preferred method for precise electroclinical analysis of seizures and other episodic disorders.

Various types of electrodes can be inserted to lie in the epidural and subdural spaces, or can be implanted stereotactically into the brain for intracranial EEG recording. They can improve localization of the epileptogenic zone. All techniques carry small but significant risks of infection, hemorrhage, and even death. Their use, therefore, is limited to selected patients who are candidates for epilepsy surgery, in whom extracranial EEG and other noninvasive tests have failed to delineate an epileptogenic zone that could be resected. Similar techniques can be used intraoperatively to guide the surgical treatment of epilepsy.

Extracranial EEG monitoring intraoperatively may be used during cerebrovascular procedures to continuously assess cerebral function and to warn of vascular compromise.

In computer EEG analysis, the EEG is first recorded in the conventional way, then filtered, digitized, and transmitted to a computer. The most common forms of computer analysis are in either the time or frequency domain. Frequency analysis usually uses Fast-Fourier transformation to give a frequency spectrum of the EEG (spectral analysis). The advantages of computer analysis lie in (1) quantification (e.g., relative activity in different frequency bands, comparison of left-right asymmetries), (2) signals analysis where tests of mathematical interaction between different EEG signals are performed (e.g., coherence measurements between different brain regions), (3) data display (e.g., display of waveform potentials or spectra in a two-dimensional representation of the head—so-called brainmapping), (4) data compression, and (5) automation (e.g., automatic detection of epileptiform discharges and seizures). This area has been growing rapidly and is expected to contribute more to routine EEG studies in coming years.

READINGS

American Electroencephalographic Society guidelines in EEG and evoked potentials. J Clin Neurophysiol 3:1, 1986

Aminoff MJ (ed): Electrodiagnosis in Clinical Neurology. 2nd Ed. Churchill Livingstone, New York, 1986

Ayala GF, Dichter M, Gumnit RJ, et al: Genesis of epileptic interictal spikes, new knowledge of feedback systems suggests a neurophysiologic explanation of brief paroxysms. Brain Res 52:1, 1973

Binnie CD, Rowan AJ, Gutter TH: A Manual of Electroencephalographic Technology. Cambridge University Press, Cambridge, 1982

Blume WT: Atlas of Pediatric Electroencephalography. Raven Press, New York, 1982

Goldensohn ES, Koehle R: EEG Interpretation. Problems of Overreading and Underreading. Futura Publishing, Mount Kisco, NY, 1975

Halliday AM, Butler SR, Paul R (eds): A Textbook of Clinical Neurophysiology. John Wiley & Sons, New York, 1987

Jasper HH: Report of the Committee on Methods of Clinical Examination in Electroencephalography. Electroenceph Clin Neurophysiol 10:370, 1958

Klass DW, Daly DD (eds): Current Practice of Clinical Electroencephalography. Raven Press, New York, 1979

Lopes da Silva F, Storm van Leeuwen W, Remond A (eds): Clinical applications of computer analysis of EEG and other neurophysiological signals. In Gevins AS and Rémond A (eds): Handbook of Electroencephalography and Clinical Neurophysiology. Revised Series. Vol. 2. Elsevier Science Publishing, Amsterdam, 1986

Lüders H, Lesser RP (eds): Epilepsy: Electroclinical Syndromes. Springer-Verlag, Berlin, Heidelberg, 1987

Niedermeyer E, Lopes da Silva F (eds): Electroencephalography. 2nd Ed. Urban & Schwarzenberg, Baltimore, 1987

Nunez PL: Electric Fields of the Brain. Oxford University Press, New York, 1981

Schwartzkroin PA, Wheal H (eds): Electrophysiology of Epilepsy. Academic Press, London, 1984

Tyner FS, Knott JR, Mayer WB Jr: Fundamentals of EEG Technology. Vol. 1. Raven Press, New York, 1983

Tyner FS, Knott JR, Mayer WB Jr: Fundamentals of EEG Technology. Vol. 2. Raven Press, New York, 1989

USEFUL TESTS IN HEREDITARY METABOLIC DISEASE 7

Hereditary metabolic diseases with defined biochemical abnormalities are an important and growing class of neurologic diseases. There are many more recognized hereditary diseases that have been described clinically and pathologically, but for which the underlying biochemical lesion is not known (e.g., Kufs disease). Diagnostic approaches to some of these will be discussed in the next chapter.

Most of the diseases now recognized as metabolic are autosomal recessive. However, with the notable exception of a few disorders such as Wilson's disease, which can have a rather characteristic combination of clinical features and associated laboratory abnormalities, they are difficult to diagnose. In addition to being rare, they show great variability in phenotype and generally lack specific clinical features. The biochemical abnormalities underlying them often demand assays in specialized laboratories. With advances in molecular genetics, linkage studies and locus-specific probes may even replace some of the more straightforward biochemical assays for autosomal recessive disease, particularly for identification of heterozygotes.

Autosomal dominant diseases (e.g., Huntington's disease, familial Alzheimer's disease, neurofibromatosis, Charcot-Marie-Tooth disease) are more common, but less well understood. The underlying biochemical lesions are not known, but it is clear that soon closely linked gene probes will be available for diagnosis in appropriate kindreds. Linkage analysis for Huntington's disease is already available for presymptomatic diagnosis.

This chapter begins with a very brief outline of current clinical biochemical approaches to the diagnosis of autosomal recessive disease and an introduction to a few basic concepts of clinical molecular biology. The subsequent sections are intended as a short guide to tests currently in use for diagnosis of several adult-onset autosomal recessive metabolic diseases. All are rare.

When a patient who may have such a rare disease is first seen, it is usually impossible to establish an accurate and brief enough differential diagnosis for all of the appropriate tests to be ordered at once. The correct differential diagnosis often becomes apparent only as the clinical picture evolves. Thus, appropriate samples (e.g., urine, leukocytes, biopsies) should be obtained and stored to allow later study. This chapter provides an initial guide for such a workup.

BIOCHEMICAL TESTS IN DIAGNOSIS

The metabolic basis of autosomal recessive and X-linked metabolic diseases can generally be appreciated by using two simple biochemical paradigms. The first, two-stage paradigm is that one gene codes for one peptide, and peptide synthesis parallels gene dose. Thus, a homozygotic or hemizygotic state for a deleterious mutant allele leads to symptoms by causing a deficiency of the protein (or, more strictly, the peptide) encoded by the abnormal locus. For example, a mutant locus in a gene coding for an enzyme may reduce total tissue enzyme activity. In fact, all of the autosomal recessive diseases with defined biochemical causes result from deficiencies of enzyme activity. One way to diagnose these diseases, therefore, is to assay tissue for the appropriate enzyme: it is established by finding an abnormally low activity.

McArdle's disease, which is a deficiency of muscle glycogen phosphorylase (see *Hereditary Metabolic Disease Presenting Primarily as Myopathic Disorders*) is an example of this type of disorder. Low activity of muscle phosphorylase prevents rapid breakdown of glycogen during anaerobic exercise conditions. This leads to an energy crisis in the exercising muscle that is clinically characterized by easy fatiguability and electrically silent muscle cramps. This disease also illustrates the importance of recognizing that tissue-specific isozymes may be selectively affected in disease. Only the muscle phosphorylase isozyme is affected; hepatic glycogenolysis is normal. The diagnosis can be established histochemically by an absence of phosphorylase activity in muscle biopsy specimens.

In contrast, tissue-specific isozymes do not seem to exist for some of the enzyme deficiencies associated with the lipidoses. These are systemic diseases. For example, in Niemann-Pick disease types A and B (in which there is a deficiency of sphingomyelinase, which hydrolyses sphingomyelin to its components ceramide and phosphocholine), abnormal lipid storage can be demonstrated in neurons of brain, spinal cord, and gut and in histiocytes in liver, spleen, and bone marrow. Therefore, tissue for study in a diagnostic workup can potentially be obtained from several sites more accessible than the CNS. The most generally useful cells for enzyme assays are leukocytes and culture fibroblasts.

The second general biochemical paradigm for understanding hereditary metabolic disease is that metabolic pathways may often be treated as a linear sequence of reactions:

$$A \xrightarrow{1} B \xrightarrow{2} C \xrightarrow{3}$$

In such a simple system, an abnormally low activity of enzyme 3 will give rise to accumulation of precursors A, B, and C as well as an abnormally low concentration of the end product D. Thus, presence of increased levels of A, B, and C identify a deficiency of enzyme 3, whereas increased levels of A alone imply a deficiency of enzyme 1, and so on. Diagnosis can be made by measuring the abnormally elevated concentrations of the intermediates in the reaction sequence. These may be found in specific tissues or serum or may be excreted in the urine or feces. For example, the hepatic porphyrias can be diagnosed from the pattern of increased excretion of intermediates in the heme biosynthetic pathway. Decreased concentrations of normal end products are seen in disorders of glycolysis or glycogenolysis (e.g., glycogenosis types III, V, and VII and phosphoglycerate kinase deficiency). The venous lactate concentration should rise after ischemic forearm exercise, and this rise is reduced or absent in these disorders.

Biochemical diagnoses are essential for hereditary metabolic disease. An important lesson apparent from review of these disorders is that either patients with different phenotypes may have the same apparent enzyme deficiency or patients with different enzyme defects may manifest the same phenotype. Later in the chapter biochemical approaches to diagnosis of hereditary metabolic disease affecting the nervous system will be outlined; however, it is beyond the scope of this book to attempt full clinical descriptions of the disorders or of assay methods. Readings listed at the end of the chapter should be consulted for such clinical information.

MOLECULAR BIOLOGIC APPROACHES

Molecular biology and genetics will probably assume preeminence in the next decade for diagnosis of hereditary diseases. There are now probes that are tightly linked or specific for the locus of both autosomal dominant (e.g., Huntington's disease) and X-linked (e.g., Duchenne muscular dystrophy) diseases for which traditional biochemical markers are not available. Antenatal diagnosis early in pregnancy with chorionic villus biopsy is possible. A particular power of the techniques with X-linked diseases is that they can also be used to identify carriers.

Descriptions of these methods may be found in a number of sources, cited at the end of the chapter. Here only a sketch of the two basic approaches will be given, describing how such tests can be developed either (1) when the abnormal protein responsible for a disease is known and isolated or (2) when it is completely unknown. The success of these approaches lies in the fact that it is often easier to identify an abnormality in the genome than in a specific protein.

If the abnormal protein is known, the responsible gene can be identified after only partial sequencing of the protein. A radiolabeled (^{32}P) synthetic oligonucleotide probe that hybridizes uniquely with the gene can be constructed from the known correspondence between the nucleotides and the amino acid sequence (the genetic code). The probe can be hybridized with electrophoretically separated fragments of DNA complementary to cell messenger RNA (cDNA) (Southern blot). Sensitivity can be greatly increased by selectively amplifying the gene of interest from a patient's tissue using the polymerase chain reaction.

The segment of cDNA that hybridizes with the probe can often be identified as coming from a normal or abnormal gene on the basis of its electrophoretic mobility. Although substitutions or deletions of a few bases might, in principle, lead to changes in migration for short cDNA fragments, in reality this is relatively insensitive. The major factor determining migration is the pattern of fragmentation of the cDNA by restriction endonucleases.

Restriction endonucleases are bacterial enzymes (e.g., Hind III, Bam) that make internal breaks in DNA when different, short, and highly specific base sequences are recognized. Large deletions from a gene (or occasionally even point mutations) lead to changes in splicing pattern and thus in electrophoretic mobility of the fragments recognized by a given oligonucleotide probe. In familial amyloid neuropathy, for example, a single substitution of methionine for valine at position 30 of the protein transthyretin arises from change of an adenine for a guanine in the transthyretin gene. This base change leads to a new restriction site for the endonuclease NsiI, giving rise to a readily identifiable extra fragment on the Southern blot.

A different approach is used with diseases in which the abnormal protein is unknown. (Actually, abnormal allele would be more accurate, as any allele, including those for "controller" regions of DNA, can be affected.)

Most of the dominantly inherited neurologic diseases such as Huntington's disease currently fall into this category. This approach is based on the idea in classic genetics of searching for linkage of random genetic markers to a given phenotype. Classic genetic markers include the discrete blood groups (e.g., ABO, Lutheran, Duffy) and human major histocompatibility complex (HLA) antigens. The only essential requirements for such markers is that they occupy specific and fixed loci in the human genome.

Until recently the problem with this approach was that too few classic marker loci had been identified to allow tight and informative linkages to be established with other genes in all areas of the genome. However, the discovery of restriction fragment length polymorphisms (RFLPs) has changed that. As mentioned earlier, bacterial restriction endonucleases cleave DNA wherever characteristic, short sequences occur. Such restriction sites are usually formed by stretches of DNA composed of repetitive sequences with variable numbers of repeats. These sequences (known as *introns*) do not code for proteins or have other known functions, so variations in their sequences appear to have no deleterious consequences. Their use as markers stems from the fact that these regions show considerable polymorphism among individuals. Southern blots prepared using DNA fragmented by restriction enzymes can demonstrate this polymorphism (restriction fragment length polymorphism or RFLP) when suitable probes are used. These RFLPs are inherited as simple mendelian codominant traits (expressed only in the genotype) and may be used in genetic analysis just as classic markers.

Linkage of a marker to a given phenotype must be expressed quantitatively. The linkage is expressed with respect to a recombination fraction (θ), which is an indirect measure of the distance between the marker and disease genes. If the two gene loci are on different chromosomes (unlinked) $\theta = 0.5$. However, if they are on the same chromosome, θ will be less than 0.5. The closer the physical distance between the two loci, the lower the probability of recombination events disrupting the linkage and the smaller the recombination fraction. If a marker is very tightly linked ($\theta < 0.05$) to the locus for a disease-producing allele, presence of the marker alone can be used to infer with high probability that the abnormal allele is also present in a patient. This approach is already useful in presymptomatic diagnosis of later onset diseases such as Huntington's disease, familial Alzheimer's disease, neurofibromatosis, and myotonic dystrophy.

The recombination fraction between a candidate marker gene (or RFLP) and a disease-producing gene can be calculated from statistical analysis of data from many kindreds describing the association of the candidate marker gene (or RFLP) and the disease phenotype. Results are commonly assessed using a log of the odds (LOD) score, an expression of the probability that two genes are linked. Linkage is established if the LOD score is greater than 3, corresponding to odds in favor of linkage of greater than 1,000 to 1. An LOD score of −3 or less rather definitely rules out any likelihood of linkage. The LOD score becomes more significant as the database used to generate it increases in size.

To be diagnostically useful, a marker must also be polymorphic enough to be informative for linkage. A marker is informative in a given kindred only if it is uniquely associated with the disease phenotype in a particular kindred. For autosomal dominant disease, at least one parent must be doubly heterozygous for the marker and the abnormal, disease-producing allele, for that marker to be informative. Thus, if one is considering typing a kindred to search for markers, the most efficient method is to type the parents first. However, when tissue from them is not available, their genotypes can be inferred from those of their offspring. The use of randomly generated genetic markers to assess linkage is not an end in itself, but merely a step toward more direct methods based on use of a genetic marker within the disease-producing gene. Problems with linkage studies include that (1) there is always some degree of recombination (and, therefore, uncertainty in diagnosis) between the marker and disease loci and (2) linkage studies demand analysis of DNA from a kindred large enough to ensure the usefulness of the marker.

HEREDITARY METABOLIC DISEASES PRESENTING PRIMARILY WITH CNS DYSFUNCTION

Diagnostic tests for hereditary metabolic diseases presenting primarily with CNS dysfunction are outlined in Table 7-1.

Lysosomal Disorders

Niemann-Pick Disease

Niemann-Pick disease types A and B result from a deficiency of lysosomal sphingomyelinase, the enzyme catalyzing hydrolysis of sphingomyelin to ceramide and phosphocholine. This autosomal recessive deficiency leads to accumulation of lipids in lysosomes in neurons and glia as well as in macrophages of the reticuloendothelial system (leading to hepatosplenomegaly and splenomegaly). Niemann-Pick disease types C and D are phenotypically similar, but clinical symptoms do not correlate with sphingomyelinase deficiency. In fact, sphingomyelinase activity may even be normal. Several different clinical presentations for this apparently biochemically heterogeneous disorder have been identified. The juvenile onset form is characterized by progressive dementia, dystonia, spasticity, and incoordination with seizures, usually leading to death by mid adolescence. The adult form primarily affects the reticuloendothelial system, but may be accompanied by cerebellar ataxia or more generalized progressive neurologic deterioration. The diagnosis in all cases is suggested by foamy-appearing, lipid-laden cells in the bone marrow (''sea blue histiocytes'') and, in cases with neuronal involvement, often the ganglion cells of the rectal mucosa. The lysosomal (identified by acid phosphatase staining and presence of a surrounding membrane by electron microscopy) lipid accumulations have a positive Schultz reaction for cholesterol, unlike the morphologically similar bodies of Gaucher's disease.

A specific biochemical diagnosis for types A and B can be established by assaying sphingomyelinase activity in fibroblast cell cultures, leukocytes, or a liver biopsy specimen showing the characteristic pathologic changes. Assaying with [^{14}C]choline-labeled sphingomyelin is more sensitive than the more easily performed assay using a fluorescent analogue of sphingomyelin. The diagnosis of types C and D is made with demonstration of a marked impairment ($<$10 percent of normal activity) or esterification of exogenous cholesterol by cultured fibroblasts. This abnormality is not found with Niemann-Pick types A and B.

Krabbe's Disease

Krabbe's disease is an autosomal recessive leukodystrophy caused by a deficiency of lysosomal galactocerebroside-β-galactosidase. Galactocerebrosides and their sulfated derivatives are major components of myelin. With deficient galactosidase activity there is accumulation of a toxic intermediate (psychosine) in the galactocerebroside degradation pathway that leads to oligodendroglial cell death. Because glial cell death occurs as intermediates accumulate, storage of large amounts of lipids is not seen in the CNS as with other lipidoses. Involvement of the brain may be patchy. The classic biopsy finding is so-called globoid cells in the white matter, with areas of demyelination and astrocytic gliosis. The rare adult form may result from a defect at a different locus than in the neonatal disease. Patients present with a progressive spastic gait disorder, cortical blindness, and optic atrophy. Galactocerebroside-β-galactosidase activity is deficient in serum, leukocytes, and cultured fibroblasts. There is a risk of false-positive results with the serum assay, as the normal serum activity is low and the enzyme activity is not stable. Assays with both the ra-

Table 7-1. Diagnostic Tests for Hereditary Metabolic Diseases Presenting Primarily with CNS Dysfunction

Disease	Biochemical Defect	Tissue for Enzyme Activity Assay	Other Diagnostic Tests
Lysosomal Disorders			
Gaucher's disease (glucosylceramide lipidosis)	Glucocerebrosidase deficiency	Leukocytes, cultured fibroblasts	Lipid-laden histocytes (bone marrow and liver), increased serum acid phosphatase
Niemann-Pick disease (sphingomyelin lipidosis)	Sphingomyelinase deficiency in some forms	Leukocytes, cultured fibroblasts, liver biopsy	Sea-blue histiocytes in bone marrow and liver showing positive Schultz reaction for cholesterol
Krabbe's disease (galactosyl ceramide lipidosis)	Galactocerebroside–β-galactosidase deficiency	Serum (unreliable), leukocytes, cultured fibroblasts	Globoid cell, demyelination, and gliosis in brain biopsy
GM_2 gangliosidosis	Hexosaminidase A deficiency	Serum, leukocytes (preferred), cultured fibroblasts	
Sialidosis	Neuraminidase deficiency	Leukocytes, cultured fibroblasts	Thin layer chromatography (TLC) of urine for oligosaccharides
Mannosidosis	Acidic α-mannosidase deficiency	Serum, leukocytes, cultured fibroblasts	TLC of urine for mannose-rich oligosaccharides, PAS-positive vacuolation of lymphocytes and cells in bone marrow
Metachromatic leukodystrophy (sulfatide lipidosis)	Arylsulfatase A deficiency	Serum, urine, leukocytes, cultured fibroblasts	Increased urinary sulfatides by TLC, Schwann cell inclusions of metachromatic lipids on nerve biopsy, increased CSF protein, slowed nerve conduction velocities

Peroxisomal Disorder				
Adrenoleukodystrophy	Possibly lignoceroyl-coenzyme A synthetase		—	Plasma assay for increased C26 VLCFA and C24:C22 fatty acid ratio; abnormality also present in cultured skin fibroblasts
Idiopathic Disease				
Wilson's disease	Defective incorporation of copper into apoceruloplasmin	Serum		Often low serum uric acid and phosphate, low serum copper, high urinary copper excretion, and increased copper in cultured fibroblasts or liver biopsy by neutron activation analysis
Other				
Abetalipoproteinemia	Apolipoprotein B deficiency		—	Acanthocytosis, abnormal PT, PTT in some, serum cholesterol (<100 mg/dl) and triglycerides (<30 mg/dl) low, apolipoprotein B deficiency by immunologic assay

PT, prothrombin time; PTT, partial prothrombin time.

diolabeled natural substrate and a chromogenic synthetic substrate are possible. Although not a recognized problem in this disease, it is important to bear in mind that different defects of protein structure may lead to diagnostically useful differences in catalytic activity with different substrates.

Gaucher's Disease

Gaucher's disease, which results from a deficiency of lysosomal glucocerebrosidase activity, leads to accumulation of glucocerebrosides in cells of the reticuloendothelial system. In some forms, glucocerebroside accumulation is found in the CNS. The usual adult form does not involve the nervous system, but cases of a late-onset juvenile form have been described in adults. This juvenile form is characterized by a progressive seizure disorder, tremor, dementia, and gait disturbances associated with hepatosplenomegaly. Bone marrow shows lipid-laden histiocytes with acid phosphatase and PAS-positive staining (indicating the presence of reducing sugars) of the storage bodies. The Schultz reaction for cholesterol is negative, distinguishing it from Niemann-Pick disease. Abnormal elevation of the specific plasma glycolipids can be established by high performance liquid chromatography (HPLC) methods.

A specific biochemical diagnosis is established by assay of glucocerebroside activity in leukocytes or cultured fibroblasts. Interpretation of the assay is complicated by the presence of multiple isozymes: total activity can be normal in individuals who have a deficiency only of a single isoenzyme. Cultured fibroblasts are preferred for assays, especially for heterozygote detection.

Gangliosidoses

Gangliosides are *N*-acetylneuraminic acid-substituted glycosphingolipids. At least 10 types of gangliosides are found in the adult brain. They differ in the number and position of the *N*-acetylneuraminic acid and hexose (glucose and galactose) groups. Catabolism occurs by stepwise removal, first of *N*-acetylneuraminic acid molecules and then of sugars from the nonreducing end by specific exohydrolases. The gangliosidoses develop due to deficiencies of these exohydrolases and the abnormal accumulation of lipids proximal to the site of catabolic block. Thin-layer chromatography can be used to identify abnormal urinary oligosaccharide excretion in the urine in some forms.

GM_2 gangliosidosis resulting from a deficiency of hexosaminidase A is the most important of these diseases in adult neurology. The infantile form

(Tay-Sachs disease) has been well described because of the high frequency of the mutant allele among certain cultural groups. GM_2 gangliosidosis can present in adults as a syndrome of cerebellar dysfunction and anterior horn cell disease.

Hexosaminidase A is present in most tissues. Serum, leukocytes, and cultured fibroblasts are suitable for assays, with the leukocyte assay producing fewer false-positive results. Positive results should be carefully repeated for confirmation. False-positive results have been described during pregnancy, with diabetes, or with severe tissue injury. Consistent differences in assay results have been found using the synthetic fluorogenic substrate and the natural ganglioside (GM_2). This probably reflects heterogeneity of the specific enzymatic defect.

Sialidosis

Sialidosis is strictly a juvenile onset disease, but deserves mention because adult neurologists may be called on to evaluate epilepsy in adolescents. The more common clinical type can present as a progressive myoclonus epilepsy, with decreasing visual acuity and possibly ataxia or mild mental retardation. A cherry red macula is seen on funduscopic examination. The diagnosis may be suspected by finding increased sialylated oligosaccharides (by 100-fold or more) in urine using thin-layer chromatography. It is confirmed by finding a deficiency of lysosomal α-neuraminidase in leukocytes or cultured fibroblasts.

Mannosidosis

Mannosidosis is a systemic disease that results from a deficiency of acidic α-mannosidase. Postmortem studies demonstrate neuronal loss and demyelination in the brain, where neurons swollen with PAS-positive lysosomes may be found. Clinically, the juvenile- and the milder adult-onset forms are characterized by dementia, partial deafness, cataracts, and, often, bony deformities. Thin-layer chromatography of urine demonstrates increased levels of mannose-rich oligosaccharides. A bone marrow biopsy may show lymphocytes filled with carbohydrate-rich (PAS-positive) vacuoles. Definitive diagnosis is established by demonstration of a severe reduction of acidic-mannosidase activity in serum, leukocytes, or cultured fibroblasts.

Metachromatic Leukodystrophy

The name metachromatic leukodystrophy reflects these diagnostic pathologic findings: metachromatic staining occurs when certain cationic dyes (such as toluidine blue) shift their absorption spectra (and thus change their color) when in association with anionic groups such as those of the sulfatides. The sulfatides accumulated in metachromatic leukodystrophy are sulfated forms of the cerebrosides, primarily galactosyl cerebroside. Arylsulfatase A is the lysosomal enzyme responsible for the first stage in their breakdown. Accumulation of sulfatides in oligodendroglial cells impairs their function and leads to breakdown of their myelin sheaths. Unlike the juvenile form, adult metachromatic leukodystrophy can have a very prolonged course, characterized by spastic ataxia, dementia, and a demyelinating peripheral neuropathy.

There are increased sulfatides in urine even with the heterozygote state. These can be detected qualitatively by the characteristic metachromatic reaction of the lipid extract or by thin-layer chromatography. In clinically affected individuals, a sural nerve biopsy will show a variable degree of demyelination and metachromatic material in phagocytes and Schwann cells. Both homozygotes and heterozygotes will be deficient in arylsulfatase A activity. The assay is complicated by the presence of a related enzyme, arylsulfatase B. Activity is most easily measured using a chromogenic substrate. The serum assay is less reliable for clearly distinguishing heterozygotes from normals. Activity in leukocytes or cultured fibroblasts is more reliable. The gold-standard assay is the rate of hydrolysis of the ^{35}S-labeled sulfatide by cultured fibroblasts.

A childhood form of the disease is associated with normal arylsulfatase activity, but a deficiency in a cerebroside sulfate sulfatase activation factor.

Peroxisomal Disorders: Adrenoleukodystrophy

Peroxisomes are intracellular organelles that constitute a specialized compartment for a broad range of catalytic processes. Adrenoleukodystrophy (ALD) is an X-linked recessive disorder thought to be caused by an inability of peroxisomes to appropriately degrade very long chain fatty acids (VLCFA) that are present in trace quantities in the usual diet. Accumulation of VLCFA appears to trigger an inflammatory response. The adrenal glands and cerebral white matter are affected. The less common adult form may present as a myeloneuropathy or a progressive dementia with personality changes, ataxia, and pyramidal signs. Neurologic symptoms are accompanied or preceded by adrenal dysfunction in most.

Biochemical diagnosis is made by demonstrating increased VLCFA in plasma or cultured fibroblasts using HPLC. Patients with ALD show a twofold to tenfold increase in the concentration of hexacosanoic acid (C26:0) and an abnormally high (>1.1) ratio of tetracosanoic (C24:0) to docosanoic (C22:0) acids. Heterozygotes have less marked abnormalities. The assay is difficult and should only be performed in experienced laboratories. If overt Addison's disease (primary adrenal failure) is not present, an abnormally low ACTH response can usually be demonstrated.

Wilson's Disease

Wilson's disease is an autosomal recessive disease of copper metabolism clinically characterized by the combination of hepatic cirrhosis and neurologic abnormalities. Symptoms may begin between 5 and 40 years of age. Two neurologic syndromes are classically recognized, both of which can be accompanied by disorders of thought processes (psychiatric symptoms). The more common presentation is with flapping tremors. More rarely, a dystonic form associated with spasticity and bulbar dysfunction (a memorable combination of drooling, dysarthria, and a cheerful-appearing expression) can be seen. Slit-lamp examination should invariably demonstrate Kayser-Fleischer rings in cases with neurologic symptoms. The characteristic brown rings result from copper deposition in the cornea. Copper deposition also occurs in other tissues, notably the basal ganglia.

Routine clinical laboratory studies may demonstrate mild renal dysfunction, including hematuria. Baseline renal function studies are important because they allow clear documentation of any impairment induced later with penicillamine treatment. A mild hemolytic anemia may be present.

Central to the diagnosis is demonstration of low serum ceruloplasmin, low total serum copper, and high urinary copper excretion. Serum ceruloplasmin levels normally vary with age (higher in children). Decreased ceruloplasmin is an incidental finding in hypoproteinemic states. It also accompanies the nephrotic syndrome, protein-losing enteropathy, malnutrition, and malabsorption states as well as the extremely rare, neonatal-onset Menkes disease. Quantitative urinary copper excretion correlates roughly with disease duration in Wilson's disease and may be normal early in the disease. More sensitive is measurement of an abnormally high penicillinase-induced copper excretion, although this can also occur with the nonspecific increased copper storage associated with other forms of cholestatic hepatic disease.

The most sensitive test (useful for presymptomatic patients) involves measurement by neutron activation analysis of abnormally high copper in cultured fibroblasts or liver biopsy specimens. (For the latter, fixation in alcohol is recommended.)

HEREDITARY METABOLIC DISEASES PRESENTING PRIMARILY AS MYOPATHIC DISORDERS

Diagnostic tests for hereditary metabolic diseases presenting primarily as myopathic disorders are outlined in Table 7-2.

Muscular Dystrophies

The diagnosis of muscular dystrophies in index cases is primarily clinical, aided (especially in late-onset cases) by muscle biopsy results. Serum creatine phosphokinase (CPK) is frequently elevated—always in Duchenne dystrophy, but variably in the more indolent, later-onset myopathies. The identification of the gene for dystrophin, the abnormal protein in Duchenne and Becker dystrophies, has improved carrier detection and potentially allows prenatal diagnosis. Assay for dystrophin in muscle biopsy specimens may allow more certain diagnoses and better assessment of prognosis early in the course of the clinically heterogeneous Becker dystrophies. Markers tightly linked to the gene for myotonic dystrophy on chromosome 19 promise similar developments for this disorder in the near future.

Defects in Energy Metabolism

Defects of Glycogenolysis and Glycolysis

Abnormal Lysosomal Glycogen Metabolism: Acid Maltase Deficiency

Acid maltase deficiency (glycogenosis type II) is the common name for the autosomal recessive deficiency of lysosomal α-1,4-glucosidase. This enzyme is present in all tissues and catalyzes hydrolysis of linear oligosaccharides to glucose in a pathway distinct from the energy-producing pathway of glycogenolysis. The deficiency state leads to accumulation of glycogen in lysosomes in affected tissues.

In adults, the disease presents as a chronic progressive myopathy, involving both proximal and distal muscles with prominent respiratory muscle involvement. A definitive diagnosis is made by muscle biopsy. Serum CPK may be elevated. Noninvasive, specific screening tests are assays for glucosidase activity, which is decreased in the disease in leukocytes and urine. A more sensitive assay is performed on cultured fibroblasts.

Abnormal Glycogenolysis: McArdle's Disease and Debrancher Enzyme Deficiency

McArdle's disease (muscle phosphorylase deficiency, glycogenosis type IV) was the first clearly defined hereditary metabolic disease of muscle. There is more than one isozyme of phosphorylase and the deficiency is

Table 7-2. Diagnostic Tests for Hereditary Metabolic Myopathies

Disease	Biochemical Defect	Enzyme Activity Assay	Other Biological Tests
Acid maltase deficiency (glycogenosis type II)	α-1,4-glucosidase deficiency	Urine, leukocyte, or cultured fibroblasts (most sensitive)	Increased serum CPK, frequently nonspecific increase in urinary oligosaccharides
Debrancher deficiency (glycogenosis type III)	Amylo-1, 6-glucosidase deficiency	Leukocytes or cultured fibroblasts	Increased serum CPK, abnormal ischemic lactate test possible
McCardle's disease (glycogenosis type V)	Muscle phosphorylase deficiency	Muscle	Increased serum CPK, exercise-induced myoglobinuria, abnormal ischemic lactate test
Glycogenosis type VII	Muscle phosphofructokinase deficiency	Erythrocytes (partial deficiency), muscle	Increased serum CPK, abnormal ischemic lactate test
Myoadenylate deaminase deficiency	Muscle myoadenylate deaminase	Muscle biopsy (not in cultured muscle)	Increased CPK common, normal ischemic lactate, low increase in venous ammonia and hypoxanthine levels with exercise

specifically for the muscle isozyme. Clinically, the disease is characterized by the onset of exercise intolerance in adolescence. Later, patients note painful muscle cramps with exercise. Severe exercise may lead to myoglobinuria. Appropriate pacing of exercise allows increased tolerance with development of a second wind.

The easiest noninvasive screening test is the ischemic forearm exercise test, also known as the ischemic lactate test. The patient is allowed to rest supine for 30 minutes in order to avoid possible artifactual elevation of the baseline serum lactate by muscle activity (in patients who do *not* have complete phosphorylase deficiency). A sphygmomanometer cuff is then placed around the upper arm and an intravenous catheter, equipped with a three-way stopcock to allow easy withdrawal of blood samples, is placed in an antecubital vein that drains the deep forearm muscles. Blood is drawn (10 ml in an ethylene-diamine tetra-acetic acid (EDTA)-containing green top tube) for the resting serum venous lactate (normal value less than 2 mmol/L). The patient is asked to squeeze a rubber bulb. (Some laboratories use a defined work protocol to improve reproducibility.) The sphygmomanometer cuff is then inflated above arterial pressure, making the forearm ischemic, and the patient is asked to begin to squeeze the bulb rapidly and vigorously. It is important to encourage maximal effort: good cooperation is essential as the ischemic exercise becomes painful with severe fatigue of the forearm. The patient is asked to exercise to exhaustion, which should occur in about 1 minute. The sphygmomanometer cuff is then deflated rapidly and the patient's arm is kept at rest. Further samples of blood for lactate assay are drawn at 30 seconds, 1 minute, and 4 minutes after exercise. Normally lactate concentration rises by at least two, and often three or four times after a good effort. An elevation of less than 1.5 times resting levels (with a good effort during exercise) indicates a defect of muscle glycogenolysis or glycolysis.

Phosphorus magnetic resonance spectroscopy is an even more reliable noninvasive test for this disorder, and for other glycolytic defects, but currently is available only at specialized research centers. Muscle biopsy is usually performed for histologic and histochemical diagnosis and differentiation of McArdle's disease from other glycolytic enzyme defects that have a similar morphologic appearance. The histochemical reaction for phosphorylase is easily performed on cryostat sections. Other glycolytic enzyme defects have been described (e.g., the muscle phosphofructokinase isozyme, phosphoglycerate kinase, and muscle lactate dehydrogenase deficiencies) that result in a positive or blunted ischemic lactate test and myoglobinuria, but they are extremely rare. Engel and Banker (1986) can be consulted for details.

The presence of myoglobinuria may be confirmed at the bedside by a positive dipstick reaction for heme in a freshly voided urine specimen, combined with demonstration of the absence of microscopic hematuria. Laboratory spectrophotometry can distinguish myoglobinuria from hemoglobinuria.

Debrancher enzyme (amylo-1,6-glucosidase; glycogenosis type III) deficiency presents in adults as a chronic progressive myopathy characterized by muscle wasting and weakness without cramps. The deficient debrancher enzyme catalyzes hydrolysis of the 1,6-branch points in glycogen. Recall that glycogen, a complex glucose polymer, is constructed like a bush, with long limbs of linear 1,4-linked glucose polymers interrupted by 1,6-branch points.

Nonspecific tests for the disease include increased urinary oligosaccharides and serum CPK. Hyperlipidemia may be present. The ischemic lactate test should be abnormal. The specific diagnosis is established by demonstrating deficient hydrolytic activity for liberation of glucose from limit dextrin in a muscle biopsy specimen. Further assays of hydrolytic activity with different substrates tested with different tissues allow further classification of this disorder: at least two tissue-specific polypeptides (so-called liver and muscle subunits) contribute to this multimeric protein.

Muscle Carnitine or Carnitine Palmitoyl Transferase Deficiencies

Abnormalities of muscle carnitine uptake or carnitine utilization are related to the mitochondrial cytopathies (see *Hereditary Metabolic Diseases Presenting Primarily As Neuropathies*) because fatty acids are transported into mitochondria for oxidation as carnitine acyl esters.

Systemic carnitine deficiency is a severe multisystem disorder presenting in early childhood and will not be discussed here. Muscle carnitine deficiency, which may present in adults as progressive weakness with episodic exacerbations triggered by exercise or changes in diet, is different clinically and biochemically from the systemic deficiency. In muscle carnitine deficiency, the serum CPK is often elevated. Myoglobinuria can occur, but it is not usually a prominent feature.

Muscle biopsy shows increased lipid globules in muscle fibers. The diagnosis is established by demonstrating increased neutral lipid in a muscle biopsy specimen and by measurement of reduced total carnitine in muscle (in the absence of other metabolic defects involving fatty acid metabolism). Serum carnitine may be normal or low. Primary carnitine deficiency results from a defect in transport of carnitine into muscle, as opposed to the many secondary carnitine deficiencies that result from more distal blocks in fatty acid oxidation and abnormally increased carnitine sequestration as carnitine-fatty acid acyl esters. For the purpose of identifying the latter disorders, plasma and urine may be sent for coupled gas chromatography—mass spectrometry to identify abnormal elevations of organic acids, the nature of which may define the site of the primary metabolic defect. Differentiation of primary from secondary carnitine deficiencies is important.

Carnitine palmitoyl transferase isozymes catalyze formation of the carnitine-fatty acyl ester in the cytoplasm and its hydrolysis in the mitochondrial matrix. A syndrome of recurrent weakness with muscle pain and intermittent myoglobinuria has been described in patients with carnitine palmitoyl transferase deficiency. The abnormal isozyme has been found in all tissues studied (liver, cultured fibroblasts, leukocytes, platelets, and muscle). Diagnosis is difficult because there are no morphologic changes on muscle biopsy and it is necessary to demonstrate deficiency of activity of the enzyme.

Myoadenylate Deaminase Deficiency

Deficiency of the muscle isozyme of myoadenylate deaminase is the most common of the autosomal recessive metabolic myopathies. The clinical syndrome begins with adolescent or adult onset of abnormal fatigability and pain in the muscles. A venous lactate-ammonia assay may be used to diagnose the disorder. The procedure is similar to the ischemic lactate test. Venous blood samples (10 ml; sent on ice in EDTA-containing green-topped tubes) are drawn before and after exhausting exercise for assay for ammonia (and usually lactate). The test must demonstrate an adequate rise in venous lactate (to approximately 4.5 mmol/L). The maximal rise in ammonia concentration is somewhat delayed relative to lactate. In a normal response the ammonia concentration increases approximately 1.5 percent as much as lactate. An increase of ammonia concentration of less than 0.7 percent of the lactate concentration increase is clearly abnormal. Histochemical assay for myoadenylate deaminase activity on cryostat sections from muscle biopsy is also possible. It should be noted, however, that adenylate deaminase deficiency can be found in asymptomatic persons.

Periodic Paralysis

The biochemical abnormalities responsible for the periodic paralyses are not known at present, but they will be mentioned because of their association with characteristic electrolyte changes. Hypokalemic periodic paralysis is an autosomal dominant disorder (with variable penetrance, especially in women) of recurrent, often diurnal (worse in the night or on awakening and improving through the day) weakness with exacerbations sometimes triggered by relatively heavy intake of carbohydrates or salt. Symptoms usually begin before age 20. During acute attacks, serum potassium decreases dramatically, often reaching a level as low as 1.5 mEq/L. Urinary potassium excretion is low, appropriate to the low serum concentration. Between attacks, the serum potassium concentration is normal. A different syndrome of hypokalemic paralysis is associated with hyperthyroidism in Oriental males. Hypokalemic periodic paralyses are distinguished from other hypokalemic states by not being associated with total body potassium depletion. With evidence for marked total potassium depletion (correction needing >100 mEq potassium) or renal excretion in excess of 20 mEq/day with a serum potassium concentration of less than 3 mEq/L, investigations to identify potassium wasting states (secondary hypokalemic paralysis) should be undertaken. Attacks of hyperkalemic periodic paralysis may be precipitated in susceptible individuals by glucose loading (2 g/kg orally or IV over 60 minutes) with insulin (10 to 20 U regular insulin subcutaneously). Salt loading (NaCl 2 g orally each hour for 4 hours) may be combined with the glucose test. Response to provocative testing can be monitored using the compound motor action potential (CMAP). With progressive weakness, the CMAP first decreases in amplitude until eventually the muscle may become electrically inexcitable. Serum potassium concentrations measured before and after onset of weakness should show a significant decrease.

Hyperkalemic periodic paralysis is also autosomal dominant. Attacks of weakness may be brief, but can last for days and be accompanied by myalgia. Serum potassium concentration is increased relative to that between attacks, but may remain within normal limits. Attacks may be provoked in the laboratory by oral administration of 2 to 10 g of potassium chloride (check for significant contraindications to potassium administration and monitor the ECG during such a challenge).

HEREDITARY METABOLIC DISEASES PRESENTING PRIMARILY AS NEUROPATHIES

Few known hereditary metabolic diseases present primarily as pure neuropathies. The majority of neuropathies result from acquired systemic metabolic abnormalities. The metabolic defects underlying the most common hereditary neuropathies (e.g., hereditary motor and sensory neuropathy [HMSN] type I) have not yet been described. It is important to search for other neurologic signs when a hereditary neuropathy is suspected, as several of the disorders considered in other sections of this chapter (e.g., adrenoleukodystrophy, metachromatic leukodystrophy, and mitochondrial cytopathies) may have associated neuropathies.

Diagnostic tests for hereditary metabolic diseases presenting primarily as neuropathies are outlined in Table 7-3.

Hepatic Porphyrias

Of the various hepatic porphyrias that have been described, only three present with neurologic symptoms: intermittent acute porphyria, hereditary coproporphyria, and variegate porphyria. These disorders result from specific enzyme deficiencies in the heme biosynthetic pathway and the secondary build-up of biosynthetic intermediates. Phenotypic manifestations of these enzyme deficiencies are unusual because they show autosomal dominant inheritance. The characteristic intermittent exacerbations are due to factors (e.g., drug ingestions) that increase activity of the proximal, rate-limiting enzyme in the heme biosynthetic pathway, δ-aminolevulinic acid synthase. Attacks are clinically characterized by abdominal pain, mental disturbances, and signs and symptoms of peripheral nerve dysfunction. The skin of patients with variegate porphyria (and many with the rarer hereditary coproporphyria) characteristically shows photosensitivity. However, clinical differences do not otherwise distinguish the neuropathic types reliably: biochemical tests are needed to establish the specific diagnosis.

During an acute attack, urine concentrations of α-aminolevulinic acid and porphobilinogen (which change in parallel) are dramatically elevated and can be determined, even with the relative insensitive, qualitative Ehrlich's test. Between attacks, concentrations may be normal. As predicted by the more distal locations of the deficient enzymes in hereditary coproporphyria and variegate porphyria, greater numbers of intermediates in the heme biosynthetic pathway are excreted in abnormally elevated amounts with exacerbations of these forms of the disorder. Hereditary coproporphyria can be identified by elevated urinary coproporphyrin excretion during exacerbations and variegate porphyria by excretion of several ether-insoluble porphyrin peptides. The larger intermediates are also excreted in feces. Fecal porphyrin excretion is only minimally elevated during attacks of intermittent acute porphyria. However, large amounts of coproporphyrin are found in feces during attacks of hereditary coproporphyria and increased coproporphyrin, protoporphyrin, and ether-insoluble peptides are seen with variegate porphyria. Excretion of these compounds in feces may be elevated, even between attacks.

Diagnosis of latent porphyrias is ideally based on establishing the specific enzyme deficiency. The deficiency of porphobilinogen deaminase in intermittent acute porphyria can be assayed in erythrocytes, leukocytes, or cultured fibroblasts. The coproporphyrin oxidase deficiency of hereditary coproporphyria is expressed in leukocytes and skin fibroblasts. A specific enzyme deficiency responsible for variegate porphyria has yet to be established. Note that toxic porphyrias can occur (e.g., with lead intoxication).

Fabry's Disease

Fabry's disease is an X-linked deficiency of the lysosomal enzyme α-galactosidase A. This enzyme catalyzes hydrolysis of galactosyl ceramides. The hemizygote state leads to accumulation of neutral glycosphingolipids in neurons, vascular endothelial cells, and smooth muscle. The clinical syndrome begins in childhood or adolescence with episodic dysesthetic crises (burning feet), progressing to constant discomfort, characteristic angiokeratomas of the skin, corneal opacities, renal insufficiency, and early cerebral or cardiac infarctions.

An elevated erythrocyte sedimentation rate (ESR) may accompany the early dysesthetic crises. Signs of renal insufficiency, such as isosthenuria and proteinuria, may precede neurologic symptoms and should be sought. The renal sediment may show characteristic birefringent lipid globules, having the appearance of Maltese crosses. Analysis of plasma and urine by high performance liquid chromatography (HPLC) can be used to identify the abnormally abundant glycolipids in both patients and heterozygotes. Biopsy of kidney or skin of affected patients may demonstrate refractile lysosomal lipid inclusions. The diagnosis is confirmed by determination of α-galactosidase A deficiency in leukocytes or cultured fibroblasts. A serum assay has been developed but is less desirable as the serum enzyme activity is unstable. Heterozygotes (carriers) will show enzyme activities intermediate between those of normals and affected individuals. Care must be taken when attempting to confirm the heterozygote state using cultured fibroblasts, as activity can increase with time in culture. A decrease in enzyme activity has been reported in some individuals showing no signs of disease in themselves or their families.

Refsum's Disease

Refsum's disease is a very rare autosomal recessive disorder of early onset (<20 years old) that is characterized by the tetrad of sensorimotor peripheral neuropathy, retinitis pigmentosa, cerebellar ataxis, and increased

Table 7-3. Diagnostic Tests for Hereditary Metabolic Diseases Presenting Frequently as Neuropathies

Disease	Biochemical Defect	Enzyme Diagnostic Test
Hepatic Porphyrias		
Acute intermittent porphyria	Porphobilinogen deaminase deficiency	1. Increased urinary δ-aminolevulinic acid and porphobilinogen with acute attacks 2. Decreased porphobilinogen deaminase activity in erythrocytes, leukocytes, or cultured fibroblasts, even with latent disease
Hereditary coprophyria	Coproporphyrinogen oxidase deficiency	1. Increased fecal excretion of coproporphyrin III and urinary δ-aminolevulinic acid, porphobilinogen, and coproporphyrin with acute attacks 2. Decreased coproporphyrinogen oxidase in leukocytes and cultured fibroblasts
Variegate porphyria	Unknown	1. Continuous increased fecal excretion of ether-insoluble porphyrins 2. Increased urinary excretion of δ-aminolevulinic acid, porphobilinogen, and ether-insoluble porphyrins with acute attack

Amyloidosis		
Familial amyloidosis	Transthyretin structure	1. Birefringent, congo red staining deposits in blood vessels and nerves with nerve, skin, or rectal biopsies; axonal degeneration in nerve 2. May have conduction block on ECG 3. May show active urinary sediment, proteinuria, and isosthenuria
Others		
Fabry's disease	α-Galactosidase A deficiency	1. α-Galactosidase activity in serum or leukocytes 2. Neuronal or vascular neutral lipid deposits in rectal or renal biopsies
Refsum's disease	Phytanic acid α-hydroxylase deficiency	1. Increased serum phytanic acid by gas-liquid chromatography 2. Deficiency of hydroxylase activity in cultured fibroblasts

CSF protein. Other associated features have also been described. The biochemical defect is a deficiency of phytanic acid β-hydroxylase, the first step in oxidation of phytanic acid. Phytanic acid is a C-20 branched chain fatty acid present in trace quantities in foodstuffs. Accumulation of phytanic acid occurs in axons and Schwann cells as well as elsewhere in the body.

Serum phytanic acid levels can be measured by gas-liquid chromatography and are very high. The normal concentration is low (less than 0.3 mg/dl), but in patients with Refsum's disease it may rise to constitute between 5 and 30 percent of total serum fatty acids. The enzyme abnormality persists in cultured fibroblasts. Fibroblasts from affected individuals may have less than 5 percent of the normal capacity for phytanic acid oxidation, despite unimpaired palmitate oxidation.

HEREDITARY METABOLIC DISEASES PRESENTING PRIMARILY WITH EARLY CEREBROVASCULAR ACCIDENTS

Several inherited diseases predispose to cerebrovascular disease. Diabetes mellitus, sickle cell anemia, and familial hypercholesterolemias are among the more common ones. Unusual syndromes that may be suggested by a history of recurrent deep venous thrombosis and pulmonary embolism or other venous thrombotic complications include protein C and S deficiencies and antithrombin III deficiency. Proteins C and S are vitamin K-dependent glycoproteins that work together to limit coagulation by degrading activated clotting factors IVa and VIIIa. Antithrombin III binds to thrombin and other serine proteinases to inhibit their activity, also limiting thrombus formation. There is no effective general screening test for these coagulation disorders. They can only be diagnosed by specific assays for amounts of the factors present and their activities. Fabry's disease is another rare cause of early strokes (see *Hereditary Metabolic Diseases Presenting Primarily As Neuropathies*).

Individuals with homocystinuria have long been recognized to have an increased tendency to develop arterial or venous thrombosis (sometimes triggered by angiography). They also may show mental retardation, seizures, skeletal deformities, and lens dislocations. The disease is autosomal recessive and secondary to a deficiency of cystathionine β-synthetase activity. It has been suggested that heterozygotes who are otherwise asymptomatic may also be at increased risk for vascular events.

The easiest screening test for homocystinuria (homozygote or heterozygote) is using the cyanide-nitroprusside test to assay for increased homocystine in urine. It is not specific, however, as other disorders of the transulfuration pathway, including vitamin deficiencies, can lead to increased homocystine excretion. More reliable is a serum amino acid assay. Serum homocystine and methionine concentrations are elevated in the serum, whereas cystathionine and cysteine concentrations are greatly reduced. Sensitivity can be increased by prior methionine loading, which should increase serum homocystine concentration. Plasma for this assay must be deproteinized rapidly to prevent binding of homocystine to proteins, thus artifactually lowering its concentration. Definitive diagnosis is made by demonstration of decreased cystathionine β-synthetase activity in cultured fibroblasts.

MITOCHONDRIAL CYTOPATHIES

Mitochondrial cytopathies are unusual in their mode of inheritance and the variability of phenotypic expression. Although often sporadic, they may show a maternal pattern of inheritance. They can present as encephalopathies, myopathies, and neuropathies (sometimes with systemic abnormalities such as heart block or renal disease), even within the same kindred. Clinical features of adult-onset disease include various combinations of cerebellar ataxia, external ophthalmoplegia, myopathy, myoclonus epilepsy, pigmentary retinopathy, optic atrophy, recurrent encephalopathy or strokelike episodes, dementia, sensorimotor polyneuropathy, and deafness. Specific syndromes have been identified (DiMauro et al., 1985).

Biochemical defects associated with these phenotypes have been found, notably in enzymes of the mitochondrial electron transport chain. Some of the polypeptides of these proteins are coded by the mitochondrial genome, which is maternally transmitted. However, defects of the nuclear genome can also be responsible for mitochondrial dysfunction. Abnormalities of the mitochondrial genome have been identified in some patients, which can be used for identification of asymptomatic carriers of the abnormal genetic material.

Nonspecific abnormalities that may be found include an elevated serum CPK or myopathic electromyography (EMG) pattern. In some patients (usually those with more severe myopathies), the resting venous serum lactate and lactate/pyruvate ratio may be elevated. Care must be taken when performing this test to avoid false-positive results, which may be obtained if patients move too much before the blood draw. The patient should be resting supine for at least 30 minutes before the blood is drawn. The test sensitivity may be increased by a well-defined exercise protocol followed before the blood is drawn; however, this demands careful supervision and planning so that comparable and well-defined amounts of work may be obtained from both normal controls and myopathic patients. Gas chromatography–mass spectrometry of urine for organic acids may define abnormal patterns of substrate use, suggesting a metabolic block to oxidative metabolism.

Diagnosis in most centers relies on biopsy of affected muscle and demonstration of characteristic ragged-red fibers with modified Gomori-trichrome stain. Electron microscopy shows ultrastructural abnormalities of the mitochondria. The activities of enzymes of the respiratory chain can be assayed in mitochondria from the muscle biopsy and specific deficiencies have been found, but these assays are technically difficult to perform reliably and require larger biopsy samples. Genetic analysis may show mitochondrial DNA deletions or point mutation in some cases.

READINGS

Benson PF, Fenson AIH: Genetic Biochemical Disorders. Oxford University Press, Oxford, 1985

Boers GHJ, Smals AGH, Trijbels FJM, et al: Heterozygosity for homocystinuria in premature peripheral and cerebral occlusive arterial disease. N Engl J Med 313:709, 1985

Caskey CT: Disease diagnosis by recombinant DNA methods. Science 236:1223, 1987

DiMauro S, Bresolin N: Phosphorylase deficiency. p. 1585. In Engel AG, Banker BQ (eds): Myology: Basic and Clinical. McGraw-Hill, New York, 1986

Eisenstein BI: The polymerase chain reaction: A new method of using molecular genetics for medical diagnosis. N Engl J Med 322:178, 1990

Engel AG: Periodic paralysis. p. 1843. In Engel AG, Banker BQ (eds): Myology: Basic and Clinical. McGraw-Hill, New York, 1986

Exner T, Rickard KA, Kronenberg H: A sensitive test demonstrating lupus anticoagulant and its behavioral patterns. Br J Hematol 40:143, 1978

Fink JK, Filling-Katz MR, Sokol J, et al: Clinical spectrum of Niemann-Pick disease type C. Neurology 39:1040, 1989

Harding AE, Rosenberg RN: Molecular genetics and neurologic disease: basic principles and methods. p. 1. In Rosenberg RN, Harding AE (eds): The Molecular Biology of Neurological Disease. Butterworths, New York, 1988

Hoffman EP, Kunkel LM, Angelini C, et al: Improved diagnosis of Becker muscular dystrophy by dystrophin testing. Neurology 39:1011, 1989

Kolodny EH, Cable WHL: Inborn errors of metabolism. Ann Neurol 11:221, 1982

Ott J: A short guide to linkage analysis. p. 19. In Davies KE (ed): Human Genetic Disease: A Practical Approach. IRL Press, Oxofrd, 1986

Poulton J, Gardiner RM: Non-invasive diagnosis of mitochondrial myopathy. Lancet 1:961, 1989

Rowland LP, Wood DS, Schon EA, DiMauro S: Molecular Genetics in Diseases of Brain, Nerve and Muscle. Oxford University Press, New York, 1989

Schafer AI: The hypercoagulable states. Ann Intern Med 102:814, 1985

Scrivner CR, Beaudet AL, Sly WS, Valle D: The Metabolic Basis of Inherited Disease. 6th Ed. McGraw-Hill, New York, 1989

ROLE OF BIOPSIES IN NEUROLOGIC DIAGNOSIS 8

Stirling Carpenter

Biopsies are performed mostly in diseases for which there is no other specific diagnostic test. Occasionally, they function as a screening device when the clinical picture is not specific enough to suggest a limited number of diagnoses or are used to provide extra reassurance in the face of a positive biochemical test. The primary tissues biopsied for diagnosis of neurologic disease include skin, skeletal muscle, sural nerve, bone marrow, rectal mucosa or the appendix (the latter two for their autonomic plexuses), and, of course, brain.

PREPARATION

Several different types of preparations can be used, each having advantages and disadvantages. Cryostat sections are quick and versatile. They do not require preliminary fixation, and extraction of tissue components is minimal. A wide range of stains and antibody reactions, as well as enzyme histochemistry, can be performed on these sections. However, freezing and cutting must be meticulous to avoid unacceptable artifacts. Cryostat sections have particular application to the study of muscle biopsies.

Paraffin sections are widely and routinely used in the study of tissues. The repertory of stains applicable is large and well documented, but while being processed the tissues are exposed to solvents that remove certain lipid components such as triglycerides. Most antibody reactions can also be performed on paraffin-embedded tissue, although the type of fixation may be critical.

Preliminary fixation is necessary to preserve structure. Most commonly the tissue is fixed in buffered 10 percent formalin (actually 4 percent formaldehyde). Formalin is inexpensive, penetrates relatively quickly into tissues, and is well known; but it causes considerable tissue shrinkage and distortion and, if not well buffered, reacts with hemoglobin to produce acid hematin. Buffered gluteraldehyde, particularly at 2 to 2.5 percent concentration, preserves morphology well, but it penetrates tissue relatively slowly and is expensive. It is thus suitable only for relatively small specimens. In addition, gluteraldehyde tends to make paraffin sections brittle and hard to cut. Mixtures of formalin and gluteraldehyde have been proposed and may have considerable advantages, although modifications in embedding procedures may be necessary to take advantage of them. Fixation in Bouin solution, which contains picric acid, is advantageous for some stains and antibody reactions. Various proprietary fixatives are also available.

Plastic or resin sections of gluteraldehyde-fixed tissue produce the best morphologic preservation. Semithin sections are cut at 1 μm in thickness. If stained with paraphenylene diamine, phase microscopy should be used. If stained with toluidine blue, bright field microscopy is adequate. Resin section blocks must be relatively small to allow proper infiltration of the tissues, and the range of stains possible is limited because many do not penetrate the resin sufficiently and removal of resin is tedious. Immunocytochemistry for some antigens is possible after epoxy resin embedding. One method involves removal of the resin. Colloidal gold tagging and scanning electron microscopy can be combined for low power localization. Low-temperature resins are necessary for preservation of certain antigens.

Smears and touch preparations of unfixed tissue are used, particularly in diagnosis of tumors in brain or in bone marrow biopsies. Whole mounts of squash preparations of skeletal muscle are used in supravital studies of terminal nerve twigs and motor endplates.

Teased fiber preparations of peripheral nerves are extremely useful in the study of nerve biopsies. They provide the best method for detecting segments of demyelination and remyelination. They allow the measurement of successive lengths of internodes, which vary in normal and regenerated fibers and in demyelinating conditions. They also allow a view in continuity of considerable stretches of single axons so that the various types of swelling of axons or myelin sheaths can be appreciated.

The tissue is first fixed, preferably in 2 percent buffered gluteraldehyde, and then postfixed for 24 hours in osmium tetroxide, which stains the myelin black. They are then softened in glycerin. A method for axonal staining is also available. Teasing of nerve fibers is time-consuming, tedious, and exacting.

SKIN BIOPSY

Skin biopsy is useful in the diagnosis of certain storage diseases, in neuroaxonal dystrophy, and in some cases of mitochondrial cytopathy. The possibly useful preparations include both semithin and ultrathin resin sections, cryostat sections, and paraffin sections. The most useful type of preparation depends on the disease being considered.

Storage Diseases

In Lafora's disease characteristic PAS-positive inclusions are seen in the peripheral cells of sweat gland ducts with cryostat and paraffin sections. They are also visible on resin sections, but less so because the area sampled is smaller and sections are thinner. Electron microscopy is not necessary. Inclusions can also be seen in myoepithelial cells of apocrine glands from the axilla, and occasionally in eccrine myoepithelial cells. A negative skin biopsy appears to rule out the possibility of Lafora's disease if the eccrine ducts are adequately represented.

Batten's disease (ceroid-lipofuscinosis) is one of the most common recessive hereditary CNS diseases, the most common neuronal storage disease, and the least understood. At present there is no biochemical test to identify it. Three or four different forms have been described that differ in age of onset, rapidity of deterioration, and to some extent in the ultrastructural pattern of storage deposits. Symptoms include seizures and ataxia followed by mental and motor deterioration. Pigmentary retinal degeneration, which may be the first sign, occurs in almost all cases, except those with adult onset.

Definite diagnosis depends on biopsy with electron microscopy. Cryostat sections with acid phosphatase reactions may be useful as a screening method, but they are by no means diagnostic. The deposits in skin are too small to be reliably detected on paraffin sections. A major problem in the diagnosis of Batten's disease from skin is the ubiquity of lipofuscin in many cell types and the tendency of some pathologists to interpret normal lipofuscin deposits as a sign of disease. Despite the name of ceroid-lipofuscinosis, ordinary lipofuscin is of no diagnostic importance, since lipofuscin granules can be seen in eccrine secretory cells of normal infants by the age of 2 years.

In infantile cases (Santavuori's disease) electron microscopy shows membrane-bound granular osmiophilic deposits, which are present in a great variety of cell types but particularly in eccrine secretory cells and smooth muscle. On semithin resin sections they have considerable density so that they are visible in these cell types by phase microscopy. Patients with late infantile Batten's disease (Jansky-Bielschowsky disease) have onset of symptoms between the ages of 2 and 4 years. The ultrastructural pattern is of curvilinear bodies that show a fine lamination at high magnification. Many cell types are involved, including fibroblasts, endothelium, smooth muscle, and even basal epithelial cells; whereas large aggregates are present in eccrine secretory cells.

Juvenile patients with Batten's disease vary in their initial manifestations and ages of onset. Early juvenile cases may begin as early as 4 years with seizures, whereas the Spielmeyer-Vogt type begins around the ages of 8 or 10 with visual problems. This juvenile group is also characterized by considerable variation in the degree of involvement of various cell types in the skin. A superficial biopsy that does not include the eccrine secretory cells, therefore, is inadequate. The so-called fingerprint profiles, which are the most characteristic pattern found in most cell types, are generally visible on semithin sections. However, occasionally patients without Batten's disease have typical fingerprint profiles accumulating in eccrine secretory cells. Thus confirmation of involvement of a second cell type, such as eccrine duct cells or smooth muscle or skeletal muscle, is mandatory for positive diagnosis. A few juvenile patients with Batten's disease will be found to have deposits with the ultrastructural characteristics of granular osmiophilic deposits, similar to those in the infantile form. These patients tend to show rather marked involvement of eccrine secretory cells and smooth muscle.

The problem of diagnosis from skin in the adult form of neuronal ceroid-lipofuscinosis (Kufs disease) becomes insuperable because of the very limited extent of storage in these patients and because patients without the disease tend to have similar deposits in their eccrine secretory cells.

Changes in skin may also be seen in a number of other storage diseases in which well-defined biochemical defects are known. These include the infantile form of Sandhoff's disease; GM_1 gangliosidosis; fucosidosis; mannosidosis; Fabry's disease; galactosialidosis; Niemann-Pick disease type A; mucolipidosis types II, III, and IV; and glycogenosis types II, III, and IV.

Neuroaxonal Dystrophy

Neuron axonal dystrophy in its early form is marked by progressive psychomotor deterioration, hypotonia with upper motor neuron signs, and optic atrophy. The later onset form shows spasticity, ataxia, and myoclonus with less prominent cognitive signs. There is no general biologic test for neuroaxonal dystrophy, although some cases have recently been reported with a deficiency of α-N-acetylgalactosaminidase. The dystrophic changes are characteristically found at or near axon terminals. The autonomic endings in the vicinity of the eccrine secretory coils are a reliable site for finding the characteristic spheroids of this disease but they are detectable only by electron microscopy in this area. More superficial cutaneous nerve twigs may also be involved. It is not certain to what extent a negative biopsy rules out the diagnosis. No data are available to evaluate the usefulness of skin biopsy in the rarer juvenile forms of the disease.

Mitochondrial Cytopathies

In mitochondrial cytopathies, abnormal mitochondria have occasionally been found in eccrine secretory cells in cases of Kearns-Sayre syndrome or occasional cases of MERRF (myoclonus epilepsy with ragged red fibers). We have seen similar mitochondrial abnormality biopsies in two infants with intractable seizure disorders. The abnormal mitochondria show clustering and circumferential cristae. These changes must not be confused with artifactual matrix swelling of mitochondria, which occurs when fixation is slow.

SKELETAL MUSCLE BIOPSY

The skeletal muscle to be biopsied should be involved by the disease process but not in an end stage. Communication with the pathologist is important, both as an aid to interpretation and as a stimulus. Interpretation of muscle biopsies is a highly specialized subject.

Skeletal muscle may be biopsied for diagnosis of primary muscle disease or diagnosis of denervation. It is also biopsied for diagnosis of systemic disease such as vasculitis, which may affect many organ systems. It can be involved in some storage diseases, and it appears to be the biopsy site of choice in diagnosis of mitochondrial disease, even when there are no symptoms related to muscle.

Needle biopsies of muscle result in a smaller scar and are preferred in some hospitals. Open biopsies provide easier orientation of specimens, the ability to isometrically clamp the specimen, and the possibility of doing nerve and skin biopsy with the same incision.

Particularly useful preparations are cryostat and resin sections. Paraffin sections are adequate for diagnosis of vasculitis, but in other respects their usefulness is very limited. However, cryostat sections offer the advantages of better preservation of cytoplasmic integrity, the possibility of performing enzyme reactions, and better preservation of antigens for immunologic reactions. In addition, unlike paraffin sections, they are not routinely processed through lipid solvents. Nevertheless, tissue freezing and sectioning must be performed meticulously for satisfactory results.

Gluteraldehyde-fixed epoxy resin sections provide the best morphologic preservation. The portion of the biopsy intended for gluteraldehyde fixation should be removed by the surgeon in an open biopsy in a precisely oriented isometric clamp. This means that the surgeon must take two specimens, one without a clamp for cryostat sections and one in a clamp for gluteraldehyde fixation. Tissue should be left in the clamp in 2 percent buffered gluteraldehyde for 4 hours before being transferred to buffer. On a proper specimen, well-oriented transverse and longitudinal sections can be obtained. Some structures, such as vacuoles, are more easily appreciated in resin sections than on cryostat sections. The blocks also offer the possibility of performing electron microscopy on selected areas, when appropriate. A muscle biopsy studied only with paraffin sections, for all conditions except vasculitis, has barely been studied at all.

On cryostat sections, a basic battery of histochemical stains must be performed, including the modified trichrome, hematoxylin and eosin, ATPase reactions preincubated at pH 9.4 and 4.2, NADH-tetrazolium reductase, PAS, oil red O or a similar lipid stain, and an acid phosphatase reaction.

The modified trichrome and hematoxylin and eosin are advantageous as general tissue stains. The ATPase reactions are essential for accurate fiber typing. At pH 9.4, the ATPase activity of type I fibers is low, whereas that of type IIs is high. At pH 4.6, type Is and IIAs are high and IIBs are low. At pH 4.3, type Is are high and IIAs and IIBs are low. Knowledge of the fiber type distribution and the presence or absence of type-specific changes is of great diagnostic usefulness. For example, disuse atrophy and muscle atrophy secondary to steroid treatment selectively affect the type IIB fibers. Normal muscle shows a checkerboard pattern of type Is and type IIs. In cases of partial denervation with significant axonal sprouting and reinnervation (such as in a chronic peripheral neuropathy), considerable type grouping may occur, with large blocks composed solidly of type Is or type IIs. Since the ATPase is contained in the heads of the myosin fibril, the reaction also provides a view of the distribution of the myosin in the muscle fibers.

The oxidative enzyme reaction (NADH-tetrazolium reductase) helps to show the distribution of mitochondria, although the reaction product may cling also to other membranous organelles. Tubular aggregates, which are present in a syndrome of muscle cramps, are strongly positive with this reaction; target fibers, present in many denervating conditions, are most easily visualized with it. Atrophic denervated fibers tend to show an unusually strong reaction because their mitochondria come closer together as the fiber volume collapses.

The PAS stain will show excess glycogen, whereas denervated muscle fibers tend to have a low glycogen content. The lipid stain is important in detecting lipid storage disorders such as carnitine deficiency. In addition, the ragged red fibers of mitochondrial disease tend to have an excess lipid content.

We have found the Gomori acid phosphatase reaction extremely useful, although technically exacting. The pathologist must realize that ordinary lipofuscin produces a positive acid phosphatase reaction, is ubiquitous, and increases with aging and denervation of muscle. The acid phosphatase reaction is particularly useful in lysosomal storage diseases.

Other stains or reactions are performed in special circumstances. The cytochrome oxidase reaction is useful in mitochondrial disease because abnormal mitochondria tend to be negative. The menadione nitro-blue tetrazolium reaction is specific for reducing body myopathy. The reactions for myophosphorylase or phosphofructokinase can be used to rule in or rule out these forms of glycogen storage diseases.

The immunocytochemical reaction for type I major histocompatibility products on the surface of muscle fibers is of great diagnostic usefulness in inflammatory myopathies. Normal mature muscle fibers show no reaction; however, in cases of polymyositis all muscle fibers express type I products, as muscle fibers (in areas of damage) also do in dermatomyositis. The use of antidystrophin antibodies can verify a diagnosis of Duchenne or Becker muscular dystrophy. Deficiency of the Ca^{2+}-adenosine triphosphatase of the sarcoplasmic reticulum in Brodie's disease (which impairs skeletal muscle relaxation) can be displayed by use of an appropriate antibody.

Electron microscopy is particularly useful in distinguishing among various forms of inflammatory myopathy. Tubuloreticular structures are seen in endothelial cells in dermatomyositis and lupus myositis (often along with capillary necrosis), in contrast to polymyositis. The diagnosis of inclusion body myositis is confirmed by the electron microscopic finding of characteristic abnormal tubular filaments in cytoplasm or nuclei of muscle cells. It is also useful in investigation of obscure myopathies.

NERVE BIOPSY

Nerve biopsy is useful for diagnosis of specific neuropathies and for diagnosis of some diseases (particularly leukodystrophies) affecting both central and peripheral myelin. Specific diagnosis in cases of distal symmetric polyneuropathies is not often achieved by nerve biopsy, however, and so should not be an automatic part of a workup in those cases. Interpretation of nerve biopsies, like skeletal muscle biopsies, is a highly specialized field. The most useful preparations are gluteraldehyde-fixed, resin-embedded tissue. These provide accurate morphology for large and small myelinated fibers and some visualization of unmyelinated fibers. Cryostat sections are larger and deeper, which may make it easier to pick up significant numbers of ovoids of wallerian degeneration on them. In addition, it is easy to perform a variety of diagnostically useful stains, such as the PAS stain.

Teased fiber preparations are extremely useful. They can show evidence of demyelination, when it is not apparent from tissue sections. They are also quite useful in establishing the diagnosis of tomaculous neuropathy. Their preparation is relatively labor intensive. Paraffin sections of nerve can be useful and informative if the tissue is fixed in 2 percent buffered gluteraldehyde. Sudan black as a myelin stain is particularly advantageous in such sections, and the degree of clarity almost rivals that of resin sections.

The battery of stains for cryostat sections should include the modified trichrome and hematoxylin and eosin as general tissue stains. PAS is useful as a myelin stain and mandatory for detecting polyglucosan bodies. An acid phosphatase reaction is useful in showing evidence of acute myelin breakdown or in storage diseases. On the other hand, the pathologist must be familiar with the considerable number of normally occurring acid phosphatase positive sites in Schwann cells. Oxidative enzyme reactions are sometimes useful in showing dystrophic axons. The acetic cresyl violet stain is specific for metachromatic leukodystrophy.

BONE MARROW BIOPSY

Bone marrow biopsy is useful in the diagnosis of Niemann-Pick disease type C (also called type II Niemann-Pick or juvenile dystonic lipidosis). In Wright-stained smears, sea blue histiocytes can be identified, as well as cells containing numerous lucent vacuoles. Paraffin sections of the bone marrow are not useful because the characteristic lipids dissolve.

RECTAL BIOPSY AND APPENDECTOMY

Biopsy of the lower GI tract to obtain autonomic neurons can be achieved either by rectal biopsy of appendectomy. The latter offers a much greater certainty of finding neurons and may be less hazardous. Autonomic neurons are particularly relevant to the diagnosis of almost all neuronal storage diseases, except for perhaps some late-onset forms where the number of neurons involved is very small. They do not show inclusions in Lafora's disease. The autonomic plexus also displays characteristic abnormalities in axonal dystrophy, although electron microscopy is necessary to find them. Amyloid may be detected in a rectal biopsy and is characteristically identified with Congo red staining and polarization as birefringent deposits, showing optical dichroism and appearing red with light polarized in one direction and apple green when the incident light is polarized in the perpendicular direction. It can also be detected with fluorescence microscopy using a thioflavin S or T stain.

BRAIN BIOPSY

Biopsy of the brain for diagnosis, rather than for therapeutic removal of a lesion, may be indicated when other diagnostic means are exhausted. Because brain biopsy involves a loss of some presumably functional tissue and results in a scar (which could possibly become epileptogenic), a decision to perform a brain biopsy must not be taken lightly. The usefulness of the expected diagnostic knowledge must be weighed against the risks of operation and anesthesia and the possibility of inconclusive results. The patient's family must participate in the decision-making process. Brain biopsy is not likely to be useful in diseases that involve primarily subcortical structures and in those characterized only by neuronal loss and gliosis, without features more specific than the distribution of abnormalities.

Brain biopsies should in general be studied with all the resources of the pathology laboratory, including paraffin, cryostat, and resin sections. If enough tissue is available, some should be frozen for possible biochemical study. Smears of unfixed tissue are quite useful in tumor diagnosis and can show inflammatory infiltrates. They are fast and easy to perform, but the morphology of neurons is not well preserved. Cryostat sectioning should probably be omitted in Creutzfeldt-Jakob disease or human immunovirus (HIV) infection.

Communication among surgeon, pathologist, and neurologist is important, both in advance and during the operation to ensure that the tissue is properly treated. The pathologist should be present during the biopsy to divide and fix the sample promptly.

The required size of the sample may vary with the suspected type of disease or the expertise of the laboratory in dealing with minute samples. Under some circumstances, stereotaxic biopsies may be adequate.

Diseases for which brain biopsy may be needed include Alzheimer's disease, disseminated Lewy body disease, Creutzfeldt-Jakob disease, Gerstmann-Sträussler syndrome, atypical inclusion body disease, various tumors and infections (notably herpes simplex encephalitis), and various leukodystrophies without known biochemical defect, such as Alexander's disease and Canavan's disease. Biopsy may be useful (but usually more as a research tool) in other poorly characterized cortical diseases, so this list should not be considered complete.

In Alzheimer's disease the pathology consists of senile plaques and neurofibrillary tangles, both of which may be visualized using the modified Bielschowsky stain, thioflavin S or T with fluorescence microscopy, or Congo red with polarization. The parietal lobe gives the greatest concentration of lesions in the neocortex. Antibodies to components of senile plaques, such as the antibody to Alz-50, may reveal more widespread abnormality than is visible with any stain.

Generalized Lewy body disease is characterized by various degrees of parkinsonism and dementia. It may be associated with changes typical of Alzheimer's disease. The Lewy bodies appear as eosinophilic cytoplasmic inclusions, often surrounded by a slight halo. They are blue with azocarmine stain and negative with PAS stain. They stain with antibodies to ubiquitin; their periphery stains with antibodies to neurofilaments. By electron microscopy, they are seen to be formed of very dense filamentous masses.

Atypical inclusion body disease is a rare cause of the progressive myoclonus epilepsy syndrome. PAS-positive, round, homogeneous inclusions are seen in large neurons in the cerebral cortex on paraffin or cryostat sections. Unlike Lafora bodies, they do not stain with Alcian blue, and by electron microscopy they are finely granular and homogeneous, of moderate electron density, and enclosed in a membranous space.

The general diagnosis of a leukodystrophy can now be made from imaging studies. Specific biochemical tests are available for adrenal leukodystrophy, Krabbe's disease, and metachromatic leukodystrophy. The latter two can also be diagnosed from peripheral nerve biopsy. Other rare types of leukodystrophy are only pathologically defined and only appear to affect central myelin. In such instances, brain biopsy, if carefully studied, can afford a more precise definition of the disease than is possible by noninvasive clinical studies alone.

In Creutzfeldt-Jakob disease, the characteristic abnormality is spongiform change, which is a fine vacuolization of the neurophil. It must be distinguished from status spongiosus, which is the result of an increased extracellular space resulting from loss of elements of the neurophil. The vacuoles of spongiform changes are intracellular, although this may not be obvious at the level of the light microscope. It must be distinguished from artifactual vacuolization, which can follow slow fixation, and from early ischemia. The intensity may vary from region to region. Some degree of microglial infiltration, astrocytic proliferation, and neuronal loss will also generally be present.

The Gerstmann-Sträussler syndrome often presents as a progressive spinocerebellar ataxia with dementia or progressive spastic paresis with dementia. Familial cases consistent with an autosomal-dominant transmission are known. The disease has been transmitted to experimental animals, in whom it creates a spongiform encephalopathy. The disease is thus considered closely related to Creutzfeldt-Jakob disease. Pathologically, it is characterized by extremely numerous large amyloid plaques in the cerebral cortex, basal ganglia, and cerebellum. The amyloid reacts with antibodies to prion protein rather than to Alz-50.

Herpes simplex encephalitis involves fairly consistently specific regions of the brain—the medial temporal lobes, insular cortex, and cingulate gyrus. Some benefit is obtained from early treatment. There has been controversy as to whether biopsy diagnosis should be obtained before treatment. Currently, treatment is most commonly begun without pathologic confirmation of the diagnosis. Rapid diagnosis of an inflammatory process may be made from fresh smears of the brain tissue. Detection of viral antigen on smears of the brain biopsy is the most rapid means of specific diagnosis. In situ hybridization with cDNA probes can also provide a specific diagnosis. Typical inclusion bodies on paraffin sections are seen in a small minority of positive cases. Any biopsy should be cultured for viral growth, as this is probably the most sensitive diagnostic method.

In acquired immune deficiency syndrome (AIDS), the brain may be involved by lymphoma, toxoplasmosis, cytomegalovirus, progressive multifocal leukoencephalopathy, tuberculosis, syphilis, herpes simplex, herpes zoster, *Cryptococcus,* the HIV virus itself, other banal or unusual organisms, or any combination of these. Brain biopsy is particularly useful in the diagnosis of lymphoma and toxoplasmosis. Toxoplasma pseudocysts may be found around, but not in, areas of intense inflammation or tissue destruction. Hematoxylin and eosin stain reveals them as well as any method short of a reliable antibody.

READINGS

Adams JH, Urquhart GED: Early diagnosis of herpes encephalitis. N Engl J Med 297:1288, 1977

Asbury AK, Johnson PC: Pathology of Peripheral Nerve. WB Saunders, Philadelphia, 1978

Carpenter S: Skin biopsy for diagnosis of hereditary neurologic metabolic disease. Arch Dermatol 123:1618, 1987

Carpenter S: Morphological diagnosis and misdiagnosis in Batten-Kufs' disease. Am J Med Genet, suppl., 5:85, 1988

Carpenter S, Karpati G: Pathology of Skeletal Muscle. p. 39. Churchill Livingstone, New York, 1983

Hyman BT, Van Hoesen GW, Wolozin BL, et al: Alz-50 antibody recognizes Alzheimer-related neuronal changes. Ann Neurol 23:371, 1988

Karpati G, Pouliot Y, Carpenter S: Expression of immunoreactive major histocompatibility complex products in human skeletal muscle. Ann Neurol 23:64, 1988

Masters CL, Gajdusek DC, Gibbs CJ: Creutzfeldt-Jakob disease virus isolations from the Gerstmann-Sträussler syndrome with an analysis of the various forms of amyloid plaque deposition in the virus-induced spongiform encephalopathies. Brain 104:559, 1981

Masters CL, Richardson EP Jr: Subacute spongiform encephalopathy (Creutzfeldt-Jakob disease): the nature and progression of the spongiform change. Brain 101:333, 1987

Ota T, Hisatomi Y, Kashiwamuro K, et al: Histochemistry and ultrastructure of atypical myoclonus body (type II). Acta Neuropathol 28:45, 1974

Schindler D, Bishop DF, Wolfe DE, et al: Neuroaxonal dystrophy due to lysosomal alpha-N-acetylgalactosaminidase deficiency. N Engl J Med 320:1735, 1989

Sever JL, Gibbs CJ (eds): Retroviruses in the nervous system. Ann Neurol, suppl., 32:Sl, 1988

Part II

DIAGNOSTIC APPROACHES TO COMMON NEUROLOGIC PROBLEMS

As noted in Part I, we believe that evaluation of neurologic disease is an art based fundamentally on the history and clinical examination. Laboratory tests have an important but secondary role. Each test entails extra expenses and possibly morbidity for the patient. The laboratory evaluation for each patient, therefore, should be thoughtfully individualized.

In our belief, the enormous varieties of clinical presentations and the specificity of diagnosis demanded of a specialist preclude application of flow charts for guiding test ordering. This section presents a series of tables providing *basic* differential diagnoses for several common neurologic syndromes and tests that should be *considered* during their evaluation. The text elaborates briefly on our approach to these syndromes. We must emphasize that these tables of tests do not constitute lists of data that should be collected on every patient. Readers are referred to texts of general neurology (*Principles of Neurology* by Adams and Victor is our favorite) for an introduction to the full clinical evaluation of patients.

The recommendations made in Part II will meet with a variable consensus from other neurologists—some are clearly idiosyncratic. We hope, however, that our suggestions might help readers develop their own strategies for workup of different neurologic problems. The chapters are structured such that they can be read or referred to independently.

READING

Adams RD, Victor M: Principles of Neurology. Ed. 4. McGraw-Hill, New York, 1989

LABORATORY TESTS FOR EVALUATING MENINGITIS AND ENCEPHALITIS

9

Table 9-1. Differential Diagnosis of Acute Bacterial Meningitis in Adults

Normal Host
Streptococcus pneumoniae
Neisseria meningitidis
Haemophilus influenza (relatively rare in adults)
Listeria monocytogenes

Hospitalized Patients (in Addition to Above)
General
- Gram-negative species
- *Staphylococcus aureus*

With shunts or other intracranial devices
- *S. epidermidis*
- *Corynebacterium* sp.
- *Propionibacterium acnes*

Immunocompromised Patients (in Addition to Above)
Gram-negative bacteria (including *Pseudomonas* and *Acinetobacter*)
Streptococci
Anaerobes
Coagulase-negative staphylococci

Table 9-2. Differential Diagnosis of Acute Aseptic Meningitis

Viral Infection
Enteroviruses (coxsackievirus A and B, echovirus, nonparalytic poliovirus)
Mumps
Herpes viruses (herpes simplex types 1 and 2, varicella zoster)
Lymphocytic choriomeningitis
Adenovirus
HIV-1
Cytomegalovirus
Epstein-Barr virus

Nonviral Infections
Partially treated bacterial infections
Leptospirosis
Mycoplasma
Tuberculosis
Syphilis
Subacute bacterial endocarditis
Parameningeal infections

Noninfectious Causes
Drugs and intrathecal chemicals
Vasculitis
Mollaret's meningitis
Neoplasm (lymphoma, leukemia, carcinoma)

Table 9-3. Differential Diagnosis of Subacute and Chronic Meningitis

Infectious
Mycobacteria
M. tuberculosis
Spirochetal
Treponema pallidum
Borrelia burgdorfrei
Fungal
Cryptococcus neoformans
Coccidioides immitis
Parasitic
Toxoplasma gondii

Neoplastic

Vasculitis

Idiopathic Inflammatory Disorders
Sarcoidosis
Behçet syndrome

Table 9-4. Infectious Etiologies of Subacute and Chronic Meningitis of Particular Concern in Immunocompromised Patients

Tuberculosis
Cryptococcus neoformans
Toxoplasma gondii
Listeria monocytogenes
Candida
Aspergillus
Nocardia asteroides
Mycobacterium intracellulare
HIV-1

Table 9-5. Evaluation of Meningitis and Meningoencephalitis

Test	Condition	Notes
Blood Tests		
CBC with platelet count	Bacterial	Leukocytosis with increased immature granulocytes; pneumococcus and meningococous can cause DIC. Chronic meningitis or abscess associated with anemia of chronic disease.
PT, PTT	Bacterial	Coagulopathy with DIC
Electrolytes	Chronic meningitis or later bacterial meningitis	SIADH common (particularly with *Mycobacterium tuberculosis*)
BUN, Cr		Assessment of renal function important in dosing of antibiotics
ESR	Chronic inflammatory processes	Elevated
SPEP, FANA, rheumatoid factor	Vasculitides	Frequently abnormal in some vasculitides involving the CNS that may lead to chronic meningitis syndrome; more specific tests for evaluation of these disorders are described in later chapters
Angiotensin-converting enzyme	Sarcoidosis	Elevated in about 60% with sarcoidosis, a rare cause of chronic meningitis
Lumbar Puncture		Increased opening pressure frequent; leukocytosis with lymphocytic predominance in aseptic and chronic meningitides and granulocyte predominance in bacterial meningitis; increased total protein; decreased glucose in bacterial, fungal, and mycobacterial infections and carcinomatous meningitis; India ink stain for cryptococcus; cytology may identify neoplastic cells; consider requesting cell surface markers to establish clonality in suspected lymphoma or leukemia; serology and culture as described below and in Table 9-6

Serology (Blood and CSF)	Infectious meningitides and meningoencephalitides	Demonstration of virus specific IgM correlates with recent infection as does fourfold rise in titer between acute and convalescent phase sera by complement fixation; radioimmunoassay for herpes virus-specific glycoprotein; see Table 9-6 for serologic evaluation of chronic meningitis
Cultures	Bacterial	Immediate Gram stain of culture CSF and blood CSF diagnostic in most acute bacterial meningitides; rapid transport to laboratory increases culture yield
	Viral	Culture often difficult; use viral transport media; samples from throat and rectal swabs, urine (mumps) and genital lesions of use in addition to blood and CSF cultures; consult laboratory
	Chronic meningitis	Large volumes of CSF (>10 ml) should be sent to laboratory; repeated lumbar cultures may be needed for diagnosis; consult laboratory: special handling and growth conditions may facilitate isolation of specific agents; culture of early A.M. sputum and gastric washings for TB and biopsy specimens for TB and fungal infections may be used
Radiology		
Chest x-ray	Chronic meningitis	Many etiologies of chronic meningitis (e.g., cryptococcus, TB, sarcoidosis) have pulmonary involvement, important to identify, because tissue diagnosis can be relatively easy
Skull and sinus films	Bacterial meningitis, aseptic meningitis	Sinus infection may provide focus for meningitis; parameningeal focus may lead to aseptic meningitis
Head CT	Meningitis	Basal meningeal contrast enhancement and focal-enhancing lesions may be seen, particularly with carcinomatous meningitis, sarcoidosis, and tuberculosis

Continued

Table 9-5. *Continued*

Test	Condition	Notes
	Associated with meningitis	
	Abscess	Usually well-defined focal hypodensity with surrounding hypodensity edema and mass effect; ring enhancement with contrast
	Sinusitis, mastoiditis	Fluid density (sharply contrasting with bone and air); local bony erosion may be apparent
	Complications of meningitis	
	Hydrocephalus	Ventriculomegaly, periventricular hypodensity, flattening of gyri
	Venous thrombosis	Increased density within thrombosed sinus and failure to fill involved vein with contrast; local superficial gyral contrast enhancement with diffuse white matter hypodensity from edema
	Infarction	Focal hypodensity, increasing with edema; contrast enhancement after 5–7 days
MRI		Higher sensitivity for abscesses and other focal inflammatory or neoplastic lesions; locally increased signal in T_2-weighted images from edema and inflammation of meninges

Table 9-6. Staining Characteristics and Appearance of CNS Bacterial Pathogens

Staining Characteristics	Organisms
Gram-Negative	
Cocci	
Paired (intracellular and extracellular)	*Neisseria meningitidis*
Rods	
Small, occasionally in short chains	*Haemophilus influenzae*
Large	*Escherichia coli*
Gram-Positive	
Cocci	
Chains or irregular clusters	*Staphylococcus aureus*
Rodlike (occasionally coccoid)	*Listeria monocytogenes*
Lancet-shaped	
Chains or pairs (diplococci)	*Streptococcus pneumoniae*
India Ink-Positive	*Cryptococcus*

Table 9-7. Microbiologic and Serologic Tests in Chronic Meningitis

Organism	CSF Smear	Serology		Culture			Other Tests
		CSF	Blood	CSF	Blood	Other	
Mycobacterium tuberculosis	+ (AFB)	–	–	+	–	Sputum, gastric aspirate, bone marrow	TB skin test
Cryptococcus neoformans	+ (India ink)	+	+	+	–	–	CSF and serum cryptococcus polysaccharide antigen
Coccidioides immitis	+	+	+	+	–	–	
Treponema pallidum	–	+ (VDRL)	+ (FTA-ABS)	+	–	–	
Histoplasma capsulatum	–	+	+	+	–	–	Skin test not recommended as may cause positive serology
Toxoplasma gondii	–	+	+	–	–	–	Brain biopsy (abscess site)
Borrelia burgdorferi	–	+	+	–	–	–	
HIV	–	+	+	–	–	–	Circulating T-cell helper/suppressive ratio depressed (<1) with immunosuppression; polymerase chain reaction detection of HIV DNA in circulating leukocytes of Ab-negative patients
Candida albicans	+	–	–	+	+	+	Blood and other cultures usually positive only in disseminated disease
Nocardia asteroides	+	–	–	+	–	–	

Table 9-8. Differential Diagnosis of Acute and Subacute Encephalitis in Adults

Infectious

Immune-competent patients

- Viral
  - Herpes simplex
  - Togaviridae (St. Louis encephalitis and western and eastern equine encephalitis)
  - Enteroviruses
  - Rabies
- Bacterial
  - *Listeria*
  - *Mycoplasma*
  - *Legionella*
- Spirochetal
  - *Borrelia burgdorferi*
  - Neurosyphilis
- Rickettsia
  - Rocky Mountain spotted fever

Immunosuppressed patients (in addition to those above)

- Viral
  - Epstein-Barr virus
  - Cytomegalovirus
  - Varicella-zoster
  - Papovavirus
  - HIV-1
- Parasitic
  - Toxoplasmosis

Demyelinating

- Postinfectious
- Postvaccinial
- (Idiopathic) acute disseminated encephalomyelitis

Table 9-9. Other Tests to Consider in Predominantly Encephalitic Presentations

Tests	Notes
Lumbar puncture	Evaluate for signs of increased intracranial pressure from cerebral edema and meningeal inflammation; necrotizing encephalitis may show leukocytosis, red cells, xanthochromia, and increased total protein
Serology	Blood or CSF antibodies to organism
Virus isolation	Blood, CSF, brain tissue, other body fluids (e.g., significant viral titers in saliva and urine for rabies)
EEG	Relatively sensitive study in herpes simplex encephalitis showing lateralized periodic epileptiform discharges with slow waves or other focal abnormalities
Head CT	Diffuse or focal edema often better defined using contrast; HSV shows frontotemporal abnormalities and hypodensity with irregular contrast enhancement in about half of patients; probability of changes increases with disease progression
MRI	Increased sensitivity relative to CT for changes secondary to edema and demyelination; postinfectious or papovavirus encephalitis may show widespread or multifocal demyelination
Brain biopsy	Biopsy of involved areas may demonstrate viral inclusion bodies and other diagnostic changes

Further Notes

EVALUATION OF MENINGITIS

The nature of the onset, time course, and rate of progression of symptoms and signs provide important clues to the etiology of a meningitis syndrome. Acute meningitis most commonly is infectious, usually either bacterial (pyogenic) or viral in the normal host (Tables 9-1 and 9-2). Chemical meningitis can also occur acutely as an iatrogenic disorder or with rupture of intracranial cyst (e.g., colloid cyst). Although often classified as chronic menigitides, meningeal dissemination of a neoplasm or tuberculous meningitis usually presents subacutely (Tables 9-3 and 9-4). Infectious etiologies of chronic meningitis include less pathogenic organisms (e.g., fungi, parasites, and spirochetes). A number of other chronic meningitides of uncertain etiology have been well characterized clinically (e.g., sarcoidosis). Vasculitis leading to recurrent aseptic meningeal inflammation has been described but is also rare.

Acute Meningitis

Evaluation of acute meningitis (Table 9-5) is a neurologic emergency. If suspicion of purulent meningitis is high, treatment should be initiated on a presumptive basis. If treatment is withheld because aseptic meningitis is suspected, this diagnosis should be repeatedly reassessed until the acute phase of the illness has clearly resolved.

CSF Studies and Bacterial Culture

The critical distinction between pyogenic and aseptic meningitis can usually be made early with reasonable confidence after CSF examination (see Ch. 1).

Opening pressure is always elevated from cerebral edema in bacterial meningitis. A CSF cell count should be performed by the examining physician immediately after the lumbar puncture (LP). Almost all patients with untreated bacterial meningitis will have more than 1,000 cells/mm^3, whereas most (about two-third) patients with viral meningitis will have cell counts under 1,000 cells/mm^3. Polymorphonuclear leukocytes are characteristic of untreated bacterial infections but can also be seen very early with meningitis of other etiologies. A predominantly lymphocytic pleocytosis is characteristic of nonbacterial infections (viral, fungal, chemical) after the first 12 to 24 hours. In partially treated bacterial meningitis, lymphocytes may predominate as in viral meningitis. Monocytes are characteristic of *Listeria* infections.

A Gram stain of the CSF should also be performed immediately. Stain of sediment from a centrifuged CSF sample is diagnostic in 80 to 90 percent of untreated patients with bacterial meningitis (Table 9-6). The sensitivity is lower after antibiotic therapy has been started, but the test remains useful.

CSF glucose concentration is the most important biochemical study. The glucose concentration is usually normal or only slightly low in viral meningitis, but is less than 0.4 of serum glucose concentration in most patients with bacterial meningitis and is often extremely low (see Ch. 1). However, even extreme hypoglycorrhachia is not specific; for example, it may be seen acutely in chemical meningitis. Elevation of the total protein occurs with both bacterial and aseptic infections. It is generally higher and can be greater than 2 g/L in bacterial meningitis.

With known or suspected bacterial meningitis, CSF samples for bacterial culture (at least 1 ml) should be rapidly transported to the laboratory: alkalosis with a reduction in carbon dioxide tension as the sample is exposed to air may reduce viability of any microorganisms in the CSF. Blood cultures (at least two sets from separate sites) should be drawn before initiation of any antibacterial therapy.

If the CSF is nonpurulent, and particularly if there is a clinical suspicion of malignancy, it is important to obtain CSF cytologic examination. If the LP is performed outside of usual laboratory hours, precluding rapid cell concentration for cytologic studies, the CSF sample is best refrigerated immediately: cell structure may remain sufficiently intact for study for 24 to 48 hours. However, cell degradation in CSF invariably begins within hours.

When Should Lumbar Puncture Be Performed?

The most feared complication of an LP is cerebral herniation, but this problem is unlikely with patients who have a normal level of consciousness, a normal funduscopic examination, and a nonfocal neurologic examination. Others should have a computed tomography (CT) scan before an LP. Nonetheless, therapy must not be delayed by the perceived need for a CT scan; empiric treatment should be initiated if acute bacterial meningitis is suspected. Note that the absence of papilledema alone is not sufficient to ensure a safe LP in questionable cases.

A repeat LP should be considered 1 to 2 days after initiation of therapy in acute bacterial meningitis to ensure an appropriate response to treatment and a sterile CSF culture on antibiotic therapy.

In cases of suspected viral meningitis (in which there is no hypoglycorrhachia and CSF protein is less than about 1.5 g/L) associated with a predominantly polymorphonuclear leukocyte pleocytosis, a repeat LP should be performed after 8 to 12 hours. If the shift from polymorphonuclear to lymphocytic predominance has not begun, the diagnosis of viral meningitis is less likely, and the possibility of a nonviral etiology should be entertained.

Rapid Tests for Bacterial Meningitis

A number of rapid tests are available for identification of some bacterial antigens. *Streptococcus pneumoniae*, *Haemophilus influenzae*, and *Neisseria meningitides* antigens can be detected by counterimmunoelectrophoresis assay or enzyme-linked immunosorbent assay (ELISA). The advantage of specific bacterial antigen assays is that they are unaffected by the changes in membrane-staining properties that follow antibiotic therapy and lower the sensitivity of the Gram stain. However, they are relatively insensitive to *S. pneumoniae* (the most common cause of bacterial meningitis in adults) and, therefore, are more important in a pediatric population.

Serology and Culture in Viral Meningitis

Establishing the etiology of viral meningitis syndromes is generally of little help in immediate patient management, but may aid in understanding patterns of viral meningitis and in anticipating later complications in individual patients. Over two-thirds of cases of viral meningitis are due to enteroviruses (coxsackievirus A and B, echovirus). Mumps virus is the next most common cause, with lymphocytic choriomeningitis, adenovirus, Epstein-Barr virus, herpes simplex, and varicella-zoster accounting for smaller proportions. An aseptic meningitis can occur also with acute HIV infection. Especially in the immunocompromised host, cytomegalovirus (CMV) should be considered.

Viral isolation can be attempted from CSF, stool, and pharyngeal secretions. About 0.5 to 1 ml of CSF is needed. Throat swabs and stool specimens (only a few grams are needed) should be sent to the laboratory in viral isolation media to inhibit bacterial growth. The floors of any vesicular skin lesions suspected to be caused by varicella-zoster or herpes simplex should be scraped, smeared onto a microscope slide, and placed quickly in fixative. Herpetic lesions show multinucleated giant cells and sometimes intranuclear inclusions from a Tzanck (methylene blue) stain. Acute and convalescent sera should be obtained for serologic diagnosis.

Spirochetal Disease

Meningitis is one of the initial manifestations of neurosyphilis. Spirochetes cannot be cultured in the usual media. Diagnosis is based on clinical suspicion and systemic signs of primary infection and serologic diagnosis, as is discussed in Chapter 13. Simultaneous infection with human immunodeficiency virus (HIV)-1 may lead to a more prolonged and severe meningitis syndrome than is otherwise usual.

The endemic areas for Lyme neuroborreliosis, which is also associated with an early meningitis syndrome, are enlarging. Almost all patients will have positive serology for the Lyme agent (*Borrelia burgdorferi*). Both serum and CSF serology should be obtained. A major diagnostic problem in endemic areas is distinguishing patients who have developed antibodies as a result of past (usually asymptomatic) exposure from those with active disease. The reference cited at the end of the chapter from Halperin's laboratory proposes comparison of antibody titers in serum and CSF to identify intrathecal antispirochetal antibody production as a marker for active CNS disease from the Lyme agent.

Parameningeal Foci

Parameningeal foci of infection (e.g., mastoiditis) may intermittently seed the CSF, leading to florid, purulent meningitis or, by mechanisms that are less clear, may give rise to a syndrome of aseptic meningitis. The clinical history and examination are critical for their identification, as otitis, focal tenderness, signs of trauma, or other suggestive features are invariably present. Sinus films are a good screening test if a head CT has not been obtained.

Tests Useful in Monitoring Patients for Complications of Bacterial Meningitis or its Therapy

Patients with pyogenic infections must be monitored carefully for complications of infection, as well as to ensure that therapy is effective. Monitoring of electrolytes is important with bacterial meningitis because of the potential for developing the syndrome of inappropriate secretion of antidiuretic hormone (SIADH). Meningococcemia may lead to adrenal failure with the Waterhouse-Friderichsen syndrome. This can be confirmed by measurement of serum cortisol before and after ACTH stimulation. Electrolyte imbalances and hemodynamic instability may occur if untreated. Focal neurologic deficits may arise secondary to vasculitis or venous thrombosis. These are associated with focal mass effect and hypodensity from edema on plain CT (see Ch. 11). Sensorineural deafness is one of the more common complications of bacterial meningitis. When it is suspected, audiologic testing should be performed for documentation.

Subacute and Chronic Meningitis

Subacute meningitis develops relatively slowly (i.e., over the course of 1 to 4 weeks). A chronic meningitis is a syndrome in which signs and symptoms of meningeal inflammation persist for 4 weeks or more. These syndromes can be manifestations of many infectious and noninfectious diseases. Evaluation (Tables 9-3 and 9-4) often poses a special diagnostic problem due to the low titers of many of the infectious agents in body fluids and the uncertain etiologies of some syndromes.

Cerebrospinal Fluid Examination

CSF studies are the first step in evaluation. Usually lymphocytes are the predominant cell type. Polymorphonuclear cells may be found with early tuberculous, fungal, or parasitic infection. Bizarre cells with pleomorphic nuclei may be seen with a neoplastic process. A Gram stain should be performed immediately if there is any suspicion of a partially treated bacterial meningitis. An India ink stain will show the characteristic dye-excluding spheroids of *Cryptococcus*. Multiple AFB smears of sediment concentrated from a large volume (5 to 15 ml) of CSF should be performed if tuberculous meningitis is suspected.

As a general rule, the CSF glucose concentration is often low in tuberculous meningitis, frequently low with fungal infections, and sometimes low in neoplastic meningitis. CSF protein concentrations may be elevated for all forms of subacute or chronic meningitis. High protein concentrations (greater than about 1.5 g/L) may lead to secondary hydrocephalus.

Cytology

CSF cytologic examination can frequently identify neoplastic cells with meningeal carcinomatosis, leukemia, or lymphoma; but multiple LPs may be necessary. Cisternal punctures have been reported to provide a higher yield for cytology than lumbar puncture in certain conditions.

Serologic Tests

Serologic studies of the CSF are sometimes diagnostic, particularly with cryptococcus, Lyme neuroborreliosis and syphilis (Table 9-7). Blood serology may be helpful in many cases as well. Obtaining blood serology for HIV-1 should be considered.

Cerebrospinal Fluid Culture

Large amounts of CSF (15 ml) should be sent for culture. The microbiology laboratory should be notified so that fluid can be cultured in special media for fastidious organisms. Repeated LPs are frequently needed and will stimulate bulk flow of CSF toward the lumbar cistern, potentially increasing the sensitivity for detecting disease of the intracranial meninges. In extraordinary cases, consideration may be given to a cisternal puncture to obtain CSF for culture.

Brain Imaging

Imaging of the head is useful for ruling out focal mass lesions (e.g., neoplasms or abscesses) and may also directly demonstrate areas of inflammation in the basal meninges. Enhancement with CT or magnetic resonance imaging (MRI) contrast agents or abnormal hyperintense signals on T_2-weighted MRI images may be noted in areas of meningeal inflammation. This information can be used to direct a meningeal biopsy if needed.

Tests for Systemic Disease

The infectious causes of subacute or chronic meningitis are often accompanied by signs of disseminated disease. There is often primary pulmonary involvement (e.g., *Mycobacterium tuberculosis, Coccidioides*). In these cases, the chest x-ray, followed by serial sputum culture and possibly bronchoscopy (if radiologic abnormalities are present), may be diagnostic. Culture of early morning gastric aspirates may also help in diagnosis of tuberculosis. Skin testing may help with diagnosis of tuberculosis, but should not be performed for histoplasmosis as serology may be altered by intradermal antigen administration. Control antigens should always be applied as a screen for anergy.

CNS sarcoidosis is almost always accompanied by pulmonary disease.

A chest x-ray, chest CT, or a gallium scan may sometimes help to suggest this noninvasively (see Ch. 15). Biopsy of affected tissue can establish the diagnosis. Signs of systemic immune deficiency should also be sought with specific consideration of the possibility of HIV infection.

Meningeal Biopsy

If sites for meningeal biopsy are suggested by localizable findings in the neurologic examination or the imaging studies, meningeal biopsy may be considered for more direct evidence of inflammation and possibly specific etiologic diagnosis if the less invasive approaches are unsuccessful and etiologic diagnosis is critical to management.

EVALUATION OF SUSPECTED ENCEPHALITIS

The acute and subacute encephalitis syndromes are marked by prominent early mental changes, with or without focal cortical dysfunction. The initial concern is to establish whether there is an infectious cause for the encephalitis syndrome (Table 9-8). Several of the infectious causes are life-threatening but potentially reversible (e.g., herpes simplex, *Listeria*, *Mycoplasma*, *Legionella*, *Toxoplasma*). Lyme neuroborreliosis may also respond well to antibiotics, but encephalitis from this agent is relatively rare and has only recently been recognized. Immunosuppressed patients, particularly those with acquired immunodeficiency syndrome (AIDS), are susceptible to a broader range of agents, including, in addition to those mentioned above, HIV, herpes zoster, CMV, and papovavirus.

If infection is ruled out, the possibility of demyelinating disease must be considered. Early treatment with steroids may improve the natural history of these disorders.

Cerebrospinal Fluid Examination

CSF examination may show an increased opening pressure from cerebral edema. There is a variable leukocytosis, but, in general, it will be less marked for the degree of cerebral dysfunction than is seen with meningitis. Monocytes may predominate with *Listeria*. A lymphocytic pleocytosis is characteristically found with viral encephalitis or demyelinating disease.

It is important to look for red cells and xanthochromia. The presence of red cells is useful in distinguishing a primary necrotizing encephalitis from a meningoencephalitis. Red cells from an encephalitic process should show some degree of crenation because of prolonged exposure to CSF: fresh cells from trauma during the tap will all have normal morphology (see Ch. 1).

Oligoclonal bands and CSF IgG can be nonspecifically elevated in any infectious process. However, they can be particularly high in demyelinating diseases.

Microbiologic and Serologic Tests

The CSF Gram stain should not be forgotten. In *Listeria*, the CSF Gram stain may directly demonstrate the gram-positive, rod-shaped organisms. The diagnosis can be confirmed by culture.

Serology can be helpful in several instances. Complement-fixing antibodies are elevated in serum, and CSF and serum cold agglutinins may be increased with *Mycoplasma*. Specific antibodies directed against *Legionella* may be assayed in serum. Serology combined with observation of response to therapy or biopsy of a focal lesion can be used to establish the diagnosis of toxoplasmosis.

Definitive diagnosis of viral disease demands demonstration of elevated specific viral antibody titers (showing that the titers are rising from acute to convalescent sera or a transition from IgM to IgG virus-directed antibodies between acute and convalescent phase sera are more specific), isolation of the virus (rarely possible), or brain biopsy.

Brain Imaging

Brain imaging should be the initial study in patients with suspected encephalitis. Toxoplasmosis or *Listeria* can show focal ring-enhancing lesions by CT or areas of increased signal on T_2-weighted images by MRI. Viral encephalitis such as that caused by herpes simplex may show no changes early in the course or only minimal signs of edema. Eventually, CT will demonstrate diffuse, contrast-enhancing hypolucencies localized to the temporal lobe(s) in most patients. MRI changes consistent with edema in the affected area(s) provide an earlier, more sensitive marker.

EEG

The EEG may show nonspecific diffuse or focal disturbances. In herpes simplex encephalitis periodic lateralized epileptiform discharges (PLEDs) may be seen (unliterally or bilaterally) with an abnormally slow background (see Ch. 6).

Brain Biopsy

Biopsy of focal brain lesions in *Listeria* infection or toxoplasmosis should demonstrate the causative organisms or make alternative diagnoses less likely. Biopsy of an affected temporal lobe in herpes simplex encephalitis can demonstrate the classic pathologic changes of perivascular inflammation, neuronal inclusion bodies, and hemorrhagic necrosis. Immunofluorescence studies for the specific viral antigens and viral culture may be positive. In general, however, brain biopsy is not indicated for the diagnosis of a viral encephalitis. With the availability of antiviral therapy that has minimal potential morbidity, brain biopsy for diagnosis of herpes simplex encephalitis has become uncommon.

READINGS

Benson CA, Harris AA: Acute neurologic infections. Med Clin North Am 70(5):987, 1986

Gabuzda DH, Hirsch MS: Neurologic manifestations of human immunodeficiency virus: clinical features and pathogenesis. Ann Intern Med 107:383, 1987

Halperin JJ, Luft BJ, Anand AK, et al.: Lyme neuroborreliosis: central nervous system manifestations. Neurology 39:753, 1989

Hart G: Syphilis tests in diagnostic and therapeutic decision making. Ann Intern Med 104:368, 1986

Levy RM, Bredesen DE, Rosenblum ML: Opportunistic central nervous system pathology in patients with AIDS. Ann Neurol 23(suppl.):S7, 1988

Mandell GL, Douglas RG, Bennett JG: Principles and Practice of Infectious Diseases. 3rd Ed. Churchill Livingstone, New York, 1989

Reese RE, Douglas RG: A Practical Approach to Infectious Diseases. Ed. 2. Little, Brown, Boston, 1986

Swartz MN: Chronic meningitis—many causes to consider. N Engl J Med 317:957, 1987

Thurston SE: The Little Black Book of Neurology. Year Book Medical Publishers, Chicago, 1987

Wilhelm C, Ellnor JJ: Chronic meningitis. Neurol Clin North Am 4(1):115, 1986

LABORATORY TESTS FOR EVALUATING STUPOR AND COMA

10

Table 10-1. Differential Diagnosis of Stupor and Coma

Metabolic
Hypoxia
Hypoglycemia or hyperglycemia
Hyponatremia or hypernatremia
Hypercalcemia or hypermagnesemia
Acidosis (respiratory)
Uremia
Hepatic failure
Hypothyroidism
Hypophosphatemia
Thiamine deficiency
Hypothermia
Multifocal metabolic encephalopathy

Trauma
Concussion
Contusion
Hematoma (epidural, subdural, intracerebral, intraventricular)

Infection
Meningitis
Encephalitis
Severe systemic illness (toxic encephalopathy)

Intoxications
Sedatives (e.g., barbiturates, benzodiazepines, ethanol, narcotics)
Psychotropic drugs (e.g., PCP, amphetamines, tricyclic antidepressants, cholinergic drugs, lithium, phenothiazines)
Therapeutic drugs (e.g., anticonvulsants, salicylate, paracetamol, propoxyphene hydrochloride)
Toxins (e.g., ethylene glycol)

Epileptic
Postictal state
Complex partial status
Absence status

Cerebrovascular Disease
Subarachnoid or intracerebral hemorrhage
Infarction (posterior circulation or massive hemispheric)
Global hypoperfusion

Neoplasm or abscess
Mass effect
Secondary hydrocephalus

Hydrocephalus (Acute)

Idiopathic
Reye syndrome

Psychogenic unresponsiveness

(Modified from Plum et al., 1984, with permission.)

Table 10-2. Evaluation of Stupor and Coma

Test	Condition	Notes
Blood Tests		
Serum glucose	Hypoglycemia or hyperglycemia	Initial rapid fingerstick blood sugar to rule out severe hypoglycemia recommended before giving glucose and thiamine
Arterial blood gas	Hypoxia, hypercarbia, metabolic acidosis	Not only for acute respiratory distress, but also for chronic carbon dioxide retention; may give clues in poisonings, hypoperfusion states, DKA
CBC	Systemic infection	Leukocytosis from stress possible, as well as infection
	Cerebral infarction	Polycythemia, thrombocytosis, severe anemia are predisposing
Electrolytes	Hyponatremia or hypernatremia	Increased anion gap in DKA, with acidic toxins (e.g., salicylate, ethylene glycol), and lactic acidosis also suggested
Calcium	Hypocalcemia or hypercalcemia	Hypocalcemia may predispose to seizures and subsequently a postictal state; hypercalcemia causes depression of consciousness directly
Phosphate	Hypophosphatemia	Associated with severe malnutrition and alcoholism
Liver function tests (SGOT, SGPT, bilirubin)	Hepatic insufficiency	Signs of chronic hyperbilirubinemia should be sought on examination; elevated serum ammonia has an imperfect correlation with acute neurologic dysfunction
Creatine kinase	Rhabdomyolysis	Rhabdomyolysis secondary to pressure on a limb during coma may lead to secondary renal failure
Magnesium	Hypomagnesemia or hypermagnesemia	Hypermagnesemia is usually secondary to antacids, but renal failure may be contributory

Continued

Table 10-2. *Continued*

Test	Condition	Notes
Serum osmolality	Metabolic comas	Elevated in severe dehydration, hyperglycemia or with exogenous agents (e.g., ethylene glycol)
Blood ketones	DKA	Should be ordered in diabetics or if increased anion gap is found
Urine Tests		
Urine glucose	Elevated in DKA or hyperglycemic coma	
Urine myoglobin	Rhabdomyolysis	
Drug and Toxin Screens		
Serum and urine	Intoxications	Consider potential variation in pharmacodynamics of therapeutic drugs, especially in elderly adults; urine tests are, generally, more sensitive for agents excreted by the kidneys; consider (at least): Amphetamines Barbiturates Benzodiazepine Cocaine Methadone Methaqualone Opiates Phencyclidine Acetaminophen Salicylate Ethanol Methanol Ethylene glycol Opiates Therapeutic drugs
Radiology		
Skull and sinus films	Trauma	Fractures may predispose to hemorrhage, venous thrombosis and CNS infection; consider concussion with fractures
Cervical spine films	Trauma	Spinal trauma is often associated with head trauma

Continued

Table 10-2. *Continued*

Test	Condition	Notes
Head CT	Subdural hematoma	Acutely blood is hyperdense; on CT subdurals have concave inner face, convex outer face, and mass effect (obliteration of gyral markings with midline displacement); intermediate (2–4 weeks) lesions may be isodense and are better visualized with contrast infusion; chronic lesions are hypodense
	Epidural hematoma	Biconvex hyperdense lesion adjacent to the inner table of skull; because epidural hematomas expand rapidly under arterial pressure, chronic lesions are not a reasonable diagnostic possibility
	Intracerebral hematoma	See Table 11-5
	Subarachnoid hemorrhage	Increased density of CSF from blood in sulci, sylvian and interhemispheric fissures, and/or basal cisterns; secondary hydrocephalus is a common cause of later deterioration in level of consciousness
	Ischemic infarct	See Table 11-5
	Encephalitis	Patchy hypodensity from edema that may cross vascular territories; look particularly in temporal lobes; irregular enhancement with intravenous contrast
	Neoplasm	See Table 11-5
	Hydrocephalus (symptomatic)	Ventriculomegaly, periventricular white matter hypodensities (particularly around the frontal horns), and gyral effacement
MRI	Hematoma	Distinguishes CT isodense lesions well, but otherwise is less useful than CT for early lesions because of poor discrimination of acute blood
	Infarct	See Table 11-5

Continued

Table 10-2. *Continued*

Test	Condition	Notes
	Encephalitis	MRI is more sensitive than CT for defining the associated edema
EEG		
	Psychogenic unresponsiveness	Normal EEG with an occipital alpha rhythm that shows good reactivity with stimulation
	Epilepsy	Diffuse or focally accentuated slowing postictally; nonconvulsive status can be identified
	Intoxication	Progression from diffuse slowing, to slowing and depressed amplitude, to burst suppression pattern, and ultimately, a flat line EEG with increasing depth of coma
	Focal lesion (infarct, neoplasm, abscess)	Localized slowing, PLEDs, focally decreased voltage possible
	Brainstem infarct	Diffuse, unreactive alpha rhythm may be seen with coma; EEG is normal in a locked-in state
	Metabolic coma	Diffuse, symmetric changes as with intoxications; bilaterally synchronous 2–4Hz triphasic waves are classically associated with hepatic coma, but also seen in other metabolic comas

Further Notes

ACUTE EVALUATION OF THE COMATOSE PATIENT

Metabolic Disorders

Evaluation of new-onset stupor or coma represents a neurologic emergency. Appropriate, rapid treatment can prevent permanent damage in some cases. Assessment should begin with vital signs (blood pressure, heart rate, body temperature), examination of respiratory (including arterial blood gas for evidence of carbon dioxide narcosis or hypoxia) and circulatory function, estimation of serum glucose concentration by fingerstick colorimetry (Chemstrips), and consideration of possible trauma. Hypoglycemic damage can be rapid, and empiric therapy should be started before results of laboratory tests are known if it is suspected. Blood should be drawn for serum chemistries (electrolytes, glucose, blood urea nitrogen [BUN], creatinine, calcium, phosphate, bilirubin, serum glutamic-oxaloacetic transaminase [SGOT], serum glutamate-pyruvate transaminase [SGPT], creatine phosphokinase [CPK]) before glucose is administered. Wernicke's encephalopathy may be worsened by glucose administration alone, so thiamine should be given with glucose if history and signs are suggestive.

Until the etiology of coma is clear and the possibility of arrhthymias or other causes of hypotension established to be unlikely, continuous monitoring of the cardiac rhythm and frequent assessment of vital signs are essential for safe management.

Trauma

Potential trauma or infection should be considered next. Plain films of the skull remain the most sensitive test for skull fractures. If trauma has occurred, the possibility of cervical spine injury should be rapidly assessed with cervical spine films. Subdural hematomas are best visualized by head computed tomography (CT). If an acute subdural hematoma is suspected, one should look for the characteristic hyperdense band from blood, concave on the cortical face, and convex against the skull. It will be associated with a mass effect (ventricular asymmetry, compression of sulci, and possible midline shift). Intraparenchymal shearing forces accompanying head trauma can lead to intracerebral hemorrhage. Coma due to simple concussion remains a diagnosis of exclusion.

Infection

Patients with fever, leukocytosis, or meningismus will certainly be suspected to harbor infection. However, elderly patients may not manifest these signs. Therefore, evidence of systemic infection (particularly infiltrates on chest x-ray or pyuria) should be looked for in all patients. Severe systemic illnesses are often associated with obtundation. More important for the neurologist, however, is that they can also lead to secondary CNS infection. A lumbar puncture should be included in the evaluation of all patients with stupor or coma of uncertain etiology. In most cases, patients should have a CT before a decision to tap is made (see Ch. 9). All patients in deep coma should ideally have a CT before lumbar puncture (LP).

Drugs and Toxins

Overdoses of drugs or other intoxications should be identified rapidly to initiate efforts to stop absorption (e.g., active charcoal, gastric lavage). Important tests include electrolytes (elevated anion gap from salicylates, ethylene glycol), hepatic enzymes such as SGOT and SGPT (e.g., elevated in acetaminophen overdose and other chemical causes of hepatitis), arterial blood gas, and chest x-ray (consider pulmonary edema secondary to barbiturate overdose or aspiration pneumonia).

The diagnosis can be established by confirming appropriately high levels of the intoxicant(s) in blood or urine or recovering the agent(s) from gastric contents. Urine tests are inherently more sensitive than serum tests for drugs excreted by the kidneys. Urine, therefore, should be collected immediately. Extra samples of serum and urine should be frozen in the event that the need for additional assays is suggested later in the clinical course. Clinical signs, the time course of clinical changes, the patient's apparent social milieu and habits, and known therapeutic drug use must be considered when choosing appropriate screening tests. The possibility of simultaneous intoxications with more than one substance must be considered.

Obtundation as a *secondary* consequence of a drug overdose (e.g., after seizures, hypotension, cerebral infarction, extracerebral hemorrhage) should also be considered.

Seizures

Seizures or a postictal state should always be considered as a cause of impaired consciousness, particularly if there are signs of an improving level of consciousness during the inital period of evaluation. The EEG is an important test in suspected seizure disorders, as described later.

Focal Cerebral Lesions and Subarachnoid Hemorrhage

In general, stupor or coma result from bihemispheric cortical dysfunction or damage to the deep midline structures. Focal lesions in the CNS that directly affect these pathways (e.g., basilar thrombosis) or cause global dysfunction secondary to increased intracranial pressure and brainstem distortion, therefore, can also lead to coma. CT images are essential first steps in evaluation (see Ch. 11). It should be noted that subarachnoid hemorrhage leads to obtundation disproportionate to the mass effect of the blood alone.

Small subarachnoid hemorrhages may not be seen with CT, particularly after the first day. LP should be performed in any patient with a strongly suggestive clinical history and a nondiagnostic CT scan: hemoglobin persists in the CSF for about a week after hemorrhage and bilirubin for 2 to 4 weeks. Sensitive spectrophotometric assays for the presence of bilirubin that can be used with CSF are usually available in laboratories servicing neonatal care units. Small "warning" leaks may be a prodrome to larger subarachnoid hemorrhages and are important to identify.

The high risk of vascular spasm and secondary infarction triggered by intra-arterial dye infusion after subarachnoid hemorrhages is often—and appropriately—emphasized. Because of the risk of vasospasm, patients who present with subarachnoid hemorrhage are best evaluated with angiography in the first 48 hours if early surgical intervention is being considered. Otherwise, angiography should be delayed for 2 to 3 weeks, by which time the risk of vasospasm is reduced.

THE ELECTROENCEPHALOGRAM IN EVALUATION OF COMA

The EEG is useful in the evaluation of coma. In acute evaluation of a patient it is useful for establishing the diagnosis of nonconvulsive status epilepticus. More generally, it may help in characterization of the clinical diagnosis of a seizure disorder or postictal state (see Ch. 12).

The EEG can also be useful in coma with nonepileptic etiologies. A few specific patterns are particularly significant. A normal EEG suggests either psychogenic coma if reactivity is preserved or focal brainstem dysfunction (e.g., locked-in syndrome). A burst suppression pattern suggests severe global damage. Pronounced asymmetries imply focal damage.

The prognostic significance of a single study showing diffuse abnormalities is often unclear. Serial EEGs can be useful, especially in patients in deep coma who have few signs to follow clinically. Progression to patterns showing greater synchronization of activity, more normal rhythmicity, and reactivity suggests a better prognosis.

Electrocerebral inactivity has been used as one of the criteria for brain death (see Ch. 6). For interpretation of the significance of electrocerebral inactivity in acute coma it is essential to rule out factors such as drug intoxication (e.g., phenobarbitol) or hypothermia.

MULTIFACTORIAL ENCEPHALOPATHIES

Patients (especially those who are elderly or very ill) with new onset of delirium or obtundation can present a special diagnostic problem. It is important to consider the possible effects of the interaction of multiple factors (e.g., mild hypoxia, anemia, cardiac failure, uremia, systemic infection), none of which independently would be sufficient to cause the observed changes. Sensory deprivation, insomnia, and drug withdrawal (especially from alcohol) should be considered in clinical assessment. The multifactorial "metabolic" encephalopathies are common. Unfortunately, the diagnosis remains clinical and can only be proposed after results of blood tests, CT, LP, and EEG have made more specific etiologies unlikely.

Embolism of air, blood clots, and fat are common cause of encephalopathies after cardiac or orthopaedic surgery. Air emboli commonly present as delirium. Emboli from fat or blood clots can be associated with focal neurologic signs and encephalopathy that is exacerbated by hypoxia from concomitant pulmonary emboli.

READINGS

Ede RJ, Williams R: Reye's syndrome in adults. Br Med J 296:517–518, 1988

Haddow LM, Winchester JR: Clinical Management of Poisons and Drug Overdose. WB Saunders, Philadelphia, 1983

Plum F, Posner JB: The Diagnosis of Stupor and Coma. Ed. 3. FA Davis, Philadelphia, 1984

Ropper A: Coma in the emergency room. p. 79. In Ernest MP (ed): Neurologic Emergencies. Churchill Livingstone, New York, 1983

LABORATORY TESTS FOR EVALUATING FOCAL CEREBRAL DEFECTS

11

Table 11-1. Differential Diagnosis of a Focal Cerebral Deficit

Vascular Disease
Infarction
Large vessel: anterior circulation, posterior circulation
Small vessel
Hemorrhage
Intracerebral hemorrhage
Subarachnoid hemorrhage
Subdural or epidural hemorrhage
Vascular malformation
Neoplasm
Primary CNS tumor
Metastatic tumor
Inflammatory Disease
Infection
Abscess
Encephalitis (e.g., herpes simplex)
Neurosyphilis
Demyelinating disease
Multiple sclerosis
Vasculitis
Epilepsy (Postictal)

Table 11-2. Etiologies of Stroke in the Young Patient

Cardiac Embolism
Valvular disease
Arrhythmias
Cardiomyopathy
Atrial myxoma
Right-to-left shunt
Myocardial infarction

Vascular Disease
Large vessel disease
- Premature cerebrovascular atherosclerosis (e.g., hyperlipidemias)
- Arterial dissection
- Venous thrombosis (e.g., peripartum, associated with infection or dehydration)
- Fibromuscular dysplasia

Vasculitis (e.g., SLE, polyarteritis nodosa, hypersensitivity vasculitis)
Arteriovenous malformation
Moyamoya disease

Blood Disorders
Sickle cell anemia
Hypercoagulable state
- Lupus anticoagulant
- Antithrombin III deficiency
- Protein C or protein S deficiencies

Thrombocytopenia or impaired platelet function
Polycythemia, thrombocytosis
DIC

Metabolic Disease
Diabetes mellitus
Fabry's disease
Homocystinuria (homozygous or heterozygous)
MELAS

Migraine

Table 11-3. Primary Hypercoagulable States and Tests Used in Their Evaluation

Abnormality	Test
Deficiency states Antithrombin III Factor XII Proteins C and S Plasminogen Plasminogen activator	Measure plasma levels by functional and/or immunologic assays; euglobulin lysis time can help identify fibrinolytic disorders
Lupus anticoagulant	Abnormally elevated kaolin activated PTT, false-positive VDRL, and anticardiolipin antibody may be found
Abnormal protein function	
Abnormal plasminogen	Euglobulin lysis time prolonged
Dysfibrinogenemia	Thrombin time prolonged

Table 11-4. Secondary Hypercoagulable States

Abnormalities of coagulation and fibrinolysis
- Pregnancy
- Oral contraceptives
- Malignancy
- Nephrotic syndrome

Platelet abnormalities
- Blood dyscrasia
- Hyperlipidemia
- Diabetes mellitus
- Heparin-induced thrombocytopenia

Abnormal blood flow or blood vessels
- Hyperviscosity (dehydration, sickle cell disease, increased serum proteins, blood dyscrasia)

(Modified from Schafer, 1985, with permission.)

Table 11-5. Evaluation of Focal Cerebral Defects

Test	Condition	Notes
Blood Tests		
CBC and platelets	CVA	Polycythemia, profound anemia, and DIC may predispose; may give clues to presence of infection or vasculitis
Sickle cell smear	CVA	
Electrolytes	Seizures	Hyponatremia
	CVA	Dehydration
Glucose	Hypoglycemia or hyperglycemia	May lead to focal defects in addition to global encephalopathy; hyperglycemia in diabetes predisposes to cerebral thrombosis
BUN, Cr	CVA	Indices of dehydration; uremia-induced platelet dysfunction predisposes to hemorrhage
Calcium	Seizures	Hypocalcemia
	CVA	Hypercalcemia may predispose to infarcts
PT, PTT	CVA	Elevated PTT or PT with anticoagulant use, hepatic failure, or factor deficiencies; elevated kaolin-activated PTT with lupus anticoagulant
ESR	Temporal arteritis	
	Chronic disease	Chronic infection or neoplasm may lead to secondary hypercoagulable state
VDRL	Neurosyphilis	Perform on CSF and serum. Serum FTA-ABS for patients at risk of tertiary syphilis; false-positive VDRL with lupus anticoagulant
SPEP, IEP, Cryoglobulins	CVA	Hyperviscosity syndromes may accompany paraproteinemias
CPK	CVA	Serial serum CPK measurements performed to assess for possibility of acute MI when searching for source of cardiac emboli; arrhythmias or wall hypokineses from infarction can lead to cardiac emboli; CPK must be fractionated since MM often high after strokes

Continued

Table 11-5. *Continued*

Test	Condition	Notes
Lipid profile	CVA	Should include total cholesterol, LDL, and HDL
Lumbar Puncture	Demyelinating disease	Elevated IgG, positive oligoclonal bands, and may show mild pleocytosis with acute exacerbation
	Neurosyphilis	Pleocytosis and increased protein
Radiology		
Skull film	Epidural hematoma	Local skull fracture
	Abscess	Contiguous spread of infection frequent to frontal lobes from frontal sinuses, to temporal lobes from ipsilateral maxillary sinus, to cerebellum or temporal lobe from mastoid sinus
Head CT	Ischemic infarct	Focal hypodensity developing over 1–4 days with infarct; contrast enhancement after 5–7 days
	Intracerebral hematoma	Well-defined, homogeneous hyperdense area with surrounding hypodensity from edema in the brain parenchyma
	Subdural hematoma	See Table 10-2
	Epidural hematoma	See Table 10-2
	Vascular malformation	If >1 cm in size may be visualized by CT with contrast infusion
	Neoplasm	Focal hyperdensity or hypodensity (often with surrounding hypodensity from edema); may have calcifications, contrast enhancement
	Abscess	Ring enhancement characteristic of high grade gliomas and abscesses
	Encephalitis	See Table 10-2
	Demyelinating disease	Acute large plaques may show focal enhancement with contrast
	Epilepsy	Lesions of many types (tumor, infarct, hemorrhage, gliotic scar) may provide epileptogenic focus

Continued

Table 11-5. *Continued*

Test	Condition	Notes
MRI	Ischemic infarct	Advantages over CT include more reliable visualization of early ischemic infarcts and lesions in the posterior fossa
	Subdural hematoma	Identification of CT isodense subacute hematomas is easier
	Neoplasm	Enhanced sensitivity without contrast relative to CT probably for all tumors except meningiomas; good imaging of the posterior fossa
	Epilepsy	Enhanced sensitivity relative to CT for identifying epileptogenic structural abnormalities, particularly in mesial temporal lobes
	Demyelinating disease	Plaques (acute and chronic) readily noted as areas of increased signal on T_2-weighted images
	Encephalitis	Edema identified earlier than with CT
	Vascular malformation	Flow void or relaxation time changes from adjacent hemosiderin deposits allow good sensitivity for vascular malformations; cavernous hemangiomas—frequently not seen by routine angiography—may be identified
Carotid duplex Doppler scan	Ischemic infarct	Excellent screening test for clinically significant extracranial internal carotid occlusive disease with useful visualization of wall anatomy; inferences possible about intracranial disease; newer instruments may give direct information on larger intracranial and vertebral vessels
Echocardiogram	Ischemic infarct	Good screening test for large intraventricular cardiac thrombi, hypokinetic wall segments predisposing to thrombi, valvular lesions, (rare) atrial myxomas, and septal abnormalities allowing paradoxic emboli; vegetations in endocarditis and clot in atrial appendage poorly visualized

Continued

Table 11-5. *Continued*

Test	Condition	Notes
Angiogram	CVA	Current gold standard for evaluation of vessel wall plaques and occlusive disease; other specific signs include the string sign of arterial dissection, string-of-beads pattern with vasculitis and sudden, plug-shaped occlusion accompanied by local hyperemia with an embolus
	Neoplasm	Angiography assists in differential diagnosis by defining the vascular pattern and management by defining feeding vessels
	Vascular malformation	Angiography important evaluation of most vascular lesions (except cavernous angioma); characterization possible based on flow patterns; assists in surgical management by defining feeding and draining vessels; therapeutic embolization may sometimes be attempted
Holter Monitor	Ischemic infarct	24- to 48-hour monitoring for cardiac arrhythmias with embolic stroke
EEG		
	CVA	Focal slowing, PLEDs, or focal epileptiform activity, particularly if embolic
	Migraine	Nonspecific abnormalities, sometimes lateralized
	Hematoma	Focal slowing
	Encephalitis	Periodic slow waves or mixed slow and sharp waves lateralized to affected area; may also show PLEDs
Biopsies		
Temporal arteries	Ischemic infarct	Patchy segments of inflammation (giant cells) in vessel wall in temporal arteritis
Brain	Neoplasm	All suspected neoplasms should be biopsied to establish cell type and guide therapy; differentiation from abscess may be difficult without biopsy

Further Notes

ESTABLISHING LOCATION AND ETIOLOGY

Evaluation of neurologic disease in general, and focal neurologic deficits in particular, should establish first the location and then the etiology of the disorder. One should strive not to leap to conclusions too quickly about the etiology. Cerebrovascular accidents are relatively so common that other potential causes of focal deficits are too often ignored in the differential diagnosis (Table 11-1). The possibility of focal infections (see Ch. 9), neoplasms, seizures (see Ch. 12), and demyelinating disease (see Ch. 15) should be considered in planning the evaluation. Even when it has been established that a cerebrovascular accident has occurred, the diagnosis is not established until the specific etiology of the cerebrovascular disorder has been identified with a reasonable degree of certainty.

ISCHEMIC CEREBROVASCULAR DISEASE

Age is one major factor to be considered in weighing the relative probabilities of different etiologies for ischemic strokes. Coexisting chronic diseases such as hypertension, diabetes mellitus, peripheral or cardiac atherosclerotic disease, hypercholesterolemia, or cardiac arrhythmias or infarction also provide important clues. In older patients, atherosclerotic vascular and cardiac disease (with secondary cerebral emboli) are overwhelmingly the most common causes of ischemic strokes.

Tests for the Initial Evaluation

Blood Tests

Basic blood tests that should be performed initially on all patients include the complete blood count, platelet count, prothrobin time (PT), partial thromboplastin time (PTT), renal function tests, serum glucose, and calcium. Later, fasting cholesterol and low and high density lipoprotein should be obtained. An immediate ECG with follow-up serial serum creatine phosphokinase (CPK) determinations is important to rule out myocardial infarction as a precipitant of a stroke.

Brain Imaging

In the usual North American clinical setting, every patient who presents with suspected transient ischemic attacks (TIAs) or stroke should have a head computed tomography (CT) scan (or magnetic resonance imaging [MRI]). The CT scan should be obtained immediately and urgently if a hemorrhage, cerebellar infarction, or condition demanding anticoagulation is suspected. Early or small infarcts, neoplasms or abscesses, and demyelinating disease may not be apparent on plain CT, particularly within the first 24 hours. Edema from infarction is maximal between the fourth and seventh days. Follow-up CT studies, both plain and contrast, may define acute lesions on the basis of edema and transient breakdown of the blood-brain barrier.

Angiography in Embolic Disease or Suspected Arterial Dissection

If embolic stroke is strongly suspected, performance of cerebral angiography within the initial 24 hours should be considered if the diagnosis would significantly alter management (e.g., lead to long-term anticoagulation in a patient without another clear indication, such as valvular heart disease). Cerebral emboli are lysed rapidly: 75 percent are seen in the first 48 hours, but only about 10 percent or less if angiography is further delayed.

Arterial dissection may be suspected with the onset of neurologic deficits from within a single large vessel territory associated with tenderness over the appropriate artery. A CT or MRI may show signs of one or more recent ischemic lesions within the territory of the artery. Duplex Doppler studies may demonstrate dissection in the carotid arteries but, in general, cannot be relied on for diagnosis. At present intra-arterial angiography with selective injection of dye into the artery in question is usually necessary. The classic finding is of a sudden tapering of the artery (the string sign) along the area of the dissection. MRI, which well distinguishes flowing from stationary blood or blood clots, can be used to follow the evolution of the dissection after therapy is initiated.

Carotid Duplex Doppler Studies

Patients with suspected or recognized embolic stroke (from artery to artery emboli) should all have bilateral carotid duplex Doppler studies (with particular attention paid to the characteristics of vessel wall plaques). If the duplex Doppler study suggests high-grade stenosis or total occlusion of the carotids in patients with anterior circulation events, angiography should be performed on those in whom the distinction will affect management.

The Lumbar Puncture

A lumbar puncture (LP) can be diagnostically helpful in specialized instances (e.g., suspected primary vasculitis or vasculitis secondary to basal meningitis or suspected multiple sclerosis). Patients with intracranial arterial dissections should undergo LP if immediate anticoagulation is considered: small subarachnoid hemorrhages can occur from the damaged vessel.

Further Diagnostic Tests

Evaluation for Suspected Intermittent Cardiac Arrhythmias

Patients in whom nonspecific ECG abnormalities are present or in whom there is a strongly suggestive history for cardiac infarction or arrhythmias should be considered for Holter monitoring and an echocardiogram if the etiology of the stroke syndrome remains unclear. However, routine transthoracic echocardiography usually misses the majority of blood clots in the heart, particularly those in the left atrial appendage. Vegetations in marantic endocarditis are rarely seen. Patients with documented systemic embolic sources (e.g., deep venous thrombosis) should have a special echocardiographic studies (see Ch. 2) to identify any cardiac structural abnormality that will permit right-to-left transmission of a paradoxic embolus. Ventriculography may be necessary in some cases and remains the gold standard for diagnosis of chamber abnormalities.

Cardiac ultrasound examinations can be difficult and lead to false-negative studies. We are aware of more than one case in which an atrial myxoma was missed by a competent ultrasonographer.

Evaluation for Temporal Arteritis

Temporal arteritis should be considered in elderly patients presenting with stroke, particularly if there is a history of headache, jaw claudication, or diffuse muscle pains. Dramatic elevation of the erythrocyte sedimentation rate (ESR) (around 100 mm/min by the Westergren method) is the most often described routine laboratory finding. However, temporal arteritis with a normal erythrocyte sedimentation rate (ESR) has been well documented: perhaps as many as 5 percent of affected patients may have sedimentation rates within the normal range. A mild normochromic, normocytic anemia and elevations of liver function tests may be seen. Temporal artery biopsy is needed to establish the diagnosis. Unfortunately, because involvement is patchy, there is a significant likelihood that an uninvolved segment may be taken on biopsy. Efforts should be made, therefore, to direct the biopsy using focal tenderness or external carotid angiography to identify involved segments. Biopsy of the contralateral side should be considered if the clinical suspicion is high and an initial biopsy is negative.

EVALUATION OF STROKE IN THE YOUNG PATIENT

Stroke in the young patient presents a special problem because it requires a broader differential diagnosis than that required in elderly patients. Establishing the precise etiology is also more important because prevalence of nonatherosclerotic etiologies and the longer potential lifespan increases the impact of preventive measures. Embolic strokes (particularly cardiac) and arterial dissections are relatively more common causes of stroke in young people (Table 11-2), but fixed vascular disease (e.g., from atherosclerosis) remains frequent. Thus, investigations should begin as described previously. It is only if the routine investigations fail to establish a reasonable diagnosis that more exotic etiologies should be entertained.

The percentage of younger patients with identifiable vasculitides and coagulopathies is higher than in the elderly population, but still probably under 10 percent. Metabolic disorders predisposing to stroke remain rare, even in this population. Migraine can also lead to stroke, although this must remain a diagnosis of exclusion.

Vasculitis

Cerebral vasculitis may be suspected on the basis of systemic abnormalities and involvement of other organs as described later (see Chs. 15 and 16). The diagnosis can often be confirmed by angiography. Occasionally (particularly with isolated CNS vasculitis), a brain and pia biopsy may sometimes be needed to establish evidence for small vessel disease or to confirm that multifocal vessel narrowing arises from inflammatory changes rather than other processes, such as atherosclerosis or lymphomatoid granulomatosis.

Hypercoagulable States

Diagnosis of a primary or secondary hypercoagulable state (Tables 11-3 and 11-4) should be made with the aid of a hematologist. Suspicions may be aroused by historic factors or signs in the peripheral blood smear. Primary hypercoagulable states (Table 11-3) are associated with the lupus anticoagulant and anticardiolipin antibody and deficiencies of proteins C and S and factor XII. The so-called lupus anticoagulant may give a prolonged kaolin-activated PTT (the more common measure of the partial thromboplastin time) that returns to the normal range when measured with a platelet-activated assay. The lupus anticoagulant is associated with a false-positive Venereal Disease Research Laboratory (VDRL) test. A solid phase immunoassay or enzyme-linked immunosorbent assay (ELISA) for the anticardiolipin antibody is available. Note that, although they are associated, there is not an absolute correlation between presence of the lupus anticoagulant and anticardiolipin antibody.

Specific immunologic or functional assays are available for antithrombin II, proteins C and S, and factor XII. The need for both functional and immunologic assays has been demonstrated, particularly for disorders of fibrinolysis in which both quantitative and qualitative disorders of fibrinogen and plasminogen have been found. The hematology laboratory should be contacted before ordering these tests so that blood is sent in the appropriate tubes and the laboratory is aware of any drugs that may affect the assays (e.g., warfarin, which alters protein C and S levels).

Secondary hyperviscosity states (Table 11-4) are associated with several systemic diseases. Serum protein electrophoresis and cryoglobulin levels should identify those rare patients with increased serum proteins (e.g., Waldenström's macroglobulinemia) who do not show other abnormalities.

Homocystinuria

It has been suggested that heterozygotes for homocystinuria may be at an increased risk of early stroke. Quantitative 24-hour urine homocystine excretion after methionine load and serum methionine and homocystine levels may identify this group.

PRIMARY HEMORRHAGIC DISEASE

Primary hemorrhagic disease includes intracerebral, subdural, and epidural hemorrhages. Patients presenting with any of these symptoms should be evaluated rapidly for the presence of a bleeding disorder with CBC and platelets, PT, and PTT.

Brain Imaging

Hemorrhagic disorders are in general best diagnosed by plain CT (see Ch. 10). MRI does not produce good contrast for fresh blood. However, in hemorrhages between 2 and 4 weeks old, blood may be isodense with brain parenchyma and the CT contrast poor. Definition of the lesion by CT relies on observing the mass effect (or local contrast enhancement around the clot if parenchymal). At this stage MRI can define the hematoma (and associated edema if it is intraparenchymal). The specific patterns of the hemorrhagic disorders are described in Chapter 3.

Angiography for Identification of Primary Pathology Leading to Hemorrhagic Disease

Although hypertension is the most common cause, primary intracerebral hemorrhages are frequently secondary to vascular malformations, aneurysms, or tumors (particularly malignant melanomas, choriocarcinomas, and renal cell carcinomas). In patients who are expected to survive with an acceptable neurologic impairment, aggressive efforts to identify the etiology and intervene to prevent recurrent hemorrhage should be made. MRI has an increasingly important role in localizing larger aneurysms or other vascular malformations. MRI angiography is rapidly developing and promises to be especially useful for definition of these types of lesions. However, at present, neither technique is adequate for defining the vascular anatomy well enough to guide therapy.

These patients should almost all have intra-arterial angiography. The timing of angiography depends on the nature of the suspected pathology, the clinical condition of the patient, and the plans for therapy and, therefore, should be planned in consultation with a neurosurgeon. Without angiography, identification of a tumor in a hemorrhagic lesion may be difficult acutely. Follow-up CT (with contrast) or MRI scans after 4 to 6 weeks, by which time much of the clot may have been expected to resolve, should help to identify this pathology.

Elderly patients with superficial lobar hemorrhages may have congophilic amyloid angiopathy. This disease is not amenable to surgical therapy. Thus, when this diagnosis is strongly suggested, angiography is not indicated.

NEOPLASTIC DISEASE

If brain imaging by CT or MRI identifies an intracerebral mass lesion believed to be neoplastic, the most important diagnostic consideration is distinguishing between primary and metastatic disease. A thorough history, physical examination (including rectal examination), CBC, serum electrolytes, calcium, liver function tests, urinalysis, and chest x-ray will help; however, the most rapid, direct, and potentially most useful approach is to make a tissue diagnosis by biopsy of the lesion. Stereoscopic biopsies result in very low morbidity when performed by experienced neurosurgeons. Without biopsy, the distinction between tumor and abscess is often uncertain. Angiography is usually necessary for planning surgical resection or open biopsies of tumors.

BRAIN ABSCESS

Let us reiterate a key point just made: it is usually impossible to distinguish a brain abscess from tumor without a biopsy. It is only in specific instances that biopsy should be delayed or forgone.

Establishing the Etiology of a Brain Abscess

Several important clues to the etiology of an abscess should be investigated. The majority of patients with bacterial brain abscesses have an identifiable primary site of infection: sinusitis, mastoiditis, pneumonia, congenital cardiac septal shunts, head trauma, dental infections, or endocarditis. Focal abscesses in the frontal lobes can arise from infections of the frontal sinuses, those in the anterior temporal lobes from ipsilateral maxillary sinus infection, and those in the cerebellum or more posterior temporal lobes from the ethmoid sinuses. Skull films or CT can usually identify sinus disease.

Multifocal abscesses may arise with bacterial endocarditis and should prompt investigations including CBC, ESR, urinalysis, multiple paired blood cultures over 24 hours and an echocardiogram if the physical examination suggests abnormal cardiac function, blood cultures are positive, or an artificial valve is in place. The possibility of an underlying immunosuppressed state (particularly acquired immune deficiency syndrome [AIDS]) should be considered.

Microbiologic Studies

If a brain abscess is found, material for Gram stain and culture may be obtained from culture of the primary site (e.g., during mastoidectomy for a severe mastoiditis), assiduously collected blood cultures (three paired cultures over 24 hours), or biopsy of the lesion(s) (abscess cavity, capsule, and surrounding tissue).

Frequently, bacterial abscesses have mixed flora. Aerobic organisms commonly found in brain abscesses include streptococci (including *S. pneumoniae* and *S. viridans*), *Haemophilus* species, enterobacteriaceae and *Pseudomonas* species, and in post-traumatic or postoperative cases, staphylococcus (both coagulase-negative and -positive). Anaerobic organisms (peptostreptococci, *Bacterides* species and others) may be isolated from as many as 50 percent of cases. Samples should be obtained in air-tight containers with all of the air expelled and rapidly brought to the laboratory for anaerobic culture.

In the immunocompromised host particularly and other high-risk groups (e.g., those patients from areas where parasites such as Taenia solium are endemic), consideration of fungi (phycomycetes, *Aspergillus, Nocardia*, and *Candida* species) and parasites (*Toxoplasma gondii, Taenia solium, Entamoeba histolytica*, and *Echinococcus* species) should be made. Serum and CSF serologic tests for the toxoplasmosis and cysticercosis are widely available. In some cases (e.g., suspected toxoplasmosis in an AIDS patient), consideration may be given to short-term empiric therapy while monitoring the size of the lesion by CT.

READINGS

Boers GHJ, Smals AGH, Trijbels FJM, et al.: Heterozygosity for homocystinuria in premature peripheral and cerebral occlusive arterial disease. N Engl J Med 313:709, 1985

Caplan LR, Stein RW: Stroke: A Clinical Approach. Butterworth (Publishers), Boston, 1986

Cerebral Embolism Task Force: Cardiogenic brain embolism. Arch Neurol 43:71, 1986

Cosgrove GR, Leblanc R, Meagher-Villemure K, Ethier R: Cerebral amyloid angiopathy. Neurology 35:625, 1985

DeLouvais J, Gortval P, Hurley R: Bacteriology of abscesses of the central nervous system: a multicentre prospective trial. Br Med J 2:981, 1977

Earnest MP: Emergency diagnosis and management of brain infarctions and hemorrhages. p. 127. In Earnest MP (ed): Neurologic Emergencies. Churchill Livingstone, New York, 1983

Exner T, Rickard KA, Kronenberg H: A sensitive test demonstrating lupus anticoagulant and its behavioral patterns. Br J Hematol 40:143, 1978

Grindel AB, Cohen RJ, Saul RF, Taylor JR: Cerebral infarction in young adults. Stroke 9:39, 1978

Jackson AC, Boughner DR, Barnett HJM: Mitral valve prolapse and cerebral ischcemic events in young people. Neurology 34:784, 1984

Jones HR, Caplan LR, Come PC, et al.: Cerebral emboli of paradoxical origin. Ann Neurol 13:314, 1983

Moore PM: Diagnosis and management of isolated angiitis of the central nervous system. Neurology 39:167, 1989

Raskin NH: Headache. Ed. 2. p. 317. Churchill Livingstone, New York, 1988

Samson DS, Clark K: A current review of brain abscess. Am J Med 54:201, 1973

Schafer AI: The hypercoagulable states. Ann Intern Med 102:814, 1985

LABORATORY TESTS FOR EVALUATING SEIZURES 12

Table 12-1. Differential Diagnosis of Seizures

Acquired Metabolic Disorders
Hypoglycemia
Hyponatremia
Hypocalcemia
Uremia
Hypomagnesemia

Infection
Meningitis
Encephalitis
Abscess
Systemic infection (with chronic seizure disorder)

Trauma
Contusion/hemorrhage
Early or delayed post-traumatic epilepsy

Drugs
Low anticonvulsant levels (with chronic seizure disorder)
Withdrawal (e.g., from ethanol, barbiturates, benzodiazepines, opiates, glutethimide)
Intoxication or adverse reaction
- Cocaine
- Amphetamines
- Phencyclidine
- Theophylline
- Tricyclics
- Phenothiazines
- Others

Tumors
Primary
Metastatic

Vascular Disease
Infarct
Hemorrhage
Malformations

Immunologic Disorders
Systemic lupus erythematosus
Vasculitis

Congenital Abnormalities
Perinatal encephalopathy
Neurocutaneous disorders
Identifiable structural defects (e.g., disorders of neuronal migration)

Heritable Metabolic Diseases
(e.g., hexoseaminidase deficiency, mitochondrial encephalopathy)

Primary Generalized Epilepsy
Pseudoseizures

Table 12-2. Evaluation of Seizures

Test	Condition	Notes
Blood Tests		
Serum glucose	Hypoglycemia	Check immediately with fingerstick while waiting for laboratory analysis
CBC	New onset of seizures or loss of seizure control	Systemic infections (causing leukocytosis) may lower seizure threshold for patients with other predisposing conditions (check urine and chest x-ray); CNS infections (meningitis, encephalitis, abscess) should be considered with new-onset seizures
Serum electrolytes	Hyponatremia	Lowers seizure threshold
Serum BUN, Creatinine	Uremia	Lowers seizure threshold; may cause myoclonus
SGOT, SGPT Bilirubin	Chronic seizure disorder	Hepatic toxicity seen with several anticonvulsants; hepatic insufficiency will alter anticonvulsant metabolism
Serum calcium	Hypocalcemia	Low-serum free calcium reduces seizure threshold; free serum calcium may be estimated if albumin is also measured: free calcium (mmol/L) = total serum calcium − albumin (g/dl) × 0.25 + 1.0
Serum magnesium	Hypomagnesemia	Lowers seizure threshold; found particularly in alcoholics
Free T_4, T_3	Dysthyroid state	May lower seizure threshold
Drug levels	Low anticonvulsant levels	Inadequate anticonvulsant levels most common cause of a loss of seizure control in chronic seizure disorders
	Therapeutic drug overdose	Consider particularly overdoses of tricyclics, phenothiazines, theophylline, and lithium as predisposing to seizures

Continued

Table 12-2. *Continued*

Test	Condition	Notes
	Drugs of abuse	Consider drug withdrawal (alcohol, sedatives) and intoxication (phencyclidine, amphetamines, cocaine); urine should be saved for later drug screens
ESR, SPEP anti-ds DNA, rheumatoid factor, C_3, C_4	Vasculitis	An active vasculitis (e.g., SLE) may cause seizures, but seizures would be rare as the sole manifestation; check fresh urine sediment for casts, red cells, and protein to identify renal disease
Serum prolactin	Pseudoseizures	Usually elevated after a true seizure but normal after a pseudoseizure
Lumbar Puncture		
CSF analysis	Idiopathic seizure disorder	A few lymphocytes/mm^3 may be seen after, but more than 5 to 10/mm^3 should suggest another etiology; total protein, glucose and opening pressure should be normal
	CNS infection	CSF leukocytosis is key finding; xanthochromia and red cells may accompany a necrotizing encephalitis; changes in total protein and (depending on etiology) glucose are seen; opening pressure may be increased; see Ch. 9
Radiology		
Chest x-ray	Infection	Systemic infection lowers seizure threshold; in older patients, look for evidence of malignancy
Skull x-ray	Trauma	Skull fracture or other penetrating injury
	Developmental abnormalities	Look for asymmetries in frontal and mastoid sinuses, an abnormally thick calvarium, or an unusually small middle fossa in chronic seizure disorders

Continued

Table 12-2. *Continued*

Test	Condition	Notes
	Neurocutaneous disease	Intracranial calcifications seen in tuberous sclerosis (''popcorn'' calcifications) and Sturge-Weber disease (paragyral calcifications)
CT	Trauma	Contusion and hemorrhage are possible causes of seizures; see Table 11-5
	Infection	Look for an abscess or focal edema from encephalitis; contrast infusion increases sensitivity
	Cerebrovascular disease	Seizures more common with hemorrhages than with infarcts; see Table 11-5; venous thrombosis may show the hypodensity of clot in the sinus with contrast infusion, as well as surrounding edema
	Neoplasm	See Table 11-5
	Neurocutaneous disorders	Sturge-Weber disease classically shows calcification with a paragyral pattern; hamartomas in tuberous sclerosis are hyperdense, often calcified, and nonenhancing with contrast; malignant transformation of the hamartomas is accompanied by contrast enhancement
	Developmental abnormalities	A broad range of structural abnormalities including scarring (particularly in mesial temporal lobes), disorders of neuronal migration, agenesis of the corpus callosum associated with seizure disorders are best shown by MRI
MRI	Infection	Increased sensitivity relative to CT for encephalitis
	Cerebrovascular disease	See Table 11-5

Continued

Table 12-2. *Continued*

Test	Condition	Notes
	Developmental abnormalities	Focal scarring or structural abnormalities best seen with MRI; T_2-weighted images sensitive to gliosis; multiple imaging planes are a second advantage over CT
Angiography	Vascular disease	Defines vascular malformations; "string-of-beads" pattern in vasculitis
	Neoplasm	See Table 11-5
EEG		
	Seizures	Differentiation of focal, secondarily generalized and primary generalized seizure disorder possible; for temporal lobe activity sensitivity is increased with sphenoidal or zygomatic electrode placement
	Pseudoseizures	EEG-video correlation useful; clinically generalized seizure activity without a change in the normal EEG pattern is generally diagnostic of pseudoseizures
Neuropsychological testing		Localization of cognitive defects and lateralization of speech is important if surgical therapy is planned

Further Notes

ACUTE DIAGNOSTIC EVALUATION OF SEIZURES

The diagnosis of seizures is primarily clinical, based on history and (ideally) observation of a fit. Occasionally, laboratory investigations may establish that a problem represents seizures rather than another disorder (e.g., syncope), but the main purpose of clinical laboratory investigations is to establish the etiology of a seizure disorder, the type of seizure (because of therapeutic implications of a precise diagnosis), or (in patients with chronic refractory seizure disorders appropriate for surgical therapy) to precisely localize the seizure focus.

The brief differential diagnosis in Table 12-1 is ordered approximately as we consider potential etiologies when evaluating a patient in the emergency room. Investigations must be directed first toward ruling out life-threatening problems. The patient should be immediately assessed for signs and symptoms of systemic abnormalities (particularly hypoglycemia, electrolyte imbalances, sepsis, hypocalcemia) or CNS infection (meningitis, encephalitis) that may cause seizures. Checking blood sugar with colorimetric indicator paper as blood is drawn for laboratory tests allows immediate diagnosis of hypoglycemia. A lumbar puncture (LP) should be performed to look for evidence of CNS infection in febrile patients with seizures after a CT scan to rule out mass lesions or signs of increased intracranial pressure.

Intoxication with therapeutic drugs (e.g., theophylline) or drugs of abuse (e.g., cocaine) or drug withdrawal (e.g., alcohol) should be considered. Saving initial blood and urine samples for later study may be useful as a routine procedure: often it is only later that the key drug to screen for becomes apparent.

The possibility of new focal neurologic disorders should be considered (e.g., neoplasm, stroke). Each patient with the new onset of seizures should have a head computed tomography (CT) or magnetic resonance imaging (MRI) (see below). The patient's clinical condition determines the urgency with which this should be accomplished. Persistent neurologic deficits make a scan urgently necessary.

Patients with known epilepsy will most commonly present with poor seizure control because of low anticonvulsant levels (important to compare the current level with prior levels in the same patient if available), systemic illnesses, or increased psychological or physical stress (e.g., sleep loss). It is important, therefore, to check them for signs of respiratory or urinary tract infections. However, the possibility of either new pathology or progression of the lesion that initially gave rise to the seizure disorder should be considered as well.

Signs of trauma are often, but not always, clear. Trauma significant enough to cause seizures acutely or subacutely will usually be obvious, but trauma resulting from a seizure may not be. A subdural hematoma may be present with no external manifestations of trauma. Prolonged depression of level of consciousness or focal neurologic signs following a seizure can be indications for urgent CT, even in chronic seizure disorders. If there are signs of head trauma, a cervical spine film may be important to investigate for possible spinal injury.

Many seizure disorders remain idiopathic. However, aggressive longer-term evaluation of a focal seizure disorder will often disclose evidence of an occult chronic lesion (e.g., mesial temporal scarring). Rarely, seizures in combination with other neurologic signs will be a manifestation of one of the heritable metabolic diseases (see Chs. 7 and 8).

USE OF THE EEG IN INVESTIGATION OF SEIZURE DISORDERS

The EEG is a major tool in epilepsy evaluation. However, it is important to appreciate limitations of its role (see Ch. 6). It should be remembered that not all that spikes 'fits', and not all that 'fits' spikes!

Usually only interictal, extradural EEG recordings are available for an initial seizure evaluation. Sensitivity of the EEG for interictal changes is greater sooner (within approximately 2 weeks) after a clinical seizure than later. Activation procedures (hyperventilation, photic stimulation), sleep, the use of multiple recording montages, and prolonged (often ambulatory) monitoring increase sensitivity.

The pattern of EEG abnormalities can be useful in establishing etiology (see Ch. 6). Initially, it is important to distinguish generalized from focal seizure disorders. Generalized seizure disorders with otherwise normal EEG activity and an unremarkable clinical setting are characteristic of forms of primary generalized epilepsy. Diffusely abnormal background activity would suggest a generalized structural or metabolic abnormality giving rise to so-called secondary generalized seizures.

Identification of focal abnormalities on the EEG suggests congenital or acquired structural lesions, although metabolic disorders can also cause focal abnormalities. The nature of any focal abnormalities may also provide an etiologic clue. Polymorphic, asymmetric slow waves suggest a focal subcortical lesion, for example, a tumor. Periodic lateralized epileptiform discharges (PLEDs) or related activity implies relatively acute cortical injury and may be seen, for example, after an embolic stroke or herpes simplex encephalitis.

RADIOLOGIC EVALUATION OF SEIZURES

Imaging plays a major role in the evaluation of seizure disorders. The skull film is often more sensitive than CT for abnormalities of the bone. With the acute onset of seizures and signs of trauma, evidence for skull fractures should be sought. In chronic disorders, maldevelopment of the skull may be used as a clue to underlying brain abnormalities. Radiologic signs, such as enlargement of one or both of the frontal or mastoid sinuses, abnormal thickness of the calvarium, or a small middle fossa, may give clues to unilateral or generalized abnormalities in growth.

As stated earlier, CT or MRI should be obtained on all newly diagnosed seizure disorders. A scan without contrast is useful for ruling out large mass lesions, hemorrhage, or noncommunicating hydrocephalus that would be a significant contraindication to LP and can identify many congenital structural abnormalities. For younger patients (<30 years old), a plain CT scan is often adequate for initial evaluation after a first seizure. Because of the relatively higher risk of neoplasms and stroke in the older population, all patients older than about 30 years should have an infused CT scan or MRI in their initial evaluations. Use of intravenous contrast greatly increases the sensitivity for smaller mass lesions and (after 5 to 7 days) for identification of recent infarcts.

The MRI scan has greater sensitivity for most focal or developmental causes of seizures than does CT. Better gray-white discrimination and the ability to scan in multiple image planes allows superior definition of many developmental abnormalities (e.g., cerebral dysgenesis) in secondary generalized seizures. Focal atrophy is more easily defined than with CT. Hippocampal atrophy and increased signal intensity due to mesial temporal sclerosis can frequently suggest probable lateralization of the seizure focus in complex partial seizure disorders. As moving blood gives a very low intensity signal, vascular malformations can also be visualized.

Positron emission tomography (PET) permits study of regional metabolism and identification of the areas of interictal hypometabolism that have been shown to correlate with epileptogenic areas as determined electroencephalographically. These metabolic abnormalities can occur without accompanying structural lesions apparent on CT or MRI. However, PET is too expensive (and available at too few centers) for routine use. It may have a uniquely useful role in presurgical evaluation of patients with complex partial seizures and uncertain lateralization because of the development of a mirror-focus in the opposite temporal lobe that is electroencephalographically indistinguishable from the primary focus.

MEASUREMENT OF ANTICONVULSANT LEVELS

Measurement of anticonvulsant drug levels can have a major impact on management of seizure disorders, but the information must always be used in conjunction with clinical data. The so-called therapeutic range for these drugs represents statistical summaries of the correlations between drug levels and both therapeutic efficacy and dose-related side-effects in study populations. The upper and lower limits are somewhat arbitrarily defined and cannot be interpreted as marking clear toxic or subtherapeutic levels for any individual patient.

In general, measurement of anticonvulsant levels can be helpful in three ways. First, measuring levels can identify peculiarities in drug metabolism or distribution affecting response to the drugs when they are given at usual doses. Levels can provide some index of drug compliance as well. Second, changes in drug levels in response to physiologic changes in the individual or interactions with other drugs can be assessed. Altered hepatic or renal function, impaired absorption (e.g., postgastrectomy), or malabsorption leading to decreased concentrations of serum proteins that normally bind many of the drugs may give rise to clinically significant changes in the pharmacologically active concentrations of the drugs. Changes in serum concentration may occur during pregnancy and in the immediate postpartum period. Several of the commonly used drugs (e.g., phenobarbital, carbamazepine, primidone, phenytoin) can induce each other's metabolism. Finally, measurement of drug levels can be important for diagnosing dose-related toxicity.

Routine assays measure total serum concentrations. For patients with severe hypoalbuminemia measurement of free (unbound) serum concentrations of carbamazepine, phenytoin, or valproic acid may be needed for accurate estimation of the pharmacologically active amounts.

Useful interpretation of levels for all drug assays demands information on timing of the blood sampling. In order to facilitate adjusting dosage to a level adequate to produce clinical efficacy, trough levels should be obtained by drawing blood just before a dose. Peak levels are needed for assessment of possible toxicity and should be drawn between 1 and 7 hours after administration of an oral dose, depending on the drug used and its form of administration (e.g., carbamazepine, 3 hours; phenobarbital, 1 to 3 hours; phenytoin, 4 to 7 hours; valproic acid tablets, 2 to 6 hours; valproic acid syrup, 0.5 to 1.0 hour). A patient's clinical condition, medications and their dosages, and any recent changes in the medications should also be recorded each time anticonvulsant drug levels are obtained.

Steady-state levels should be measured approximately 3 weeks after initiating therapy with anticonvulsants. If drugs are loaded intravenously (e.g., phenytoin, phenobarbital), serum levels can be measured within a day of initiation of therapy to assess the volume of distribution. In patients on chronic therapy, anticonvulsant levels should be measured about 2 to 3 weeks after any changes in dosage of individual anticonvulsants or other drugs that interact with anticonvulsant metabolism or serum protein binding.

In some cases, metabolites of anticonvulsant drugs have important anticonvulsant or dose-related toxicities. The two most important examples are carbamazepine and primidone. For carbamazepine, measurements of plasma concentrations of both carbamazepine and the breakdown product, carbamazepine-10,11-epoxide, correlate better with both efficacy and toxicity than measurement of carbamazepine concentrations alone. Primidone is metabolized in a dose-dependent fashion to phenobarbital and phenylethylmalonamide, both of which have anticonvulsant activity.

LABORATORY EVALUATION OF SEIZURE PATIENTS FOR SURGICAL THERAPY

Success of surgical treatment for epilepsy relies heavily on the skill with which appropriate patients are selected. The goal of the workup is extended from that of classification of the seizure disorder and establishing its etiology to precise localization of the seizure focus. The variety of issues that need to be addressed are discussed clearly by Andermann (1987). Initial evaluation includes imaging studies as described earlier and EEG on full medication. These tests are helpful in localizing the seizure focus and planning potential surgery.

These studies can be continued for promising patients at a specialized epilepsy surgery center. EEG localization is extended or confirmed using long-term monitoring on reduced medications to correlate ictal and interictal abnormalities. Sphenoidal electrodes are important for defining mesial temporal discharges. Intracranial electrodes may be used when surface recordings suggest bilateral independent temporal discharges and the initiating focus is not clear. The ultimate goal is to establish agreement on localization as independently determined by different modalities. Neuropsychological investigations are used to determine cerebral dominance and the functional integrity of contralateral structures in the brain to help predict whether there is acceptable risk for surgery. These investigations may include intracarotid Amytal testing for lateralization of language and memory.

EVALUATION OF PSEUDOSEIZURES

Pseudoseizures are paroxysmal behavioral alterations that may resemble seizures, but are either consciously or subconsciously controlled by the patient. They are not associated with synchronous neuronal discharges or the other electrophysiologic changes characteristic of seizures. They may be difficult to identify clinically. Many patients with pseudoseizures also experience some real seizures.

The most useful test for diagnosis of pseudoseizures is continuous video monitoring combined with EEG telemetry for periods prolonged enough to record examples of suspected pseudoseizures. Clinically generalized seizures without EEG correlates (no change in baseline activity during ictus, absence of slowing postictally) are *very* rare. A second test is measurement of serum prolactin, which shows a marked rise after an epileptic seizure but will be unchanged after pseudoseizures.

As a group, patients with pseudoseizures may have distinctive psychological and psychiatric profiles, but this cannot be relied on to establish the diagnosis in individual patients; however, neuropsychiatric evaluation may be useful for assessing prognosis and developing therapy once the diagnosis is clear.

READINGS

Andermann F: Identification of candidates for surgical treatment of epilepsy. p. 51. In Engel J Jr (ed): Surgical Treatment of the Epilepsies. Raven Press, New York, 1987

Niedermeyer E: Epilepsy Guide: Diagnosis and Treatment of Epileptic Seizure Disorders, Urban & Schwarzenberg, Baltimore, 1983

Sperling MR, Wilson G, Engel J, et al.: Magnetic resonance imaging in intractable partial epilepsy: correlative studies. Ann Neurol 20:57, 1986

Trimble MR: Serum prolactin in epilepsy and hysteria. Br Med J 2:1682, 1978

MacKichen JJ, Ferrendelli JA, Wilder BJ, (eds): Antiepileptic Drugs (Section 4). p. 209. In Taylor W, Caviness MD (eds): A Textbook for the Clinical Application of Therapeutic Drug Monitoring, Abbott Laboratories, Chicago, 1987

Troupin AS: The measurement of anticonvulsant agent levels. Ann Intern Med 100:854, 1984

LABORATORY TESTS FOR EVALUATING DEMENTIA 13

Table 13-1. Differential Diagnosis of Dementia

Pseudodementia (e.g., depression)

Metabolic and Endocrine
Nutritional (e.g., deficiencies of thiamine, vitamin B_{12}, niacin)
Organ failure (kidneys, liver)
Hypercalcemia
Hypothyroidism
Chronic hypoglycemia
Toxins and drugs

Vascular
Multi-infarct state
Subcortical arteriosclerotic encephalopathy
Vasculitis

Neoplastic/Paraneoplastic
CNS tumor
Limbic encephalitis

Trauma
Subdural hematoma
Dementia pugilistica

Infections
Viral encephalitis or sequelae of viral infection (e.g., HIV-1, SSPE)
Neurosyphilis
Creuzfeldt-Jakob disease
Opportunistic CNS infections in the immunocompromised host
Chronic meningitis

Normal Pressure Hydrocephalus

Degenerative Diseases of Unknown Etiology
Alzheimer's disease
Pick's disease
Huntington's disease
Parkinson's disease
Spinocerebellar degenerations

Heritable Metabolic Diseases (e.g., metachromatic leukodystrophy, mitochondrial disorders)

Table 13-2. Evaluation of Dementia

Test	Condition	Notes
Neuropsychological Testing	Dementia	Global cognitive impairment
	Depression	Primarily affective abnormalities
Blood Tests		
CBC	Malnutrition, or vitamin B_{12} deficiency	Anemia may be present
ESR	Chronic disease, vasculitis	
BUN, Cr	Uremia	
SGOT, SGPT, bilirubin, ammonia	Hepatic insufficiency	Consider possibility of Wilson's or Creuzfeldt-Jakob disease with combined cerebral and hepatic dysfunction
Calcium	Hypercalcemia	Often secondary to malignancy with bony involvement
TSH, free T_4	Hypothyroidism	TSH is the most sensitive index for hypothyroidism; because almost all T_4 is protein-bound, total T_4 measurements are of little value
Serum vitamin B_{12}	B_{12} deficiency	Deficiencies associated with combined central and peripheral nervous system dysfunction
Serum copper and ceruloplasmin	Wilson's disease	Rare cause of dementing illness and movement disorder in young adults; look for abnormal urinary copper excretion, liver function tests, and Kayser-Fleischer rings (see Ch. 7)
Urine		
Renal sediment	Vasculitis	Look for proteinuria and red cell casts
Urine and serum drug screens	Chronic drug overdose or toxin elevations	Must be guided by history

Continued

Table 13-2. *Continued*

Test	Condition	Notes
Serology (Serum or CSF)		
VDRL	Syphilis	Positive in early stages, but may be negative late; serum FTA-ABS remains elevated and has greater specificity than serum VDRL
HIV	AIDS	Specificity of serum test very high; a characteristic AIDS-dementia syndrome arises from HIV infection alone; opportunistic CNS infection or neoplasm may also give cognitive defects
Measles	SSPE	Frequently measles antibody/titer is greatly elevated (1:256 or greater), but not always
Lumbar Puncture		
	Chronic meningitis	Predominantly lymphocytic pleocytosis is most common, with elevated protein and often a depressed glucose; see Ch. 9
	Encephalitis	Protein frequently elevated in chronic viral encephalitis; toxoplasma antigen should be sent from CSF and serum in AIDS patients; measles antibody should be checked in young adults (SSPE); see Ch. 9
	Neurosyphilis	CSF VDRL specific but not sensitive; see Ch. 1
Radiology		
Chest x-ray	Neoplasm, chronic meningitis	Lordotic views or chest CT can increase sensitivity for lung tumors with suspected limbic encephalitis; many infectious etiologies of chronic meningitis have primary lung involvement

Continued

Table 13-2. *Continued*

Test	Condition	Notes
Head CT	Vascular	Bihemispheric, multiple, hypodense regions without mass effect, particularly in the periventricular regions and basal ganglia, may be seen with multi-infarct dementia
	Neoplastic	See Table 11-5
	Trauma	Chronic subdural hematoma (low attenuation from old blood) may resemble dementia syndrome; dementia pugilistica is associated with diffuse subcortical atrophy and cavum septum pellucidum
	Infections	See Table 11-5; communicating hydrocephalus may follow meningitis
	Degenerative disease	Alzheimer's disease shows cortical/subcortical atrophy, often most prominent in frontal and parietal lobes; in Pick's disease more selective frontal and temporal atrophy is seen
	Huntington's disease	Atrophy of the head of the caudate
	Normal pressure hydrocephalus	Periventricular hypodensity, particularly around the frontal horns, with ventriculomegaly (including third ventricle) disproportionate to any generalized atrophy
MRI	Neoplastic	See Table 11-5
	Vascular	Hyperintense signals on T_2-weighted images from chronic infarcts are associated with ventricular enlargement in multi-infarct states; patchy, periventricular hyperintensity is seen with Binswanger's disease but is nonspecific
	Infections	See Tables 9-5, and 9-9

Continued

Table 13-2. *Continued*

Test	Condition	Notes
	Normal pressure hydrocephalus	Periventricular hyperintense signals on T_2-weighted image in addition to the structural changes described for CT
EEG	Metabolic encephalopathy	Diffuse slowing or triphasic waves
	Drugs	Diffuse slowing, often profound; abnormal fast activity seen with benzodiazepines
	Vascular, infectious, or neoplastic disease	May give rise to focal periodic discharges (PLEDs) acutely with slowing in later stages; may generate a seizure focus with epileptiform activity; Creuzfeldt-Jakob disease gives a periodic spiking pattern
	Degenerative diseases	In Alzheimer's disease background activity is relatively well preserved
	Limbic encephalitis	Lateralized temporal slowing, possibly with lateralized periodic spike activity, may be seen
Biopsy		
Brain	Alzheimer's disease	Neuronal loss, neurofibrillary tangles, senile plaques
	Pick's disease	Neuronal swelling, Pick's bodies, Hirano bodies
	Creuzfeldt-Jakob disease	Neuronal loss with spongiform changes
	Encephalitis	Microglial nodules; specific changes for some viruses

Further Notes

ESTABLISHING THE DEMENTIA SYNDROME

Dementia is a progressive cognitive impairment sufficient to interfere with an individual's social interactions or occupation. Features of dementia are associated with a broad range of neurologic and systemic diseases. The list in Table 13-1 is not comprehensive, but is based on a simple classification that is relatively easy to follow. The different classes are ordered approximately as we consider them when approaching a patient.

Perhaps as many as 10 percent of patients presenting with dementia have a reversible cause. A greater percentage will have a treatable cause. Neurologic evaluation should be directed primarily at identifying this group.

It is important to establish initially that the patient is actually demented. Patients with focal disorders of expression or comprehension may be mislabeled as demented by unsophisticated observers. Sometimes more difficult to identify are patients with a primary depressive disorder and other forms of pseudodementia (focal impairments of attention or cerebral processes that may mimic more global cognitive impairment).

Several neuropsychological tests are available to help establish whether the primary problem is pseudodementia. The Folstein Mini-Mental Status Examination may be sufficient for routine office use, but it is so limited in scope that it may be misleading. Psychological consultants should be asked to administer and interpret more sophisticated tests when the clinical presentation is unclear. Serial testing of patients occasionally can be useful to provide an objective measure of response to any interventions.

EVALUATION OF THE OLDER DEMENTED PATIENT

In elderly patients, degenerative disease is the most common cause of dementia. Alzheimer's disease is found in at least 50 to 60 percent of dementing older adults. Multi-infarct states are also a common cause of dementia in this age group.

Tests for Metabolic, Endocrine, and Nutritional Disorders

Toxic and metabolic causes are the most important potentially reversible causes of the dementia syndrome and should be carefully sought. Toxic confusional states and other forms of delirium can be indistinguishable from chronic dementias, particularly in hospitalized patients observed for a relatively short time. Potential contributions of therapeutic drugs (e.g., narcotics, anti-Parkinson agents), metabolic (electrolyte abnormalities, uremia, hepatic insufficiency) and endocrine (e.g., thyroid function) abnormalities, or nutritional deficiencies (thiamine, niacin, vitamin B_{12}) should be considered (see also Ch. 10). The clinical history and examination are of great importance here. A reasonable set of screening tests includes the complete blood count (CBC), serum electrolytes, glucose, blood urea nitrogen (BUN), creatinine, serum glutamic-oxaloacetic transaminase (SGPT), vitamin B_{12} level, thyrotropin stimulating hormone (TSH), free T_4, and T_3. For hypothyroidism resulting from the most common etiologies, the serum TSH level is by far the most sensitive screen. However, note that in the rare secondary (pituitary) or tertiary (hypothalamic) hypothyroidism, the TSH is low.

The effects of these factors are extremely variable and interdependent. It is impossible, for example, to establish, in any but the crudest way, reliable indices for degrees of uremia or hepatic insufficiency below which significant cognitive impairment is unlikely in any individual.

The effects of drugs are also difficult to predict. The pharmacokinetics and the range side-effects of drugs are often profoundly different in elderly and young adults. Empiric trials of withdrawal may be necessary for establishing their CNS effects.

Brain Imaging

It is useful to obtain a head computed tomography (CT) or magnetic resonance imaging (MRI) scan to assist diagnosis of all dementing patients. Head CT is adequate for defining the presence of multiple infarcts and most other focal abnormalities not characteristic of Alzheimer's disease. Identification of diffuse bihemispheric subcortical arteriosclerotic disease leading to chronic encephalopathy (Binswanger's type disease or leukoariosis) has become more frequent with MRI. T_2-weighted images show multifocal and confluent periventricular areas of hyperintense signal, prominent particularly around the frontal horns. These changes are nonspecific, however, and may occur in asymptomatic subjects or in other diseases (e.g., normal pressure hydrocephalus). CT may show decreased attenuation in the same distribution, but is much less sensitive.

Electroencephalography

We believe an EEG can also be helpful routinely in identifying characteristics not consistent with the usual degenerative processes. In Alzheimer's disease, background activity is relatively well preserved and focal abnormalities should not be present.

Lumbar Puncture and Microbiologic and Serologic Tests

Chronic meningitides can present as dementing illness, although this is not common. A lumbar puncture (LP) is an important part of a complete evaluation and should be performed if the patient history or the clinical examination suggest. Microbiologic tests are described in Ch. 9.

Neurosyphilis has historically been an important acquired cause of dementia, although we have not seen a clear example in recent years. Serologic testing for syphilis can be confusing. The most widely used serum tests are the VDRL (Venereal Disease Research Laboratory) or RPR (Rapid Plasma Reagin) tests for the presence of nonspecific antigens associated with treponemal infection, but these are not the most sensitive tests. As many as one-third of primary or late cases will be negative in serum. False-positive serum tests are also not uncommon.

The serum FTA-ABS (fluorescent treponemal antibody absorption) test is both more specific and more sensitive. The sensitivity, even for late syphilis, approaches 100 percent; and therefore it should always be used (even initially) when tertiary syphilis is suspected clinically. Its use with CSF is controversial. A positive CSF FTA-ABS may be highly sensitive for neurosyphilis, but is not very specific. Many laboratories will not perform the test on CSF because of this. Although insensitive, the VDRL test is preferred for CSF becuse it is very specific.

Evaluation for Normal Pressure Hydrocephalus

Occasionally the troubling problem is encountered of ruling out the possibility that a patient with dementia, incontinence, and a gait disorder is suffering the potentially reversible syndrome of normal pressure hydrocephalus (NPH). In general, empiric shunt placement is not warranted, as even this "minor" neurosurgical procedure is associated with a significant number of complications.

Imaging can be suggestive, but not diagnostic. Key features to note on CT or MRI include (1) ballooning of the lateral and third ventricles (the fourth ventricle is not always proportionally enlarged, in which case it is necessary to visualize a patent aquaduct using sagittal MRI; (2) enlargement of the ventricles disproportionate to the degree of diffuse atrophy indicated by dilation of sulci over the convexity; (3) little or no gyral atrophy around the falx; and (4) transependymal edema (shown on MRI as a periventricular halo of increased signal intensity on T_2-weighted images and as decreased attenuation in the same distribution by CT, although CT is much less sensitive to the changes than is MRI).

Drainage of lumbar CSF may be performed, in an effort to lower opening pressure to 5 to 10 cmH_2O, with close observation for signs of improvement that are predictive of a good response to shunt placement. Some experts have advocated assessing compliance of the subarachnoid space by saline infusion; decreased compliance is associated with NPH.

Neoplastic Disease

Cerebral neoplasms may cause forms of pseudodementia from local cerebral dysfunction (e.g., frontal tumors). Diagnostic evaluation of these disorders is discussed in Chapter 11. Patients with neoplastic disease outside of the CNS may have secondary dementias from metabolic derangements, nutritional deficiencies, secondary systemic or CNS infection, or the rare paraneoplastic syndrome of limbic encephalitis. The EEG may show temporal epileptiform or slow-wave activity with the latter.

EVALUATION OF DEMENTIA IN YOUNGER PATIENTS

Evaluation of dementing illnesses in middle-aged or younger patients should be much more aggressive, as it is less likely that they are suffering from premature degenerative illnesses. The possibilities of acquired metabolic or toxic disorders, vascular or mass lesions (leading to a pseudodementia marked by more focal than generalized impairment of cerebral processes), or chronic CNS infection as described earlier (see Ch. 9) should be considered first. The most prominent infectious etiology of dementia is now human immunodeficiency virus (HIV) encephalopathy or HIV-related opportunistic infection (see Ch. 9). Serologic testing for HIV should be performed on all younger patients with an unexplained dementing illness.

Subacute Sclerosing Panencephalitis and Creuzfeldt-Jakob Disease

With appropriate presentations, many more rare infectious disorders, such as subacute sclerosing panencephalitis (SSPE) or Creuzfeldt-Jakob disease, should be considered. In SSPE, the EEG usually demonstrates the characteristic periodic bursts of 2 to 3 Hz high-voltage sharp waves, and measles antibody titers are often elevated in the CSF. Nonspecific markers of CNS inflammation, such as oligoclonal bands and IgG, may be very high.

Early diagnosis of Creuzfeldt-Jakob disease can be difficult because its incidence is so low. EEG is currently the most useful noninvasive test. It classically shows diffuse, periodic high-voltage synchronous sharp waves (at about 1 Hz). They often occur within 12 weeks of presentation and can eventually be seen in almost all patients. In very early or late stages, fewer individuals show this pattern.

At present, the most specific test is brain biopsy, but a high index of suspicion is necessary to justify this procedure. Neuropathologic examination shows neuronal loss, spongiform changes in the brain, and gliosis. The pathologic changes can be relatively focal, but are frequently in the temporal lobes (a common biopsy site).

The identification of specific Creuzfeldt-Jakob-associated proteins in CSF may eventually provide an improved diagnostic method.

Congenital Abnormalities and Heritable Metabolic Disease

Longstanding static or progressive neurologic problems suggest a congenital malformation or inherited metabolic disease, respectively. The range of such disorders is enormous, and we will not attempt to present them here. Inherited neurologic diseases with defined biochemical or pathologic causes leading to early dementia include but are not limited to late manifestations of autosomal recessive disorders such as neuronal ceroid-lipofuscinosis, metachromatic leukodystrophy, adrenoleukodystrophy, Gerstmann-Sträussler syndrome, Neimann-Pick disease, GM_2 gangliosidosis, and polyglucosan body disease (see Ch. 7). However, none of these diseases give rise to dementia in the absence of other neurologic signs.

READINGS

Davis LE, Schmitt JW: Clinical significance of cerebrospinal fluid tests for neurosyphilis. Ann Neurol 25:50, 1989

Gabuzda DH, Hirsch MS: Neurologic manifestations of infection with human immunodeficiency virus. Ann Intern Med 107:383, 1987

Harrington MG, Merril CR, Asher DM, Gadjusek DC: Abnormal proteins in the cerebrospinal fluid of patients with Creuzfeldt-Jakob disease. N Engl J Med 315:279, 1986

Huppert FA, Tym E: Clinical and neuropsychological assessment of dementia. Br Med Bull 42:11, 1986

Katzman R, Hussey F: A simple constant-infusion manometric test for measurement of CSF absorption. Neurology 20:534, 1970

Kiloh LG: The secondary dementias of middle and later life. Br Med Bull 42:106, 1986

McKhann G, Drachman D, Folstein M, et al.: Clinical diagnosis of Alzheimer's disease: report of the NINCDS-ADRDA Work Group Neurology 34:939, 1984

Strub RL, Black FW: The Mental Status Examination in Neurology. 2nd Ed. FA Davis, Philadelphia, 1985

LABORATORY TESTS FOR EVALUATING MYELOPATHIES 14

Table 14-1. Differential Diagnosis of Myelopathies

Compressive

Traumatic (with or without fracture/dislocation) disorders of spinal column or craniovertebral junction with:
- Disc herniation
- Spondylosis, spondylolisthesis
- Congenital anomalies, basilar invagination, abnormalities of the odontoid

Mass lesion (extramedullary or intramedullary)
- Neoplastic (e.g., epidural tumor, meningioma)
- Infectious (e.g., epidural abscess)

Hemorrhage (e.g., spinal epidural hematoma, vascular malformations, iatrogenic)

Noncompressive

Primary demyelinating disease
- Multiple sclerosis
- Postinfectious
- Postvaccinial
- Idiopathic transverse myelitis

Inflammatory
- Viral (HIV, HTLV-1, herpes simplex, herpes zoster, CMV)
- Spirochetal (syphilis)
- Other (chronic adhesive arachnoiditis, paraneoplastic)

Vascular
- Infarction
- Vascular malformation
- Vasculitis
- Postirradiation

Syringomyelia

Nutritional
- Vitamin B_{12} or E deficiency

Inherited disease
- Familial spastic paraparesis
- Myelopathy with other neurologic abnormalities (e.g., spinocerebellar degeneration, polyglucosan body disease)

Table 14-2. Evaluation of Myelopathies

Test	Condition	Notes
Blood Tests		
CBC	Vitamin B_{12} deficiency	Megaloblastic anemia
	Abscess or myelitis	Leukocytosis, often with anemia of chronic disease
PT, PTT	Epidural hemorrhage	Blood dyscrasia or anticoagulant therapy can predispose to epidural hemorrhage
ESR	Epidural abscess, vasculitis	Nonspecific
Serum vitamin B_{12} level	Subacute combined degeneration	Low serum B_{12} is also associated with a neuropathy; if low, consider a Schilling test to identify malabsorption
Serology		
VDRL	Syphilis	In tertiary stages serum VDRL may be negative, but serum FTA-ABS remains abnormal; CSF VDRL is relatively specific for neurosyphilis
Other	Inflammatory myelitis	Numerous viral causes can be considered: HIV, herpes zoster, herpes simplex, coxsackievirus A and B; Lyme disease should be considered in endemic areas; acute and convalescent titers should be obtained

Continued

Table 14-2. *Continued*

Test	Condition	Notes
Lumbar Puncture		
CSF analysis: cellularity; cytology; glucose; protein	Multiple causes	May be deferred until after imaging in many cases; if a myelogram is performed, CSF must be obtained before dye injection; increased cellularity suggests inflammation; abnormal cytology characteristic of neoplasms, particularly with xanthochromia, depressed glucose, and very high protein; lesions that compress the subarachnoid space lead to a low opening pressure (<8 mmHg); red cells with xanthochromia suggest infarction or hemorrhage
CSF oligoclonal bands	Demyelinating disease	Although supporting the diagnosis of spinal MS, they are not specific and may be seen with other inflammatory conditions, both primary (e.g., viral myelitis) and secondary (e.g., infarction)
CSF immunoglobulins	Demyelinating disease	Calculate CSF IgG index; nonspecific as oligoclonal bands
Radiology		
Skull films	Craniocervical junction abnormalities	Look for congenital deformities such as platybasia or signs of a metabolic bone disorder such as Paget's disease
Spine films	Cervical spondylosis	Look for narrowing of canal to <12 mm, osteophytes and spurs, disc degeneration, loss of normal cervical lordosis, and vertebral collapse

	Neoplastic or infectious disease	Neoplastic disease classically involves destruction of the vertebral body with either sclerotic or lytic changes; infection usually leads to disc space destruction if it affects the spine itself
	Trauma	Vertebral collapse and subluxation may be seen, particularly in association with osteoporosis
	Atlantoaxial dislocation	Particularly associated with rheumatoid arthritis; flexion/extension views define maximum movement of odontoid (normally <3 mm from posterior aspect of C1 anterior arch), which, if increased, can cause myelopathy; open mouth view of C1-C2 joint helpful
Myelography		Either myelography or MRI of spinal cord should be performed urgently in suspected rapidly progressive spinal cord compression; when ordering, recall the variable relation between the level of the spinal segment and the vertebral body (see Fig. 4-3). Thus, compression will cause a sensory level below the vertebral body involved; always obtain CSF for study before dye is injected
CT	Degenerative diseases	Canal diameter relative to that of cord is easily assessed; examination may be improved with combined use of subarachnoid dye (i.e., following a myelogram)
	Neoplastic infectious disease	Defines bony destruction and soft tissue masses

Continued

Table 14-2. *Continued*

Test	Condition	Notes
MRI	Cervical spondylosis	Sagittal images provide the best visualization of craniocervical junction with good definition of cord and CSF space in T_1-weighted images; T_2-weighed images more clearly define the CSF but may exaggerate the apparent degree of compression
	Disc protrusion	T_2-weighted images define the path of CSF flow well but often overestimate any blockage of CSF flow
	Intramedullary lesions	Intramedullary lesions are well demonstrated on T_2-images, particularly with MRI contrast agent; an associated syrinx may be defined; better than CT for intramedullary lesions
	Demyelinating disease	With cardiac gating and rapid acquisition cycles intramedullary plaques may be seen in patients with spinal MS; the majority also have cerebral white matter lesions, so a head MRI should also be ordered
	Vascular malformations	Often well visualized in sagittal views as areas of abnormally decreased signal from flowing blood (flow void)
Spinal angiography	Neoplastic	Definition of vascular supply needed for planning surgical excision of primary tumors

	Vascular malformation	Localization of lesions and characterization of blood flow can sometimes be combined with therapeutic embolization
Electrophysiologic		
Electromyography	Compressive myelopathy	Radiculopathies are frequently found at site of lesion with lateral compression of nerve roots; denervation changes over multiple myotomes can result from secondary vascular compromise
	Necrotizing myelopathy	Denervation changes in affected myotomes may identify anterior horn cell death and secondary axonal degeneration associated with necrotizing myelopathies
Somatosensory evoked potentials		Can identify posterior column dysfunction; most useful when presence of myelopathy uncertain
Visual evoked potentials	Demyelinating disease	May provide evidence for a second site of white matter abnormality (optic nerve) when multifocal CNS disease is being considered

Further Notes

EVALUATION OF ACUTE OR SUBACUTE MYELOPATHIES

Evaluation of a myelopathy must proceed quickly if symptoms are acute and progressive. Although a full differential diagnosis must be considered in ordering investigations (Table 14-1), attention must be focused initially on whether a rapidly reversible etiology can be found. In practice, this means localizing a lesion, determining whether a compressive lesion is causing the problem, and then establishing its etiology. Laboratory investigations are helpful for each of these tasks.

In addition to the general and neurologic examination, blood tests (complete blood count [CBC], Sequential Multiple Analyzer Computer [SMAC] panel, prothrombin time [PT], partial thromboplastin time [PTT], and, in older men, prostatic acid phosphatase), chest radiograph, and local spine films should be obtained to establish evidence for a possible bony structural lesion or systemic disorder that may affect plans for later procedures. A computed tomography (CT) scan, myelogram, or magnetic resonance imaging (MRI) scan of the area is indicated.

Computer Tomography of the Spine

Fine-transverse CT cuts through the spine can usually define disc herniation or bony changes well without dye in the subarachnoid space. The degree of cord compression is more directly appreciated when dye is present, making CT a useful adjunct to conventional myelography. CT can also be used to identify a spinal epidural abscess or lipomas. However, if the level of dysfunction is unclear, CT may not be useful, as it is practical to study only a limited area.

When correlating clinical and radiologic findings it is important to recall the variable relationships between the vertebral bodies, levels in the spinal cord, and root exit sites as one proceeds from the cervical to the sacral spinal cord (see Ch. 4). The area of the spinal cord adjacent to a given vertebral body in the lower cervical to lower thoracic spine supplies roots that exit one or two foramina more caudally. Cord levels T12–S5 are behind vertebral bodies T10–L2. Incomplete lesions may cause neurologic deficits at levels much more caudal to their location because of the lamination of pathways in the spinal cord.

Magnetic Resonance Imaging of the Spine

In contrast to CT, which defines bony structures best, MRI allows direct visualization of soft tissue. Pathways of CSF flow can be demonstrated in T_2-weighted sagittal images, but the degree of obstruction of CSF flow may be exaggerated in the T_2-weighted images. Both intra-axial and extra-axial neoplastic tissue, edema, demyelination, spinal epidural abscesses or lipomas, syrinx cavities, and stationary and flowing blood can all be characterized with appropriate pulse sequences and use of MRI contrast agents. Resolution is good, even in the lumbar area, with use of a surface coil. Finally, MRI is noninvasive. Thus, if available, it is the test of choice for initial evaluation of stable acute myelopathies except those suspected to result from bony compression (e.g., post-traumatic) of the cord. The suspected pathology should be discussed with the radiologist before the scan is obtained to allow for optimal imaging sequences. However, optimal resolution of nontumoral extradural lesions outside the craniocervical junction may demand CT myelography. Head MRI may be a useful test for recognition of multiple sclerosis presenting as a myelopathy.

Myelography

Metrizamide myelography has until recently been the standard method for evaluation of all lesions of the cord. Disadvantages of this procedure include the following: (1) Visualization of many lesions is imperfect (particularly for intramedullary lesions) because contrast is poor for the soft tissues and (2) introduction of dye may cause worsening of symptoms or an allergic reaction. However, because it defines bony structures so well (particularly when combined with CT), it has significant advantages over MRI for evaluation of suspected nontumoral, extradural lesions.

If myelography is performed, it is important to obtain samples of CSF at the time of myelography before dye infusion. The mild inflammatory reaction from dye after a myelogram may elevate the CSF protein and cell count for weeks.

Cerebrospinal Fluid Analysis

CSF analysis may help in the differential diagnosis, despite its lack of specificity. CSF studies are helpful particularly when demyelinating disease or meningeal carcinomatosis is suspected. Significant cellularity suggests an ongoing inflammatory process. More than about 40 leukocytes/mm^3 makes demyelinating disease less likely and more than 100 leukocytes/mm^3 makes it very unlikely. A high total protein (>70 to 100 mg/dl) makes moderate compression from degenerative changes in the spine (unless significant cord necrosis has begun) and demyelinating disease unlikely. Low glucose may be found with meningeal spread of malignancy.

EVALUATION OF CHRONIC MYELOPATHIES

Because chronic myelopathies present and evolve less dramatically, clinical signs are frequently more subtle. Laboratory investigations have a potentially wider role than in acute myelopathies; they may be important for confirming the clinical diagnosis. They may be needed for determining localization of the lesion. They are also helpful in distinguishing among a broader range of possibilities in the differential diagnosis than may be commonly encountered with acute myelopathies.

Degenerative Disease and Other Causes of Extra-axial Compression

Evaluation should begin with spine films. Normal vertebral column diameters are between 16 and 22 mm in the cervical and thoracic cord. Narrowing to less than 12 mm in the cervical cord suggests cervical spondylosis. Accompanying degenerative changes (intravertebral disc narrowing, osteophytes, spurs) are characteristic. However, abnormalities must be interpreted with caution, as the incidence of all of these changes in asymptomatic patients is relatively high. Electromyography (EMG) studies may identify focal radicular denervation that can help localize a lesion responsible for a myeloradiculopathy. Myelography with CT or MRI should be used as described earlier to confirm any suspected extradural compression.

Skull films, cervical spine films, and sagittal MRI of the cervical spine and head can define congenital or acquired lesions of the craniocervical junction (e.g., platybasia, basilar invagination, atlantoaxial dislocation).

In the absence of congenital or degenerative diseases it should be remembered that some indolent extra-axial neoplasms (e.g., meningiomas, neuromas) can present as chronic myelopathies.

Multiple Sclerosis and Infectious Encephalomyelopathies

Myelopathies that clearly do not arise from extra-axial compression may present a difficult diagnostic challenge. Inflammatory and demyelinating lesions frequently show an elevated CSF IgG, an elevated IgG index, and positive oligoclonal bands. Efforts should be made to try to demonstrate more directly multifocal inflammatory disease in the CNS, the sine qua non of demyelinating disease. An abnormal visual evoked response (VER) may give evidence for multifocal CNS disease if a single lesion is demonstrated elsewhere clinically or by MRI. MRI of the head and spine will often demonstrate lesions consistent with focal myelitis or multifocal central demyelinating disease. Because of the relatively small size of the spinal cord and movement artifacts, MRI is more likely to demonstrate evidence for demyelinating disease in the brain that in the spinal cord.

Serologic screening tests will be increasingly important as the incidence of identified infectious encephalomyelopathies increases. The possibility of HIV-related infection must always be considered now and a careful clinical search for other manifestations should be made. Patients from the Caribbean particularly should be tested for HTLV-1 antibodies. Other viral causes of encephalomyelopathies (which include coxsackievirus, echovirus, herpes simplex, cytomegalovirus (CMV), and herpes zoster) present acutely or subacutely.

Intra-axial Tumors

Intra-axial tumors (e.g., ependymomas, astrocytomas) are best seen with MRI, where they appear as areas of increased signal intensity (from tumor and associated edema) on T_2-weighted images. The bulk of the cord is almost always increased locally. Sensitivity is increased with use of MRI contrast agents. Local enlargement of the cord can be appreciated by myelography (particularly when combined with postmyelogram axial CT cuts) if MRI is not available.

The Syringomyelic Syndrome

The syringomyelic syndrome has a distinctive clinical presentation, but specific diagnosis of the underlying abnormality can be challenging. MRI is the initial test of choice, as any syrinx fluid will have significantly different relaxation properties than the adjacent spinal cord and is usually well defined by T_2-defined images. An associated tumor or craniocervical junction abnormality can also be defined using sagittal cervical cord images. However, delayed CT images of the cord after infusion of the water soluble dye into the subarachnoid space may also show a syrinx in transverse sections as a focal accumulation of dye (reaching the syrinx by diffusion) in the central cord. A more specific diagnosis may be made by needle aspiration of syrinx contents under radiologic guidance: a very high protein level, particularly in association with abnormal cytology, is characteristic of a cavitation within a neoplasm.

Vascular Malformations

Vascular malformations may be diagnosed by myelography. The diagnostic yield is increased with supine views to visualize the dorsal aspect of the cord. However, MRI is more sensitive and less invasive. Flowing blood in vascular malformations results in good contrast with surrounding normal tissue because of the MRI flow void (see Ch. 3). Spinal angiography may be necessary to define flow characteristics of malformations and to identify the local vascular anatomy in preparation for surgery or embolization. The study is ideally directed to a specific site as a complete spinal angiogram may take several hours. For this reason, as well as the risks associated with the test, it should be reserved for appropriate lesions first demonstrated by myelography or MRI.

Spinal Arachnoiditis

In patients with an appropriate history of spinal surgery, myelography, hemorrhage, infection, or intrathecal drug administration, the possibility of arachnoiditis should be considered. The inflammatory process involves both roots and cord, so EMG studies may be helpful in defining the extent of the radicular component of the disease. CT with infusion of the cord may show local meningeal and reactive tissue enhancement. MRI can demonstrate loculation of the CSF, aggregation of lumbar roots, and irregular constriction of the cord by fibrous bands.

Nutritional Deficiencies

Subacute combined deficiency is the major acquired metabolic cause of myelopathy. Laboratory characterization rests primarily on demonstration of a vitamin B_{12} deficiency and peripheral neuropathy by nerve conduction studies. Neurologic symptoms may precede hematologic manifestations. The serum vitamin B_{12} level is not always decreased. Increased urinary methylmalonic acid levels may be more specific, but the assay is difficult to perform. A Schilling test should be performed, as malabsorption of vitamin B_{12} is the most common etiology.

Malabsorption states can lead to vitamin E deficiency, usually in association with deficiencies of fat soluble vitamins. Red cells that have spiked membranes and are known as acanthocytes may be seen on wet smears of peripheral blood. Serum vitamin E levels can be measured. A malabsorption state can be established by quantitative analysis of a sample of fresh stool (usually obtained after a period of 2 to 3 days on a defined high-fat diet) for fats. Vitamin E deficiency is also found in hereditary abetalipoproteinemia. Serum cholesterol lipoprotein levels are abnormally low in this disorder and may be used as a screening test.

Inherited Diseases

Several inherited diseases present with prominent myelopathic features, although usually other signs are present on examination, suggesting more widespread disease. Idiopathic disorders, such as Friedreich's ataxia or hereditary spastic paraparesis, are currently defined primarily by clinical features. Some storage disorders such as polyglucosan body disease may show dramatically abnormal signal intensity from white matter with head MRI. A few disorders of white matter have specific, defined metabolic abnormalities (e.g., adrenomyeloneuropathy, metachromatic leukodystrophy) and can be diagnosed noninvasively. Diagnostic tests for many of these rare disorders are discussed in Chapter 7. Others, such as Kufs disease (neuronal ceroid lipfuscinosis) have characteristic pathologic abnormalities on nerve or skin biopsies (see Ch. 8). Brain biopsies may sometimes be necessary for diagnosis.

READINGS

Goldstick L, Mandybur TI, Bode R: Spinal cord degeneration in AIDS. Neurology 35:103, 1985

Miska RM, Pojunas KW, McQuiller MP: Cranial magnetic resonance imaging in the evaluation of myelopathy of undetermined etiology. Neurology 37:840, 1987

Ropper AH, Poskanzer DC: The prognosis of acute and subacute transverse myelopathy based on early signs and symptoms Ann Neurol 4:51, 1978

Vernant JC, Maurs L, Gessain A, et al.: Endemic tropical spastic paraparesis associated with human T-lymphotropic virus type I: A clinical and seroepidemiological study of 25 cases. Ann Neurol 21:123, 1987

LABORATORY TESTS FOR EVALUATING MULTIFOCAL CNS DISEASE

15

Table 15-1. Differential Diagnosis of Suspected Multifocal Nervous System Disease

Demyelinating Disease
Multiple sclerosis
Other

Vascular Disease
Embolic
  Cardiac disease
Vasculitic
  Systemic vasculitis/autoimmune disease (e.g., PAN, SLE)
  Isolated CNS angiitis

Infection
Multiple abscesses
Neurosyphilis
Lyme neuroborreliosis

Neoplasm
Metastatic tumors

Idiopathic
Behçet syndrome
Sarcoidosis

Posterior Fossa and Craniovertebral Junction Lesions
Can be confused with multifocal disease (e.g., brainstem gliomas, cerebellar tumors, extra-axial lesions, Chiari malformations)

Inherited/Metabolic Disorders
Can sometimes resemble multifocal CNS disease (e.g., leukodystrophies, multisystem degenerations, polyglucosan body disease)

Table 15-2. Evaluation of Multifocal CNS Disease[a]

Test	Condition	Notes
Lumbar Puncture		
CSF analysis	Multiple sclerosis	Minimal pleocytosis (usually <5 to 10 WBC/mm^3, sometimes up to 40 WBC/mm^3); total protein normal or only mildly elevated; glucose normal; elevated total immunoglobulins and CSF IgG index; positive oligoclonal bands
	Vasculitis	Variable findings; CSF studies may be normal or may show significant leukocytosis and elevated total protein
	Abscesses/neoplasms	CSF may be abnormal, but usually acellular and not diagnostic
	Sarcoidosis	Rare cause of CNS disease; modest leukocytic pleocytosis may be seen (eosinophilia possible); total protein usually elevated; most patients have lung involvement; serum angiotensin-converting enzyme (ACE) may also be elevated
Electrophysiology		
VER		May allow identification of dysfunction (often subclinical) of the optic pathway; sensitive to small lesions of the optic nerve and can be a useful complement to MRI
BAER		May identify and localize dysfunction of brainstem auditory pathway between cochlear nucleus and medial geniculate body
SEP		Identification of dysfunction in posterior column-medial lemniscal pathways (trigeminal-medial lemniscal pathways with trigeminal stimulation)

[a] See also Tables 11-2, 14-2, and 15-3.

Continued

Table 15-2. *Continued*

Test	Condition	Notes
Blink reflex		Responses may be abnormal with lesions between the mid-pons and the high medulla
Radiology		
Head CT	Multiple sclerosis	Large acute lesions may show contrast enhancement for several weeks
	Infarcts/vasculitis	Multifocal hypodensities consistent with infarcts (usually in territories supplied by small vessels) may be seen on a plain scan; possible contrast enhancement around recent ischemic lesions
	Abscesses	Multifocal bacterial abscesses (ring-enhancing hypodensities) may be seen with embolic disease from subacute bacterial endocarditis; immunocompromised patients may have multifocal parasitic (e.g., toxoplasmosis) or fungal abscesses
	Posterior fossa lesions	Poorly visualized by CT; look for distortion of the fourth ventricle, tumors, structural anomalies, vascular malformations
	Sarcoidosis	Basal meningeal contrast enhancement may be seen
MRI	Multiple sclerosis	Diagnostic method of choice for identification of multifocal white matter lesions, which appear as focal areas of increased signal on T_2-weighted scans; periventricular location, particularly involving the corpus callosum, is characteristic; specificity is increased when infratentorial lesions are seen; sagittal T_1-weighted images may define irregular atrophy at the corpus callosum

Continued

Table 15-2. *Continued*

Test	Condition	Notes
	Abscesses	Sensitivity to changes associated with edema is higher than with CT
	Posterior fossa lesions	Test of choice for visualization of lesions in the posterior fossa; look for tumors, structural anomalies, vascular malformations
	Craniocervical junction abnormalities	Sagittal MRI of the craniocervical junction is method of choice for visualization of this area
Angiography	Vasculitis	Characteristic string-of-beads appearance from irregular narrowing of arteries
Urodynamic Testing		
	Multiple sclerosis	Before considering these tests, urinalysis and culture and measurement of residual volumes should be obtained; urinary flow rates, cystometry, ± sphincter electromyography should then be ordered for evaluation of still unexplained urinary symptoms (see text)

Table 15-3. Blood and Urine Tests for Vasculitis in Multifocal CNS Disease

Blood Tests	Notes
CBC	Anemia (often Coombs positive), leukopenia, and thrombocytopenia may be seen
ESR	May be elevated
BUN, Cr	Elevated with secondary renal dysfunction
Serum albumin	Decreased in chronic disease, particularly when proteinuria is present
Blood cultures	Positive in subacute bacterial endocarditis

Continued

Table 15-3. *Continued*

Blood Tests	Notes
Immunologic Tests	
FANA	A screening test for collagen-vascular diseases that becomes more specific at higher titers, although several drugs (including carbamazepine, ethosuximide, phenytoin, and primidone) cause false positive tests; the pattern of immunofluorescence has some diagnostic significance (e.g., homogeneous for SLE and nucleolar pattern for Sjögren's syndrome)
Anti-ds DNA, anti Sm-antibodies	Relatively specific for SLE
Anti-Ro, anti-La antibodies	Relatively specific for Sjögren's syndrome
Hepatitis B surface antigen	Associated with polyarteritis nodosa
Circulating immune complexes	
Complement (C3, C4)	Often decreased in active disease
Urinalysis	
Renal sediment, protein excretion	Hematuria or casts often found with active renal disease; protein excretion of >0.5 g/day is abnormal

Further Notes

In younger patients, demyelinating disease is usually the primary consideration in the differential diagnosis of multifocal CNS disease; in older patients it is vascular disease. Metastatic neoplastic disease is a further major consideration. Patients who are immunocompromised, who have cardiac structural or valvular abnormalities, or who are intravenous drug abusers (to identify the major groups) are at risk for multifocal CNS abscesses. Evaluation for cerebrovascular disease, intracerebral abscesses, and neoplasms metastatic to the brain has been discussed in Chapter 11. Other infectious causes of multifocal CNS disease include spirochetal disease, evaluation of which is discussed in Chapters 13 and 16. This chapter will focus on evaluation of the other major categories of multifocal CNS disease, of which multiple sclerosis is the most common. There is considerable clinical overlap with the evaluation of myelopathies discussed in Chapter 14. The discussion of the rare inherited diseases that can cause multifocal or multisystem dysfunction given in that chapter also applies here.

MULTIPLE SCLEROSIS

The role of laboratory investigation in evaluation of suspected multiple sclerosis (MS) is to (1) provide evidence for CNS lesions at more than one site, (2) confirm or establish signs of an inflammatory response in the CNS, (3) provide further criteria for following the course of disease, and (4) make alternative diagnoses less likely.

Magnetic Resonance Imaging

The most important technique for demonstrating multifocal demyelinating lesions is magnetic resonance imaging (MRI). It is the most sensitive single test: almost all patients with clinically definite MS and somewhat more than two-thirds of those with optic neuritis as a primary manifestation of MS have multifocal white matter lesions on head MRI. The plaques of demyelinating disease are most clearly defined on T_2-weighted images. The focal areas of increased signal intensity on T_2-weighted images (secondary to edema or gliosis) are not specific for demyelinating disease, although the pattern of distribution is more so (see Ch. 3). Multifocal abscesses, tumors, or UBOs (unidentified bright objects seen in images even of normal subjects and thought to result from small vessel cerebrovascular disease) may have similar appearances. In demyelinating disease, the plaques are predominantly periventricular, but may be found widely scattered throughout both the supratentorial and infratentorial white matter. Involvement of the corpus callosum and indusium griseum is characteristic and can help to distinguish primary demyelinating from vascular diseases. Sagittal images are particularly helpful for this. T_1-weighted images can demonstrate the atrophy of the corpus callosum, which accompanies more advanced disease. Serial studies can define the evolution of individual plaques and clearly demonstrate the pattern of remitting and relapsing disease in MS.

Cerebrospinal Fluid Studies

An elevated CSF IgG index and the presence of oligoclonal bands are relatively sensitive indices of CNS inflammatory disease. An increased IgG index is found in almost two-thirds of patients with clinically definite MS, and oligoclonal bands may be found in significantly more. However, they are nonspecific. The CSF cell count may help in differentiating a primary demyelinating inflammatory response from one secondary to some other pathology. In general, more than about 10 lymphocytes/mm^3 CSF is unusual in MS, even during acute exacerbations. Widespread breakdown of the blood-brain barrier is also uncommon in demyelinating disease: the total protein in MS is usually normal or only slightly elevated. CSF studies do not help predict the group of patients presenting with acute transverse myelitis or optic neuritis who will progress to develop MS.

Evoked Potentials

The importance of electrophysiologic tests has declined with the advent of MRI. Because of their relatively low sensitivity, electrophysiologic tests are not appropriate for the evaluation of all cases of suspected MS. The visual evoked response (VER) is the most useful. It is sensitive to small lesions in the optic nerve, although extremely insensitive to even large retrochiasmal abnormalities of the type visualized so well by MRI. Thus, it may aid diagnosis by providing evidence for a second lesion in patients with myelopathy suspected secondary to demyelinating disease who do not have a diagnostic head MRI.

Brainstem auditory evoked responses (BAERs) can localize lesions in the auditory pathway. However, they are not very useful for demonstrating occult multifocal lesions: positive results in the absence of clinical signs of brainstem involvement are relatively rare. Blink reflexes and somatosensory evoked potentials (SEPs) are normally even less useful for evaluating demyelinating disease because the pathways studied are less well defined and the tests are not very sensitive to small lesions in these pathways.

Urodynamics Tests

Control of micturition involves a long pathway extending from the mesial frontal cortex through the brainstem to the lumbosacral spinal cord. Thus, urinary symptoms in MS are common. Identification of abnormalities of bladder control may assist in diagnosis and have a considerable impact on management. Patients may show areflexic, hyporeflexic, or hyperreflexic bladders. There is commonly a progression from areflexia to hyperreflexia. Patients should be referred to a urodynamics laboratory for measurement of urinary flow rates, cystometry, and, in some cases, urinary sphincter electromyography (EMG). Before urodynamics testing, urine should be examined microscopically and cultured to rule out the possibility of a bladder infection, which can lead to abnormal bladder wall irritability.

Residual volumes are high in areflexic and hyporeflexic patients, the sensation of bladder filling is impaired, and urinary flow rates are low. During the filling phase of the cystometrogram, there is evidence of a decreased sensation of bladder filling, and abnormally large filling volumes are reached with reduced spontaneous contractions. Patients with hyperreflexic bladders usually have more normal sensation and small residual volumes. In this group, the cystometrogram should demonstrate prominent, irregular bladder contractions even at low volumes. Interrupted flow recordings suggest detrusor-sphincter dyssynergia. This can be confirmed by urinary-sphincter EMG studies combined with flow measurements.

OTHER ACQUIRED DEMYELINATING DISEASES

Other examples of multifocal CNS demyelinating disease include acute disseminated encephalomyelitis and the postvaccinial and postinfectious central demyelinating syndromes. Predominantly myelopathic presentations can be seen (acute transverse myelitis) (see Ch. 14). However, in their classic forms, these disorders do not mimic MS and present as acute encephalitides or encephalomyelitides. The laboratory abnormalities are as described for MS, although there may be greater inflammatory changes in the CSF. Acute disseminated encephalomyelitis may show a greater cellularity, but even then, the pleocytosis should not be in excess of 100 leukocytes/mm^3. No tests can distinguish these nonrecurrent demyelinating diseases from MS on initial presentation. It is their temporal profile that marks them as distinct disorders.

Uncommonly, acute necrotizing leukoencephalopathies may be seen. The CSF profile is distinguished by the presence of red cells and xanthochromia, as well as a prominent leukocytosis. The major disorders in the differential diagnosis are the infectious encephalitides.

VASCULITIDES

All vasculitides that affect the CNS can produce multifocal disease. An initial evaluation of a patient with multifocal CNS neurologic signs, therefore, should include laboratory investigations directed toward identifying systemic vasculitides if there is evidence of coexisting systemic disease from the clinical history or examination. Isolated cerebral involvement is rare. Tests useful in diagnosis of vasculitis are discussed in Chapters 11 and 16.

SARCOIDOSIS

Sarcoidosis is essentially never limited to the CNS. As with vasculitis, emphasis in the diagnostic evaluation should be placed on defining systemic manifestations. Evidence for pulmonary involvement will come primarily from the chest x-ray or chest CT. A gallium scan may identify granulomas as abnormal areas of increased uptake, but it is too expensive and involves too much radiation exposure to be recommended as a routine investigation. Uveitis is relatively common and slit-lamp examination should be performed in suspected cases. Serum angiotensin-converting enzyme activity is increased in about one-half of patients. Some clinicians have recommended liver biopsy for tissue diagnosis if another site that is clearly involved by the disease (e.g., hilar nodes) cannot be found.

Tests for CNS involvement are nonspecific. A modest CSF pleocytosis is often seen. The CSF total protein concentration is usually increased to higher levels than that seen in MS. CSF angiotensin converting enzyme concentrations may be elevated. Imaging with CT or MRI may occasionally identify granulomas.

POSTERIOR FOSSA DISEASE PRESENTING AS MULTIFOCAL CNS DISEASE

Involvement of the CNS by infiltrating tumors can mimic multifocal disease, particularly when in the brainstem (e.g., infiltrating glioma). Sagittal T_2-weighted MRI, in combination with axial views, are particularly helpful in assessing the size of the brainstem when searching for mass effects from infiltrative processes in that area, and can often allow tumors to be directly visualized.

Congenital malformations of the posterior fossa (e.g., the Chiari type I malformation) causing brainstem or cervical spinal cord dysfunction late in life may also be misinterpreted as suggesting multifocal CNS disease. Skull films may demonstrate platybasia or other bony deformities. Formerly, myelography with dye extending to the foramen magnum was necessary for demonstration of abnormalities. Currently sagittal MRI views of the brainstem and cervical cord are the preferred tests. Visualization of the cerebellar tonsils is important. A Chiari type I malformation is readily identified on a sagittal MRI showing extension of the cerebellar tonsils into or below the foramen magnum.

TESTS TO CONSIDER BEFORE IMMUNOSUPPRESSIVE THERAPY

Steroids or other immunosuppressive therapy are frequently used in the treatment of patients with demyelinating disease, vasculitides, and sarcoidosis. Pretreatment assessment should include a chest x-ray, tuberculin skin test, and fasting and postprandial glucose levels to identify patients with subclinical diabetes mellitus who are more likely to develop complications of therapy.

READINGS

Fazekas F, Offenbacher H, Fuchs S, et al: Criteria for an increased specificity of

MRI interpretation in elderly subjects with suspected multiple sclerosis. Neurology 38:1822, 1988
Matthews WB: Neurologic manifestations of sarcoidosis. p. 1563. In Asbury AK, McKhann GM, MacDonald WI (eds): Diseases of the Nervous System. Vol. II. WB Saunders, Philadelphia, 1986
Miller DH, Rudge P, Johnson G, et al: Serial gadolinium enhanced magnetic resonance imaging in multiple sclerosis. Brain 111:927, 1988
Moore PM, Crupps TR: Neurologic complications of vasculitis. Ann Neurol 14:155, 1983
Paty DW, Asbury AK, Herndon RM, et al: Use of magnetic resonance imaging in the diagnosis of multiple sclerosis: policy statement. Neurology 36:1575, 1986
Poser CM (ed): Diagnosis of Multiple Sclerosis. Thieme, New York, 1984
Willoughby EW, Grochowski E, Li DKB, et al: Serial magnetic resonance scanning in multiple sclerosis: a second prospective study in relapsing patients. Ann Neurol 25:43, 1989

16 LABORATORY TESTS FOR EVALUATING DISORDERS OF THE PERIPHERAL NERVES

Table 16-1. Differential Diagnosis of Disorders of Peripheral Nerves

Neuropathies

Polyneuropathy
- Demyelinating
  - Inflammatory (Guillain-Barré, chronic inflammatory demyelinating polyneuropathy [CIDPN])
  - Abnormal protein (monoclonal gammopathy)
  - Inherited (e.g., HMSN type I, Dejerine-Sottas syndrome, metachromatic leukodystrophy)
  - Paraneoplastic
- Axonal
  - Metabolic (e.g., diabetes mellitus, uremia, vitamin B_{12} deficiency, porphyria, malabsorption)
  - Toxic (e.g., alcohol, heavy metals, solvents)
  - Drugs (e.g., vinca alkaloids, cis-platinum, isoniazid, nitrofurantoin)
  - Abnormal proteins (e.g., monoclonal gammopathy, cryoglobulinemia, amyloidosis)
  - Inherited/metabolic (e.g., HMSN type II, spinocerebellar degenerations, mitochondrial disorders)
  - Paraneoplastic (especially pure sensory neuropathy)
- Mixed
  - Metabolic: diabetic
  - Secondary axonal degeneration after primary demyelination

Multifocal neuropathy/plexopathy/radiculopathy
- Mononeuropathy multiplex/polyradiculoneuropathy
  - Vascular
    - Diabetes
    - Vasculitis (e.g., polyarteritis nodosa, connective tissue disease)
    - Large vessel occlusion (e.g., monomelic neuropathy)

Continued

Table 16-1. *Continued*

Neuropathies

- Abnormal proteins
- Inflammatory (e.g., CIDPN variant, sarcoidosis, neoplastic meningitis)
- Infectious (e.g., neuroborreliosis, syphilis, leprosy, chronic meningitis)
- Compressive (multiple entrapments)

Plexopathy
- Vascular
  - Diabetes
  - Vasculitis
- Postirradiation
- Inflammatory (e.g., postvaccinial)
- Idiopathic

Focal
- Radiculopathy/mononeuropathy
  - Compressive
  - Traumatic
  - Ischemic
  - Infiltrative

Neuronopathies

Motor neuron diseases
- Amyotrophic lateral sclerosis
- Spinal muscular atrophies

Infectious
- Herpes zoster, poliomyelitis

Metabolic
- (e.g., hexoseaminadase A deficiency, hyperparathyroidism, vitamin E deficiency)

Toxic
- (e.g., heavy metals)

Table 16-2. Evaluation of Diseases of Nerves

Test	Condition	Notes
Blood Tests		
CBC	Guillain-Barré syndrome	Lymphocytosis may be seen; atypical lymphocytes with Epstein-Barr virus infection, a trigger for Guillain-Barré syndrome
	Vitamin B_{12}	Megaloblastic anemia with deficiency state
	Paraneoplastic neuropathy	Anemia of chronic disease; various specific changes with hematologic malignancies
	Vitamin E deficiency	Wet smear should be done to look for acanthocytes
ESR	Vasculitides, systemic illness	Consider the broad range of tests that can help in diagnosis of vasculitis listed in Table 15-3
Prothrombin time	GI disease	Malabsorption of fat-soluble vitamins will lead to deficiencies of vitamins D, K, and E; prothrombin time elevated with severe vitamin K deficiency or liver disease
Glucose	Diabetes	Diabetic neuropathy (multiple forms) is the most common chronic neuropathy in the nonalcoholic population; fasting and postprandial glucose should be obtained; glucose tolerance test may reveal early diabetes (neurologic manifestations may precede overt diabetes); to assess longer term serum glucose control, the fraction of glycosylated hemoglobin (Hb_{A1c}) may be measured
SGOT, SGPT, Bilirubin	Hepatic insufficiency	Viral hepatitis may trigger Guillain-Barré syndrome; liver dysfunction may suggest a toxic or systemic disease also affecting nerves
BUN, Cr	Renal failure	Dialysis does not cure the neuropathy associated with renal disease (transplantation does)

Continued

Table 16-2. *Continued*

Test	Condition	Notes
Ca^{++}	Hypocalcemia	Paresthesias common with hypocalcemia
	Hypercalcemia	Associated with several etiologies of nerve disease including malignancies, parathyroid disease, and sarcoidosis
SPEP, IEP	Chronic inflammatory polyneuropathy/paraprotein associated neuropathy	Monoclonal protein peak present in many (IgM or IgG); SPEP may show elevation of acute phase reactants; occasionally, a small monoclonal peak missed on SPEP will be found with IEP
Serum lipoproteins	Vitamin E deficiency	Hereditary abetalipoproteinemia associated with low VLDL and LDL; vitamin E deficiency can also occur with primary malabsorption states
Free erythrocyte protoporphyrin (FEP)		Level of FEP is elevated with lead toxicity but is not specific
Parathyroid hormone	Motor neuron disease	Rare cause of motor neuropathy
Hexoseaminodase A deficiency	Motor neuron disease	Rare syndrome of motor neuropathy and ataxia
Serology		
HIV antibody	Guillain-Barré syndrome	Acute and chronic demyelinating neuropathies are associated with HIV infection
EBV antibody	Guillain-Barré syndrome	Acute and convalescent titers needed; a fourfold increase in IgG antibodies is diagnostic of active disease; monospot test is less reliable
CMV antibody	Guillain-Barré syndrome	Acute and convalescent titers needed
Hepatitis B panel	Mononeuropathy multiplex	Association between presence of Hepatitis B antibodies and polyarteritis nodosa

Continued

Table 16-2. *Continued*

Test	Condition	Notes
FTA-ABS	Polyradiculoneuritis	Active neurosyphilis is usually associated with CSF pleocytosis; CSF VDRL may be positive
Borrelia burgdorferi antibody	Polyradiculoneuritis, mononeuritis multiplex	Usually occurs at later stage of infection; a significant serum titer (>1:256) is needed; specificity for active disease is increased by demonstrating intrathecal antibody production
Urine Tests		
Urinalysis	Vasculitides	Systemic vasculitides often associated with hematuria (see Table 15-3)
Aminolevulonic acid, porphobilinogens	Hepatic porphyrias	During attacks levels of intermediates of heme biosynthesis are increased; qualitative test is less sensitive than 24-hour quantitative measurement; urine should be protected from light and frozen for transport; diagnosis can be confirmed by enzyme assays on leukocytes or erythrocytes (see Ch. 7)
Urine for heavy metal (As, Pb, Hg)	Toxic neuropathies	Urinary excretion of heavy metals may continue for a prolonged period after ingestion; serum levels are the definitive tests for Pb and Hg, but less reliable for As
Lumbar Puncture		
CSF analysis	Guillain-Barré syndrome	CSF studies are normal early; elevation of protein without significant pleocytosis (<10 WBC/mm^3) develops over 1–3 weeks
	Chronic inflammatory demyelinating polyneuropathy (CIDPN)	Increased protein, with minimal pleocytosis may be seen; CSF protein levels may be useful for following disease activity; elevated CSF IgG may also be found

Continued

Table 16-2. *Continued*

Test	Condition	Notes
Electrophysiologic Tests		
EMG and nerve conduction studies	Demyelinating neuropathies	Slowing of nerve conduction velocities; dispersion of CMAP (may be marked with acquired neuropathies, and classically not seen with inherited neuropathies); prolongation of F-wave latencies; prolonged or absent H reflexes; EMG signs of denervation may occur with secondary axonal degeneration; decreased recruitment seen
	Axonal neuropathies	Decreased CMAP and SNAP; increased spontaneous activity, decreased recruitment, and polyphasic potentials in denervated muscles; absent or minimal changes in conduction velocities until very severe
	Mononeuropathy multiplex	Both demyelinating and axonal electrophysiologic characteristics may be seen in an asymmetric, multifocal pattern not necessarily corresponding to usual sites of compression
	Mononeuropathy	Focal slowing, dispersion and possibly conduction block with demyelination; secondary axonal degeneration leads to decreased distal SNAP amplitudes and denervation changes in muscles
	Radiculopathy	Denervation within myotomal territory (including paraspinal muscles) with preserved SNAPs in the setting of significant sensory loss distinguish radiculopathies from plexopathies or peripheral nerve lesions
Radiology		
Plain films of spine spondyloysis	Radiculopathy	Note canal width, presence of spondolysis, spondylolisthesis or narrowing of foramina, local bony destruction (suggesting malignancy) or disc destruction (suggesting infection)

Continued

Table 16-2. *Continued*

Test	Condition	Notes
Axial CT of spine	Radiculopathy	Look for evidence of bony destruction, narrowing of foramina, or protrusion of discs; radiologist must be guided by the clinical examination; particularly useful after myelography, allowing dye from the latter to define the subarachnoid space
Myelography	Radiculopathy	Look for compression of dural sac or lack of filling of root sleeves; disc herniation (not apparent on plain films) can be defined; roots proximal to a compressive lesion may be thickened
MRI spine	Radiculopathy	Subarachnoid space, discs, and soft tissues are fairly well visualized; differentiation between severely degenerated (low water content) and normal discs possible with T_2-weighted images; focal compressive soft tissue masses (e.g., neuromas) well defined
Skeletal survey	Polyneuropathy	Osteosclerotic multiple myeloma is associated with neuropathies; more rarely they are seen with other myelomas
Body CT	Plexopathy or mononeuropathy	Directed CT studies may identify mass lesions at the sites of dysfunction; contrast infusion allows vascular structures to be used as landmarks
Body MRI	Plexopathy or mononeuropathy	As with CT, imaging the site of the lesion may identify masses or infiltrative lesions
Biopsies		
Muscle	Axonal neuropathy	Group atrophy; diagnostic vascular inflammatory infiltration may be found with vasculitides

Continued

Table 16-2. *Continued*

Test	Condition	Notes
	Demyelinating neuropathy	Normal until secondary axonal degeneration begins
Nerve	Axonal neuropathy	Axonal degeneration
	Demyelinating neuropathy	Demyelination with secondary axonal degeneration in areas of severe demyelination; presence of macrophages confirms an inflammatory basis
	CIDPN	Demyelination, secondary axonal degeneration, and onion bulbs occur with cycles of demyelination and remyelination
	Amyloidosis	Congo red staining, bi-refringent amyloid deposits, and axonal degeneration
Bone marrow	Monoclonal gammopathy	Abnormal cellularity, developmental arrest of specific clones of cells may be seen
Abdominal fat aspirate, rectal mucosa biopsy	Amyloidosis	Characteristic amyloid deposits may be identified by experienced pathologists on needle aspirate of fat with this minimally invasive procedure; rectal mucosa biopsies are excellent for identification of amyloid but can be associated with significant morbidity

Further Notes

The clinical history and examination are essential for suggesting peripheral nerve dysfunction. The first step toward establishing the etiology is to classify the neuropathy as a radiculopathy, plexopathy, polyneuropathy, mononeuropathy, mononeuropathy multiplex, or a combination of these. Laboratory studies (especially nerve conduction studies, electromyography [EMG], and nerve/muscle biopsy) are important to both confirm the presence of a neuropathy and help characterize it.

When using laboratory tests in the evaluation of neuropathies, it is important to bear in mind that it is not unusual for significant symptoms of peripheral nerve dysfunction to occur without any recognizable changes on electrophysiologic tests or even biopsy.

POLYNEUROPATHIES

The first step in laboratory characterization of a polyneuropathy is to determine whether dysfunction arises predominantly from axonal degeneration or demyelination. Advanced demyelinating disease with secondary axonal degeneration can be clinically indistinguishable from a primary axonal degenerating neuropathy. Electrophysiologic tests (sometimes in conjunction with nerve biopsy) provide a means to discriminate these.

As discussed in more detail in Chapter 4, axonal neuropathies are characterized electrophysiologically by diminished compound motor action or sensory nerve action potentials. There is often a recognizable gradient, with the more distal nerves affected more severely. By contrast with the action potential amplitudes, conduction velocities are normal or only moderately reduced even in later stages.

Demyelinating neuropathies show conduction velocity slowing (sometimes dramatic) even with relatively little evidence of distal axonal loss. The latter is established by demonstrating that distally innervated muscles show relatively mild or minimal denervation changes by EMG relative to the degree of conduction slowing. Among the demyelinating neuropathies it is important to distinguish the acquired forms from the congenital. Acquired demyelinating neuropathies show increased temporal dispersion of the compound motor action potential (a finding that is reliable if the potential amplitude is greater than about 1 mV). They may also show conduction block. Conduction block in a motor nerve is inferred if there is a decrease in the compound motor action potential amplitude with little evidence for axonal loss to muscles in the field of innervation. Congenital demyelinating neuropathies (e.g., hereditary motor and sensory neuropathy [HMSN] type I or Charcot-Marie-Tooth disease) are distinguished from acquired disease by showing profound, uniform slowing (to < 30 m/sec), usually without blocking or dispersion.

Polyneuropathies with Metabolic Causes

Diabetic Neuropathies

Along with (toxic) alcoholic neuropathies, diabetic neuropathies are the most common types of neuropathies assessed in a general neurologic practice. Diabetic neuropathies may pose a difficult diagnostic problem for several reasons. First, the clinical presentation is variable, including in addition to symmetric polyneuropathies, mononeuritis multiplex, plexopathies, and radiculopathies. Second, a small fiber sensorimotor neuropathy may give rise to significant symptoms with no abnormalities or only minimal changes in the sensory nerve action potentials (SNAPs), compound muscle action potentials (CMAPs), or nerve conduction velocities (NCVs). Third, electrophysiologic characteristics of both axonal degeneration or peripheral demyelination may be found. Finally, the neuropathy can precede overt clinical diabetes. An oral glucose tolerance test may be warranted in patients with suspected diabetes mellitus if the diagnosis is not clear after measurement of preprandial and postprandial blood sugars and glycosylated hemoglobin (hemoglobin A_c levels).

If a diabetic neuropathy is suspected, efforts should be made to determine whether there is autonomic nervous system dysfunction. Several easy tests can be performed to assess autonomic dysfunction: measurement of resting heart rate, ECG monitoring to follow modulation of heart rate during lying and standing, deep breathing, and the Valsalva maneuver (see Ewing and Clark, 1987). Specialized laboratory tests available for assessment of autonomic function include the sympathetic skin responses (that reflect the activation of piloerector muscles in sweat glands in response to small electric shocks), measurement of skin electrical resistance (another index of sweating response), plethysmography (to measure changes in limb blood low during maneuvers that change sympathetic tone), and microneurography (for direct recording from autonomic fibers). These specialized tests are best performed and interpreted in centers experienced in their use.

Uremic Neuropathies

Uremia is another relatively frequently encountered metabolic cause of polyneuropathies. Uremia leads to a primarily axonal degenerating neuropathy. Although measurement of serum blood urea nitrogren (BUN) and creatine can identify renal insufficiency, it is impossible to directly correlate degrees of uremia with nerve damage. Like other metabolic factors adversely affecting neuronal function, the presence of uremia probably makes nerves more susceptible to damage from other causes.

Polyneuropathies Secondary to Nutritional Deficiencies

Among nutritional deficiencies causing neuropathy, vitamin B_1 (thiamine), and B_{12} (cyanocobalamin) deficiencies are the most common. Serum vitamin B_{12} levels must be measured if a deficiency is suspected, as neurologic complications can precede megaloblastic changes in red cells or hypersegmentation of polymorphonuclear granulocytes on the peripheral smear. A thiamine deficiency state can be confirmed by measurement of decreased red blood cell transketolase activity.

Vitamin E deficiency presents as a syndrome of neuropathy and cerebellar degeneration, usually associated with malabsorption states. Determination of the prothrombin time (to assess possible deficiency in the fat-soluble vitamin K), which can be prolonged in malabsorption states, is an indirect screening test. Measurement of serum vitamin E levels and 24-hour fecal fat excretion (which is increased in states in which fats and fat-soluble vitamins are malabsorbed) are more specific diagnostic tests.

Porphyrias

In appropriate clinical settings (e.g., intermittent exacerbations of often painful neuropathy associated with abdominal pain and additional features such as predominantly proximal weakness or acute personality changes), urine porphobilinogen and δ-aminolevulonic acid should be ordered to evaluate the possibility of porphyria (neurologic manifestations may be seen with acute intermittent porphyria, variegate porphyria, or coproporphyria). These and other intermediates of the heme biosynthetic pathway are elevated in serum and urine during acute exacerbations. Concentrations my be normal at other times. Tests for further characterization of the form of the porphyrias are discussed in Chapter 7.

Toxic Neuropathies

Most of the toxic neuropathies usually encountered are identified on the basis of the clinical history, but laboratory testing has an important role in evaluating heavy metal poisoning. Clinical features can guide selection of tests (e.g., GI symptoms, tremor, and ataxia for mercury [Hg]; encephalopathy with neuropathy for arsenic [As]; or a wrist drop for lead [Pb]). Quantitative 24-hour urinary excretion is the test of choice for arsenic poisoning (although hair or nail arsenic content will remain elevated for much longer periods after acute ingestions) and is useful with mercury and lead poisoning, but less reliable for the latter. More than one determination should be attempted if the clinical suspicion is high as excretion can fluctuate from day to day. Samples of urine should be collected over 24 hours in acid-washed plastic containers. However, only a 50 ml aliquot needs to be sent (frozen) to the laboratory for analysis if the total 24-hour volume is noted. Serum zinc protoporphyrin levels increase with lead intoxication and are a better screening test for lead toxicity. Blood levels for lead and mercury are the definitive tests for these intoxications. Symptoms may be ascribed to lead intoxication when blood levels exceed 30 μg/dl and zinc protoporphyrin levels exceed 140 μg/dl.

Acquired Demyelinataing Neuropathies

Acute Inflammatory Demyelinating Polyneuropathy (Guillain-Barré Syndrome)

Guillain-Barré syndrome is the most commonly encountered acute demyelinating polyneuropathy. It should be recognized early since severe weakness and respiratory insufficiency may develop rapidly. The earliest electrophysiologic changes are in nerve conduction studies, which may show prolongation of distal motor latencies and F-wave latencies and often dispersion of the CMAPs. Later in the progression of an attack, severe slowing of motor nerve conduction velocities may be seen with prolongation of the distal motor latencies (sometimes to more than three times normal). Although sensory symptoms are common, electrophysiologic abnormalities in the sensory nerves are much less marked than in motor nerves. Up to 20 percent of patients with Guillain-Barré syndrome have abnormalities on initial presentation that are undetectable electrophysiologically with routine studies. This is usually attributed to predominantly proximal (root) involvement.

In general, CSF studies may contribute little to the initial diagnosis in an acute presentation. The characteristic albuminocytologic dissociation—a rise in total protein with minimal pleocytosis (<10 lymphocytes/mm^3)—usually occurs between 1 and 3 weeks after the onset of symptoms. In typical cases lumbar puncture (LP) may be deferred for this period or may not even be necessary.

Nerve conduction studies and EMG are helpful for establishing prognosis in the Guillain-Barré syndrome. The earliest (within 2 to 4 weeks) useful predictor of a poor outcome is distal CMAP reduction to <20 percent of normal. EMG findings of spontaneous activity demonstrate secondary axonal degeneration. When serial nerve conduction velocity measurements are obtained, it may be observed that conduction velocities worsen as the clinical syndrome resolves, a sign that nerves previously showing complete conduction block are again beginning to conduct impulses over the length being studied.

The Guillain-Barré syndrome may be triggered by infectious agents, including viral hepatitis, cytomegalovirus (CMV), Epstein-Barr virus (EBV), and *Mycoplasma*. (Serologic studies showing a fourfold rise in titer between acute and convalescent phase sera or, for *Mycoplasma*, cold agglutinins in high and rising titers may help in establishing etiology for epidemiologic purposes.) HIV-1 is an emerging cause of both acute and chronic inflammatory polyneuropathies, and serology (see Ch. 9) should be evaluated in all patients at risk because of the importance of establishing infection with this agent. No reliable distinguishing characteristics of HIV-1 are associated with acute demyelinating polyneuritis, although in some patients the acute presentation is associated with a CSF lymphocytoc pleocytosis.

Chronic Inflammatory Demyelinating Polyneuropathy

Chronic inflammatory demyelinating polyneuropathy (CIDPN) is characterized by a chronic or relapsing demyelinating neuropathy associated with elevated CSF protein and absent or minimal pleocytosis. LP, therefore, is a critical part of the investigation of any possible CIDPN. The limits of the syndrome are poorly defined and include patients with primarily proximal (root) pathology who do not have clear evidence for more distal demyelination by nerve conduction studies. The nerve biopsy defines a more homogeneous group when it shows inflammatory cells in the nerve and signs of chronic demyelination and remyelination ("onion bulbs") usually with secondary loss of myelinated fibers.

Neuropathies Associated with Abnormal Circulating Proteins

Both primary axonal degenerating and demyelinating neuropathies may be associated with identifiable abnormal circulating immunoglobulins. These disorders do not have unique clinical presentations, so serum protein electrophoresis and immunoelectrophoresis should be obtained for all patients with unexplained neuropathies. Small monoclonal peaks are more easily missed with the serum protein electrophoresis test alone. Immunoglobulin quantification may be helpful. If a monoclonal protein is found, the patient should be evaluated for the presence of a hematologic disorder (e.g., multiple myeloma) with a peripheral smear, radiologic skeletal survey, and bone marrow study. Presence of abnormal light chains in urine can be associated with multiple myeloma. Neuropathy is also well described in association with (otherwise) benign monoclonal gammopathies (usually IgM kappa). Prominent polyclonal gammopathies should also be investigated in the setting of a peripheral neuropathy, but it is often a challenge to determine their clinical significance.

Patients with a neuropathy and an osteosclerotic myeloma who have additional clinical signs, such as organomegaly, enlarged lymph nodes, or skin lesions (e.g., hyperpigmentation, peripheral edema, or an abnormal patch of hair below the knees), should undergo endocrine function tests (including TSH, free T_4, T_3, and 8 AM and 4 PM cortisol) to identify the rare disorder known as POEMS (syndrome of polyneuropathy, organomegaly, endocrine abnormalities, M-protein and skin lesions; see Bardwick et al., 1980).

When a cryoglobulin-associated polyneuropathy (also rare) is suspected (e.g., distal dysesthesias worsened by cold weather), care must be taken to maintain blood drawn for the cryoglobulin assay near 37°C until arrival in the laboratory; cooling to room temperature will precipitate the cryoglobulins.

Polyneuropathies Caused by Collagen Vascular Diseases

Collagen vascular diseases are frequently associated with assymmetric polyneuropathies. The diagnosis of connective tissue disease is based on characteristic involvement of other organ systems (particularly exocrine glands in Sjögren's syndrome, the kidney and skin in systemic lupus erythematosus [SLE], and joints in rheumatoid arthritis, for example). The physical examination and clinical history are critical for recognizing these disorders.

Laboratory tests are useful in establishing the diagnosis in an appropriate clinical setting. An active renal sediment, elevated urinary protein excretion, and elevated serum BUN and creatinine may identify disease of the kidney. Wegener's granulomatosis may be suspected with evidence for abnormal renal function and skull or sinus radiographs showing thickening of sinus membranes or with a chest x-ray demonstrating pulmonary interstitial inflammation or hemorrhage.

The abnormal systemic immune response of autoimmune disease may be associated with leukocytosis, anemia, thrombocytopenia, and increased erythrocyte sedimentation rate [ESR], fluorescent antinuclear antibodies [FANA] titers, and serum immunoglobulins. Higher (>2+) FANA titers are more specific for immunologic disease. Interpretation depends on the binding pattern observed in the assay. For example, a rim pattern is seen with the anti-ds DNA antibodies associated with idiopathic SLE and a homogeneous pattern with the antihistone antibodies of drug-induced lupus. A speckled pattern is less specific. Specific circulating antibodies are associated with other diseases: anti-Ro and anti-La antibodies in Sjögren syndrome, anti-ds DNA and anti-Ro antibodies with idiopathic SLE, rheumatoid factor with rheumatoid arthritis, anti-centromere antibodies with the calcinosis, Raynaud's phenomenon, esophageal dysmotility, sclerodactyly, and telangiectasia (CREST) syndrome, and anti-RNP and anti-Sm (ENA) antibodies with mixed connective tissue disease. Active vasculitis with immune complex deposition is often accompanied by circulating immune complexes and decreased serum complement (C_3, C_4).

Sjögren syndrome, which results from involvement of the exocrine glands, may be suspected if there is reduced tearing by the Schirmer test. Technetium-99 scintigraphy is another method for demonstrating reduced exocrine gland function.

Biopsy of affected tissue (e.g., sinus mucosa, lung, kidney, nerve, muscle, or, perhaps easiest, lip salivary glands in Sjögren syndrome) can confirm the diagnosis of a connective tissue disease.

Biopsy in Neuropathy Diagnosis

Nerve biopsies can be important for evaluating polyneuropathies, particularly those that remain undiagnosed after less invasive investigation (see Ch. 8). The sural nerve has a small sensory field and can be biopsied with little morbidity (patients may complain of dysesthesias over a small strip along the lateral aspect of the foot immediately after the biopsy, but the discomfort usually resolves completely over 30 days, leaving only a small area of decreased sensation). The specimen can demonstrate axonal loss associated with axonal degeneration from primary axonal or severe demyelinating neuropathies. Specific fiber calibers may be affected. Demyelination is apparent as thinning of myelin sheaths and reduction in the number of well-myelinated nerves. Inflammatory cells may be seen. A chronic disorder associated with remyelination will show irregular, thickened foci of myelin around some nerves ("onion bulbs").

An abnormal congophilic, birefringent (apple-green in color when viewed with a polarizing microscope) amyloid infiltrate may be seen in the sural nerve in association with axonal degeneration in amyloid neuropathy. Abdominal fat needle aspirate or (with greater potential morbidity) rectal mucosa biopsy may demonstrate the same type of amyloid deposits.

With leprosy the skin biopsy may demonstrate the acid-fast bacilli of *Mycobacterium leprae* and, in the tuberculoid form, granulomas. The latter may be seen to invade cutaneous nerves. Nerve biopsy may demonstrate granulomas, sometimes with caseation, in tuberculoid leprosy. Lepromatous leprosy can show edematous nerves with inflammatory infiltrates and bacilli.

Muscle biopsy can also provide some clues in the diagnosis of neuropathies. Grouped atrophy with target fibers follows axonal loss. Vasculitic processes may cause arteritis with inflammation and necrosis in walls of small vessels in muscle. Diagnosis can also follow from biopsy of another affected organ as described in the previous section (e.g., the kidney in Fabry's disease or SLE).

FOCAL NEUROPATHIES

The most likely etiologies for focal neuropathies depend on the site of dysfunction. It is useful first to confirm the clinically suspected pattern of dysfunction (involving a myotome or dermatome, portion of a plexus, or territory of a peripheral nerve) with electrophysiologic tests. Focal dysfunction or damage of the root proximal to the dorsal root ganglion may give prominent denervation of muscles supplied without leading to decreased sensory nerve action potential amplitudes (see Ch. 4). Lesions of a nerve plexus or peripheral nerve cause both denervation changes and decreased sensory nerve action potentials. Nerve conduction studies and EMG should be used to evaluate the possibility of an underlying polyneuropathy, as such patients may be at increased risk of superimposed focal neuropathies.

Focal neuropathies that do not occur at common sites of entrapment or compression may arise from any of the causes of mononeuropathy multiplex described below or, rarely, from local tumors. After clinical and electrophysiologic localization of the site of dysfunction, local imaging using computed tomography (CT) (with intravenous contrast infusion) or magnetic resonance imaging (MRI) can help identify abnormal mass lesions. This imaging may also help guide any planned surgical intervention.

Nerve conduction studies and EMG have an important role in the evaluation of patients with focal traumatic mononeuropathies. If compound motor and sensory nerve action potential amplitudes measured across the site of trauma are initially normal or only slightly reduced, significant nerve damage is ruled out. After 2 to 4 weeks, denervation changes measured by EMG will establish whether axonal degeneration has occurred. Lack of significant improvement of abnormal signs after sufficient time for axon regrowth (6 to 12 months) implies a poor prognosis for recovery of function.

Cranial mononeuropathies or multiple cranial mononeuropathies can be caused by disorders leading to mononeuritis multiplex or local tumors, as well as by several pathologies unique to the cranial nerves. The most common cranial mononeuropathy is idiopathic Bell's palsy. Blink reflex measurements can be used to electrophysiologically localize the lesion to the ipsilateral seventh cranial nerve (efferent arc), but unless the clinical diagnosis is uncertain, this investigation is usually unwarranted. Between 10 and 14 days after the onset of symptoms, electrophysiologic study of the facial nerve and weak facial muscles (e.g., obicularis oris) may help to establish prognosis: a CMAP amplitude less than 10 percent of that on the other side or marked denervation changes on EMG predict a relatively poor prognosis for recovery of function. Recurrent or bilateral seventh nerve palsies should prompt investigations for sarcoidosis, Lyme disease, demyelinating disease, or local tumors such as an acoustic neuroma. MRI is the preferred technique for viewing the cerebellopontine angle. If MRI is not available, a CT with intravenous contrast infusion may be used, although sensitivity is lower because of bone artifacts in the posterior fossa. Audiologic studies, brainstem auditory evoked response (BAER), and skull films may be helpful in some instances to further characterize abnormalities. Inflammatory or infiltrative diseases of the basal meninges, including particularly tuberculosis, CNS lymphoma, carcinomatous meningitis, and granulomatous, fungal, or parasitic disease, may be evaluated by CSF analysis and imaging of the basal meninges by MRI or CT with intravenous contrast.

Evaluation of third nerve palsies is an extensive topic that will be discussed only briefly here. Clinical signs (e.g., involvement of other cranial nerves) can usually localize the lesion. A pupil-sparing palsy suggests an intrinsic lesion, which should prompt an investigation similar to that for generalized mononeuritis multiplex, as described later. However, extrinsic compressive lesions are not reliably ruled out by clinical signs alone. Imaging of the head with fine cuts through the superior orbital fissure and cavernous sinus using CT with intravenous contrast infusion or MRI are reasonably sensitive to large vascular abnormalities and will show most mass lesions. (Some, for example, meningioma en plaque, may be more difficult to identify.) Aneurysms, particularly of the posterior communicating artery, can be reliably shown only by contrast angiography at present, although in the near future this may prove to be an area for application of MRI angiography.

MONONEUROPATHY MULTIPLEX

Diagnosis of mononeuropathy multiplex is particularly important, because it may signal the presence of a serious systemic disease. The first step in the evaluation is to make certain that the patient does not have multiple compressive neuropathies. Patients with underlying polyneuropathies may be especially prone to this complication. Some polyneuropathies (e.g., from chronic inflammatory polyneuropathies or lead) may present asymmetrically, appearing clinically similar to mononeuritis multiplex. Of the true mononeuritides multiplex, leprosy is the most important cause world-wide, but diabetes and vasculitis are the most commonly encountered causes in North America and Europe. Less common causes include Lyme disease, sarcoidosis, cryoglobulinemia, and amyloidosis (for carpal tunnel syndrome).

Vasculitides

As has been stressed before, manifestations of vasculitis are variable and, in general, systemic. Usually evidence for involvement of more than one system can be found. For example, polyarteritis nodosa usually involves respiratory, renal, and gastrointestinal vasculature, in addition to any involvement of the nerves; Wegener's granulomatosis involves the respiratory tract and kidney; and Sjögren syndrome arises from exocrine gland dysfunction. As described earlier in discussion of connective tissue disease, the abnormal systemic immune response is often reflected in hematologic parameters, elevation of acute phase reactants, and high titers of specific circulating antibodies. Hepatitis B surface antigen is found in a majority of patients with polyarteritis nodosa. Analysis of urine sediment, renal function tests, and chest and sinus x-rays have already been discussed as noninvasive tests for involvement of the renal and respiratory systems with vasculitis. Direct demonstration of the vasculitis is sometimes possible by angiography or biopsy. Characteristic microaneuryms may be found with abdominal angiography in polyarteritis nodosa.

Sarcoidosis

Sarcoidosis is an idiopathic, systemic granulomatous disease and a rare but well-characterized cause of mononeuritis multiplex. Diagnosis depends first on establishing the presence of noncaseating granulomas in an appropriate clinical setting and second on ruling out other causes of granulomatous disease. The most important tests are the chest x-ray (bilateral hilar adenopathy is present in most, but may require verification by CT of the mediastinum), slit-lamp examination for the characteristic uveitis, serum angiotensin converting enzyme (the test is insensitive, but levels approximately two or more times normal are relatively specific), and biopsy of involved tissue. A gallium nuclear medicine scan showing abnormal uptake in the lungs is consistent with the presence of granulomas, but this test is very nonspecific. Mediastinal lymph nodes or any skin lesions are the most common sites of directed biopsy, but blind biopsies may be attempted of the liver (granulomas may be found in about 75 percent of patients with sarcoidosis, although their presence is nonspecific), conjunctiva, lip salivary glands or nerve and muscle. CSF findings are nonspecific with CNS involvement, but mild leukocytic pleocytosis and increased protein are seen in most.

Lyme Neuroborreliosis

Lyme disease is now more frequently recognized as a cause of mononeuritis multiplex. In general, this is just one presentation of a more generalized radiculoneuritis that can be defined electrophysiologically, if not by signs and symptoms. Rising serum Lyme disease titers may establish the diagnosis. However, the peripheral neuropathy usually comes at a later stage of the disease. A serum Lyme titer of 1:256 or greater may be significant, but is always difficult to interpret in an endemic area where many asymptomatic individuals have developed circulating antibodies. Nervous system involvement may be specifically identified by finding CSF antibody titers higher than those in the serum (Halperin et al., 1989).

MOTOR NEURONOPATHIES

Amyotrophic lateral sclerosis is the most commonly encountered motor neuronopathy in adult neurology clinics. Diagnosis is primarily clinical and based on the constellation of upper and lower motor neuron dysfunction. Electrophysiologic tests can be supportive by revealing evidence of widespread signs of motor denervation and collateral reinnervation (polyphasic, giant potentials, spontaneous activity) in the absence of significant abnormalities of nerve conduction except that with atrophy the CMAP amplitude decreases.

Great emphasis should be placed on evaluating the patient thoroughly to make certain that other diagnoses are unlikely. Most important is ruling out the possibility of a polyradiculopathy. The probability of motor neuron disease is increased if denervation and reinnervation changes are found in muscles in the face and tongue, where they cannot be due to degenerative disc disease. Thoracic radicular compression is unusual; so EMG changes consistent with chronic denervation and reinnervation in thoracic paraspinous muscles increase the likelihood of motor neuron disease. Noninvasive studies to look for evidence of root compression include plain films of the spine (look for evidence of diffuse degenerative disease, spondylosis, and narrowing of the foramina), CT of the spine (the radiologist should be directed to image the specific levels where denervation changes have been found), and spinal MRI. If these studies are inconclusive a myelogram may be useful, although we anticipate that the quality of MRI studies may soon make this test unnecessary. The radiologist must be made aware that dye should be allowed to run all the way to the foramen magnum. Rare cases of foramen magnum lesions, cervical spondylosis, hyperparathyroidism, hexoseaminidase A deficiency, multiple sclerosis, dysimmune and paraneoplastic states, immunosuppression-responsive syndrome of multifocal block (see Krarup et al., 1990), and lead toxicity have been described with presentations similar to amyotrophic lateral sclerosis.

Presence of lower motor neuron findings alone that cannot be ascribed to radiculopathy or polyneuropathy may represent a spinal muscular atrophy syndrome.

READINGS

Asbury AK: Disorders of peripheral nerve. p. 321. Asbury AK, McKhann GK, McDonald IW (eds): In Diseases of the Nervous System. Vol. I. WB Saunders, Philadelphia, 1986

Bardwick PA, Zvaifler MH, Gill GN, et al: Plasma cell dyscrasia with polyneuropathy, organomegaly, endocrinopathy, M protein and skin changes: the POEMS syndrome. Medicine 59:311, 1980

Brown WF, Bolton CF (eds): Clinical Electromyography. Butterworth (Publishers), Boston, 1987

Choucair AK, Ajax ET: Hair and nails in arsenical neuropathy. Ann Neurol 23:628, 1988

Cornblath DR, Mellits ED, Griffin JW, et al: Motor conduction studies in Guillain-Barré syndrome: description and prognostic value. Ann Neurol 23:354, 1988

Dyck PJ, Oviatt KF, Lambert EH: Intensive evaluation of referred unclassified neuropathies yields improved diagnosis. Ann Neurol 10:222, 1981

Dyck PJ (ed): Diabetic Neuropathy. WB Saunders, Philadelphia, 1987

Dyck PJ, Thomas PK, Lambert EH, Bunge RP (eds): Peripheral Neuropathy. 2nd Ed. WB Saunders, Philadelphia, 1984

Ewing DJ, Clarke BF: Diabetic autonomic neuropathy: A clinical viewpoint. p. 66. In Dyck PJ, Thomas PK, Asbury AK, et al (eds): Diabetic Neuropathy. WB Saunders, Philadelphia, 1987

Halperin JJ, Little BW, Coyle PK, Battwyler RJ: Lyme disease: cause of a treatable peripheral neuropathy. Neurology 37:1700, 1987

Halperin JJ, Luft BJ, Anand AK: Lyme neuroborreliosis: central nervous system manifestations. Neurology 39:753, 1989

Krarup C, Stewart JD, Summer AJ, et al: A syndrome of asymmetric weakness with motor conduction block. Neurology 40:118, 1990

Lewis RA, Summer AJ: The electrodiagnostic distinctions between chronic familial and acquired demyelinative neuropathies. Neurology 32:592, 1982

Moore PM, Cripps TR: Neurologic complications of vasculitis. Ann Neurol 14:155, 1983

Parry GH: Peripheral neuropathies associated with human immunodeficiency virus infection. Ann Neurol 23 (suppl):S49, 1988

Schaumberg HH, Spencer PS, Thomas PK: Disorders of Peripheral Nerves. FA Davis, Philadelphia, 1983

Stewart JD: Focal Peripheral Neuropathies. Elsevier Science Publishing, New York, 1987

Yi-lan W, Pei-kun L, Zi-quang C, et al: Effects of occupational lead exposure. Scand J Work Environ Health 11(suppl. 4):20, 1985

Westermark P, Stenkvist B: A new method for the diagnosis of systemic amyloidosis. Arch Intern Med 132:522, 1973

17 LABORATORY TESTS FOR EVALUATING DISEASES OF THE NEUROMUSCULAR JUNCTION

Table 17-1. Differential Diagnosis of Neuromuscular Transmission Defects

Myasthenia Gravis
Associated with thymoma
Not associated with thymoma

Lambert-Eaton Syndrome
Associated with malignancy (mostly small cell lung cancer)
Not associated with malignancy

Toxins
Botulism
Aminoglycosides

Table 17-2. Evaluation of Neuromuscular Transmission Defects

Test	Condition	Notes
Blood Tests		
T_3, Free T_4, TSH	Myasthenia gravis	Association with autoimmune thyroid disease
Anti-ACh receptor antibodies	Myasthenia gravis	Elevated titer of anti-ACh-receptor antibodies specific for myasthenia gravis; titers may be used to follow therapeutic response; seronegative myasthenia gravis occurs in 10–15% of generalized cases and up to 40% of purely ocular cases
Antistriated muscle antibodies	Myasthenia gravis	Presence of these antibodies increases probability of an associated thymoma (positive in about 90% with thymoma and 30% without)
Blood, feces, and gastric contents for mouse neutralization test	Botulism	Any possibly contaminated food and stool should also be collected appropriately for anaerobic culture for *Clostridium botulinum*; immunofluorescence staining may identify organism in stool
Radiology		
Chest x-ray	Myasthenic syndromes	Look for an anterior mediastinal mass suggesting thymoma or evidence of lung cancer (in LEMS)

Continued

Table 17-2. *Continued*

Test	Condition	Notes
CT medistinum	Myasthenia gravis	Better than chest x-ray for evaluation of possible thymoma
	Lambert-Eaton myasthenic syndrome (LEMS)	Small cell lung cancer is the malignancy most strongly associated with LEMS; chest CT needed if suspicious lesion present on chest x-ray
Electrophysiology		
Standard EMG	Myasthenia gravis	Usually normal except in very severe disease or myasthenia combined with other myopathy
Repetitive stimulation of motor nerve	Myasthenia gravis	Characteristic decremental response with postexercise repair
	LEMS	Initially low amplitude CMAP with increment (>100% increase is diagnostic) on repetitive stimulation or after exercise
	Botulism	Mild incremental response to repetitive stimulation
Single-fiber EMG	Neuromuscular transmission defect	Abnormal jitter and blocking; sensitive but not specific

Further Notes

There are relatively few recognized acquired disorders of function of the neuromuscular junction (Table 17-1). Except for myasthenia gravis they are uncommon. In adult neurology, the major concerns are primarily the autoimmune disorders of myasthenia gravis and the Lambert-Eaton myasthenic syndrome (LEMS). The latter is a misnomer in the sense that the syndrome presents more like myopathy than myasthenia. The clinical presentation of botulism with acute GI problems and weakness associated with dilated, unreactive pupils is distinctive. Rare congenital disorders of the neuromuscular junction encountered in neonates are not considered here.

When myasthenia gravis or the myasthenic syndrome is suspected, there are three specific diagnostic tasks: (1) directly confirming dysfunction of neuromuscular junction or reducing the probability of alternative diagnoses, (2) establishing whether other contributing diseases (e.g., thymoma, dysthyroid state, lung carcinoma) are also present, and (3) making certain that there is no respiratory impairment. Laboratory tests can ease or refine clinical assessment in each of these areas.

THE TENSILON TEST

The initial goal of laboratory investigation is to try to confirm the presence of disease at the neuromuscular junction. Objective clinical signs, such as ptosis, limitation of extraocular movement, or clear proximal weakness, are indications for a Tensilon (edrophonium chloride) test with suspected myasthenia gravis. Stable intravenous access should be achieved with an indwelling catheter in a peripheral vein, and a baseline examination should be performed. An initial injection of 1 to 2 mg of edrophonium chloride should be given. If there is no response in 1 to 2 minutes, an additional 3 to 4 mg should be injected. The patient should then be examined for improvement in symptoms 30 to 60 seconds later. In the absence of a positive response, more edrophonium chloride can be injected over a 3- to 6-minute period to a total dose of 10 mg. Titration of the edrophonium chloride for a response is useful, as the symptoms of some patients may actually worsen at higher doses. A positive response will last only a few minutes. In cases where significant functional overlay is suspected, single-blind trials with either edrophonium chloride or saline may be tried. Unfortunately, the side effects of edrophonium chloride (nausea, dizziness, bradycardia, and blurred vision) preclude a truly blinded study.

Particular care should be taken with patients who have a history of cardiac conduction abnormalities because of the risk of sudden augmentation of vagal tone. A syringe of atropine sulfate (0.5 to 1.0 mg) should be immediately available for emergency use if severe bradycardia develops during the test.

With this and other laboratory tests for disease of the neuromuscular junction, while a positive result can confirm the diagnosis of myasthenia gravis, a negative result does not rule it out. Some patients, particularly those who are elderly with purely ocular myasthenia, may have no laboratory abnormalities confirming neuromuscular junction disease. In such cases, a clinical diagnosis must be made.

NEUROMUSCULAR TRANSMISSION TESTS

Repetitive Nerve Stimulation

Repetitive stimulation studies can identify dysfunction of the neuromuscular junction. These involve electrical stimulation of a motor nerve with short trains shocks at 2 to 4 Hz while measuring the amplitudes of the resulting compound motor action potentials. The normal response is little or no change in compound muscle action potential (CMAP) amplitude during such repetitive stimulation. However, with patients who have myasthenia gravis, a decrement in the response (>10 percent is significant) after 1 to 2 seconds of stimulation may be seen. The decrement is repaired after a short period (10 to 30 seconds) of voluntary contraction of the muscle. In contrast, patients with Lambert-Eaton syndrome (or botulism) will show an augmentation of the CMAP amplitude (>25 percent is suggestive and >100 percent is diagnostic) after a short period of voluntary contraction. Ideally, the most involved muscles are chosen for study, but this approach can be difficult, particularly with suspected ocular myasthenia. A negative study from a convenient distal muscle (e.g., abductor digiti minimi) should be followed by an attempt with a more proximal muscle (e.g., trapezius or facial muscle). Proximal muscle studies are more sensitive, but results from proximal muscles are more difficult to interpret because of artifacts arising from inability to stabilize the muscle and the electrodes.

Single-Fiber Electromyography

Single-fiber electromyography (EMG) is the most sensitive electrophysiologic test for disorders of neuromuscular transmission. Disorders of the neuromuscular junction can be identified by finding increased jitter (see Ch. 4) and blocking during voluntary activation of motor units. However, increased jitter and blocking can be found also with neuropathies and in myopathic disorders involving segmental necrosis and reinnervation.

IMMUNOLOGIC AND THYROID FUNCTION TESTS

Myasthenia gravis and the LEMS are associated with abnormal circulating antibodies. Circulating antibodies in the LEMS have only recently been identified, and assays are still confined to a few research centers. Assays for autoantibodies in myasthenia gravis have some clinical use. Antiacetylcholine receptor antibodies are assayed by measurement of the amount of solubilized human muscle acetylcholine receptors (labeled with radioactive bungarotoxin) that is precipitated by goat antihuman IgG after incubation with test serum. Antireceptor antibodies defined in this way are found in a majority of patients with myasthenia and almost all patients with generalized myasthenia. Pure ocular myasthenia is more frequently seronegative than is generalized myasthenia. Antiacetylcholine receptor antibody titers do not correlate with the severity of disease among patients as they are polyclonal and, in different patients, recognize different idiotypes on the acetylcholine receptor.

Other autoantibodies are common in myasthenia. Of clinical importance are antistriated muscle antibodies, which are found in about one-third of all myasthenics, but in about two-thirds of those who have thymomas.

Myasthenia gravis is frequently associated with a dysthyroid state that can worsen symptoms. Thyroid function tests (thyrotropin stimulating hormone [TSH], free T_4, T_3) should be routinely obtained on all patients after diagnosis.

RADIOLOGIC INVESTIGATIONS

Radiologic investigations are important for evaluation and planning of treatment. All patients with myasthenia gravis should have a chest x-ray and computed tomography (CT) scan of the mediastinum to look for signs of a thymoma. About 10 percent of patients with myasthenia gravis will have a thymoma. The risk is greater in older patients and for males. Because thymectomy is not recommended for all elderly patients with myasthenia gravis, as it is for younger patients, periodic follow-up chest x-rays should be obtained for this group.

Patients with LEMS should have a chest x-ray to look for evidence of a lung neoplasm (small cell carcinoma is the most common associated neoplasm) or other occult neoplasms. Patients should be closely followed in subsequent years for development of cancer, even if initial studies are negative.

PULMONARY FUNCTION TESTS

Diseases of the neuromuscular junction are frequently accompanied by respiratory compromise. Respiratory function tests should always be obtained initially in generalized myasthenia. Particular care must be taken to follow respiratory function in elderly patients begun on immunosuppressive therapy, as dramatic exacerbation of their weakness may occur with steroid treatment.

The progression of pulmonary dysfunction in neuromuscular disease begins with limitation of maximum inspiratory and expiratory forces. These are measures of power in the respiratory muscles, particularly the diaphragm. Analysis of the spirometric flow-volume curve may improve discrimination of early weakness (see for example Vincken et al., 1987). Neuromuscular disease can lead to a pattern of restrictive pulmonary disease with decreased vital capacity and compliance.

Systemic illnesses (even minor viral respiratory tract infections) can cause dramatic exacerbations of weakness with myasthenia gravis. Any patient who presents with sudden worsening of symptoms should be thoroughly evaluated for infection (particularly respiratory and urinary tract infections).

MICROBIOLOGIC TESTS IN BOTULISM

Cases of suspected botulism demand rapid evaluation as progression can be limited by administration of antitoxin. Tests for toxin and culture are not usually performed by hospital laboratories, so the Public Health Laboratory must be contacted. Specimens of stool (25 g or more), serum (at least 5 ml), gastric contents and food should be kept cool (on dry ice for prolonged transfers) when being sent to the reference laboratory. Obviously, with the delay microbiologic investigation introduces, clinical examination and EMG are central to the initial evaluation.

READINGS

Newsom-Davis J: Diseases of the neuromuscular junction. p. 269. In Asbury AK, McKhann GK, McDonald IW (eds): Diseases of the Nervous System. Vol. I. WB Saunders, Philadelphia, 1986

Vincken WG, Elleker MG, Cosio MG: Flow-volume loop changes reflecting respiratory muscle weakness in chronic neuromuscular disorders. Am J Med 83:673, 1987

LABORATORY TESTS FOR EVALUATING SUSPECTED MUSCLE DISEASE 18

Table 18-1. Differential Diagnosis of Muscle Disease

Inflammatory
Dermatomyositis
Polymyositis
Inclusion body myositis
Infection (e.g., toxoplasmosis, trichinosis, HIV-1, coxsackievirus)
  Idiopathic (sarcoidosis)

Endocrine
Hyperthyroidism or hypothyroidism
Hypercortisolism (e.g., steroid myopathy)
Vitamin D deficiency
Vitamin E deficiency

Metabolic
Myoadenylate deaminase deficiency
Mitochondrial myopathies
Acid maltase deficiency
Glycolytic defects
Periodic paralyses
  Hypokalemic
  Hyperkalemic
  Normokalemic

Toxic (e.g., alcohol, phencyclidine, heroin, amphetamine)

Dystrophies
Dystrophin-related (e.g., Duchenne, Becker)
Autosomal dominant (e.g., fascioscapulohumeral, oculopharyngeal)
Autosomal recessive (e.g., limb-girdle syndromes, distal muscular dystrophy)
Myotonic disorders (e.g., myotonic dystrophy, myotonia congenita)

Other Congenital Myopathies (e.g., central core disease, nemaline body myopathy)

Table 18-2. Evaluation of Muscle Weakness

Test	Condition	Notes
Blood Tests		
CBC	Parasitic infection	Eosinophilia
	Polymyositis, dermatomyositis	Anemia of chronic disease may be seen
Electrolytes	Hypercortisolism	In severe cases hypokalemia, hypochloremia, and mild metabolic acidosis
	Periodic paralysis	During weakness, low serum [K^+] is found in the hypokalemic form and frequently elevated [K^+] in hyperkalemic form; between attacks serum [K^+] is normal
CPK	Myopathies and muscular dystrophies	Elevation associated with fiber necrosis
Serum phosphorus		Low values associated with weakness in chronic alcoholism and severe vitamin D deficiency
Venous lactate and pyruvate	Mitochondrial cytopathies	Venous [lactate] and [lactate]/[pyruvate] ratio may be elevated at rest; abnormal increases with exercise
ESR	Polymyositis, dermatomyositis	Frequently elevated, particularly in myositis associated with connective tissue disease
TSH, T_4, T_3	Dysthyroid state	Myopathy occurs with both hyper- and hypothyroidism
Serum cortisol	Cushing's syndrome	Most commonly iatrogenic

Continued

Table 18-2. *Continued*

Test	Condition	Notes
Serology		
Jo-1 antibodies	Polymyositic, dermatomyositis	Relatively specific for autoimmune myositis; consider also the autoantibodies associated with collagen-vascular disease (anti-Sm, anti-dsDNA in SLE; anti-Ro, anti-La in Sjögren and ENA in mixed connective tissue disease)
Anti-HIV antibody		In addition to an inflammatory myopathy, myopathies secondary to cachexia and azidothymidine (zidovudine) should be considered
Anti-cysticercosis, trichinosis serum antibodies	Inflammatory myopathy	Rising titers most specific for acute disease
Radiology		
Limb films	Cysticercosis, trichinosis	Calcified cysts may be found in muscle; head CT may demonstrate intracranial lesions in cysticercosis
Electrophysiologic Tests		
ECG	Duchenne dystrophy	Cardiomyopathy causes deep Q waves in limb and left chest leads
	Myotonic dystrophy, mitochondrial myopathies	Conduction blocks and arrhythmias are common
	Glycolytic defects and acid maltase deficiency	Hypertrophic cardiomyopathies are found in acid maltese deficiency (infantile form) and debrancher enzyme deficiency
	Periodic paralyses	ECG changes secondary to changes in serum $[K^+]$ are seen; during hyperkalemia T waves are peaked and during hypokalemia they flatten

EMG	Myopathies (general)	Increased recruitment in weak muscles; polyphasic potentials may be seen; abnormal (usually short) motor unit potential duration
	Polymyositis	Prominent spontaneous activity (fibrillations, positive sharp waves, high frequency discharges); these are not seen with steroid myopathy unless very severe
	Myotonic disorders	Myotonic discharges
Respiratory Function Tests		
Maximum static inspiratory and expiratory pressures at functional reserve capacity	Myopathy (general)	Most sensitive spirometric parameters for detecting respiratory muscle weakness
Vital capacity		Neuromuscular disease can give restrictive pulmonary pattern
Arterial blood gas		Respiratory muscle weakness leading to hypoventilation gives elevated PCO_2
Biopsy		
Muscle biopsy	Polymyositis	Segmental myonecrosis, interstitial or perivascular inflammatory exudates
	Dermatomyositis	Perifascicular atrophy and loss of capillaries
	Endocrine myopathies	Type II atrophy
	Muscular dystrophies	Necrosis and regeneration with connective tissue proliferation; inflammatory exudate may be seen in fascioscapulohumeral dystrophy

Continued

Table 18-2. *Continued*

Test	Condition	Notes
	Acid maltase deficiency (glycogenesis type III), glycolytic defects	PAS-positive (glycogen)-containing vacuoles
	Mitochondrial cytopathies	Ragged red fibers, lipid droplets, and abnormal mitochondrial distribution; ultrastructural appearance of mitochondria is abnormal, often with paracrystalline deposits
Special Tests		
Ischemic forearm exercise test	Glycolytic defects	Low or absent increase in venous lactate after ischemic exercise
	Myoadenylate deaminase deficiency	Low or absent increase in ammonia after exercise (with normal venous lactate changes)
Glucose load (2–3 mg/kg p.o. or IV) with subcutaneous insulin (10–20 U)	Hypokalemic periodic paralysis	Acutely precipitates attacks of weakness
Oral potassium load (2–10 g of oral potassium chloride elixir), given slowly over several hours	Hyperkalemic or normokalemic periodic paralysis	Acutely precipitates attack; monitor ECG for possible cardiac arrhythmias

Further Notes

When a patient presents with complaints of weakness, easy fatigability, or muscle pain, the initial problem is to identify the component of the motor system at which dysfunction is occurring: upper motor neuron, the anterior horn cell (neuronopathy) or its axon (neuropathy), the neuromuscular junction, or the muscle itself (myopathy or dystrophy). The clinical history and examination are the most important guides to classification of the disorder.

LABORATORY TESTS SUGGESTIVE OF PRIMARY MUSCLE DISEASE

The two most important initial laboratory tests for establishing a myopathic process are the serum creatine phosphokinase (CPK) and electromyography (EMG). Elevated CPK is a nonspecific marker of breakdown of the integrity of the sarcolemma. This occurs with muscle fiber necrosis and is prominent with inflammatory muscle diseases, the muscular dystrophies, and certain metabolic disorders.

Frank rhabdomyolysis can occur and is marked by the presence of myoglobinuria. Myoglobinuria is characteristic of deficiencies of glycolytic or glycogenolytic enzymes (in which the myoglobinuria lessens with fasting) and carnitine palmitoyltransferase deficiency (in which the myoglobinuria becomes more severe with fasting). With metabolic stresses (e.g., exercise, fasting, fever) myoglobinuria can become so great that it can lead to renal failure. When suspected, urine myoglobin should be checked both in the laboratory and at the bedside: a urine dipstick test for blood will change color in a diffuse pattern with myoglobinuria. In contrast, the individual red blood cells of hematuria give a speckled pattern to the colorimetric paper.

The EMG is a relatively nonspecific test for any muscle disease, except perhaps the myotonic disorders. Abnormalities characteristic of myopathies have been described in Chapter 4. As there is differential involvement of muscle groups in most myopathic processes, clinical examination should identify those most involved for EMG studies. Increased recruitment in weak muscles (with fasciculations and positive sharp waves if segmental fiber necrosis has occurred) is found with some myopathies. Abnormalities of motor unit potential duration (MUPD) may often be found even with mild disease. The clearest cases are those in which the MUPD is abnormally short. (The normal duration is about 10 to 15 msec and is age and muscle group dependent.) However, an abnormally prolonged MUPD also occurs with muscle disease. Increased insertional activity is characteristic of inflammatory myopathies and acid maltase deficiency. Myotonic discharges are characteristic of myotonic dystrophy.

Specific diagnoses often require muscle biopsy. As biopsy is an invasive procedure and is not always helpful, it is worthwhile to obtain other appropriate tests first. Often interpretation of changes in the muscle biopsy may depend on other laboratory findings. This is particularly important in the endocrine myopathies, for example. These are identified by establishing the underlying hormonal imbalance either directly or indirectly. (Depending on the condition suspected, thyrotropin-stimulating hormone [TSH], free T_4,T_3, A.M. cortisol, adrenocorticotrophic hormone-[ACTH] stimulated cortisol release, serum electrolytes, Ca and phosphate may be useful—the clinical history, particularly if it involves steroid treatment, should not be ignored.)

INFLAMMATORY MYOPATHIES

Inflammatory myopathies are common acquired causes of myopathic weakness. Laboratory tests helpful in initial recognition are serum CPK (frequently elevated), erythrocyte sedimentation rate (ESR) (can be elevated, particularly in syndromes associated with collagen-vascular diseases), the EMG, and muscle biopsy. With polymyositis, in addition to focal fiber necrosis and infiltration of small round inflammatory cells, muscle fibers may show sarcolemmal expression of major histocompatibility complex (MHC) determinants not normally found on muscle (see Ch. 8). Muscle biopsies in dermatomyositis show inflammatory changes less frequently, but perifascicular muscle fiber atrophy should be seen.

Once either of these disorders is identified, a further diagnostic question is whether there is an underlying systemic disease. Polymyositis or dermatomyositis can both be found in association with systemic vasculitides (rheumatoid arthritis, systemic lupus erythematosus [SLE], mixed connective tissue disease [MCTD] and others). The renal sediment (freshly obtained) should be examined for evidence of coexisting renal disease.

Active vasculitis may be accompanied by decreases in plasma complement (C_3,C_4) levels. Abnormal circulating autoantibodies characteristic of these diseases (e.g., rheumatoid factor, anti-ds DNA) can suggest specific disorders in some cases. In adults, there is a significant association of dermatomyositis with malignancy. In the absence of localizing signs or symptoms on careful examination, complete blood count (CBC), electrolytes, liver function tests, alkaline and acid phosphatase, urinalysis, chest x-ray, stool for occult blood and possibly evaluation of the GI tract (by sigmoidoscopy or barium enema) should be an adequate initial screen. The patients should be followed closely subsequently, as myositis may precede manifestations of a primary neoplasm by years.

There are other forms of inflammatory myopathies. Inclusion body myositis is not uncommon and may present as a syndrome of slowly progressive proximal and distal myopathic weakness in older patients. The CPK is usually elevated; EMG may show prominent fibrillation potentials and short polyphasic motor units. The pathognomic red rimmed vacuoles with angular fibers should be seen in the muscle biopsy.

Myopathies in patients with acquired immunodeficiency syndrome (AIDS) are still poorly understood. There is an inflammatory myopathy that appears to respond to antiviral treatment. However, both azidothymidine (AZT) and the cachexia induced by the disease may also cause myopathies.

Other causes of inflammatory myopathies are very rare. Sarcoidosis (see Ch. 15) can lead to muscle granulomas associated with more widespread inflammation. Infectious causes of inflammatory myopathies (e.g., toxoplasmosis, cysticercosis or trichinosis) should be considered. These are usually associated with prominent myalgia. Eosinophilia is often present and serum antibody titers are usually elevated (although these must be interpreted cautiously in individuals from endemic areas). Chronic lesions in muscle will calcify and can be seen on x-ray of the involved muscles. If active cysticercosis is suspected, stool should be examined for eggs of *Taenia solium* and a head CT should be obtained. Definitive diagnosis of trichinosis may demand demonstration of the larvae of *Trichinella spiralis* or calcified cysts in a muscle biopsy from an involved site.

TOXINS AND DRUGS

Toxins and drugs may lead to acute and chronic myopathies. A few examples will be cited. An acute alcoholic myopathy is characterized by painful onset of muscle necrosis after high alcohol intake. Rhabdomyolysis ensues with very high serum CPK, hyperkalemia, and myoglobinuria with the consequent risk of renal failure. A subacute painful myopathy is associated with administration of high doses of clofibrate. The pathology shows scattered fiber necrosis and regeneration and is nonspecific. Focal necrosis with secondary fibrosis at the sites of injection can be seen with a variety of agents, including narcotics. Rarely, inflammatory myopathies can be associated with idiosyncratic systemic vasculitic responses to procainamide, phenytoin, or D-penicillamine.

HERITABLE AND OTHER METABOLIC DISORDERS

Heritable metabolic disorders of muscle are discussed in Chapter 7. Myoadenylate deaminase deficiency can be diagnosed by a lactate-ammonia exercise test showing a rise in venous ammonia of less than 0.7 percent of that for lactate. Histochemical stains of a muscle biopsy specimen can confirm the diagnosis. Disorders of glycolysis may be diagnosed by an inappropriately low rise (< 1.5 times the resting level) in venous lactate after adequate ischemic forearm exercise. Specific enzyme deficiencies can be identified histochemically after muscle biopsy. Acid maltase deficiency may be suspected in syndromes of chronic progressive proximal myopathy associated with prominent spontaneous activity at rest on EMG. Muscle biopsy shows abnormal acid phosphatase staining. Some laboratories can assay for the glucosidase enzyme deficiency in leukocytes, cultured fibroblasts, or urine. Disorders of mitochondrial energy metabolism are usually sporadic, but can be familial. More severely affected patients show abnormally elevated resting venous lactate. At present the most widely used diagnostic abnormality is the presence of ragged red fibers in the muscle biopsy when stained with a modified Gomori-trichrome stain. Mitochondrial DNA analysis is becoming more important, however.

PERIODIC PARALYSES

Patients with periodic paralysis usually have diagnostic abnormalities of serum potassium during episodes of weakness (serum potassium concentration is normal between episodes). In hyperkalemic periodic paralysis diagnostic increases in serum potassium concentrations may be found with episodes of weakness, although values still remain within the normal range. In hypokalemic periodic paralysis, whereas serum potassium concentrations are often below the normal range (and may be very low, e.g., 1.5 to 2.5 mM), a relative decrease may also be diagnostic when associated with weakness. Serum CPK is usually normal. EMG studies demonstrate small or absent CMAPs and inexcitability of paralyzed muscles even to direct electrical stimulation.

Provocative testing may be necessary to establish the diagnosis. The episodes of weakness and shifts in body potassium can be precipitated by glucose-insulin (in hypokalemic periodic paralysis) or potassium chloride (in hyperkalemic periodic paralysis) challenges (Engel and Banker, 1986). Serum potassium concentrations should be measured before and after such challenges. For safety, the ECG should be monitored during provocative testing. Quantitative serial measurement of CMAP amplitudes can provide confirmation of muscle inexcitability.

MUSCULAR DYSTROPHIES

Diagnosis of muscular dystrophies has been predominantly clinical until recently. Duchenne dystrophy is invariably associated with very high levels of serum creatine phosphokinase activity (on the order of 10 times normal), but much more modest and sometimes normal serum creatine phosphokinase activity may be seen with more indolent dystrophies. Muscle biopsy is important for confirming the clinical diagnosis. The muscle biopsy shows scattered fibro-fatty replacement, muscle fiber necrosis, and absent dystrophin antibody staining of the sarcolemma. For Duchenne muscular dystrophy, prenatal diagnosis and carrier state detection can now be made by molecular genetic analysis. Prognosis in the heterogeneous group of Becker muscular dystrophy and differentiation from other clinically similar autosomal recessive or dominant disorders may be predicted by assay of dystrophin levels and molecular weight in biopsied muscle.

For later-onset muscular dystrophies, diagnosis still relies primarily on clinical assessment for the significance of the patterns of muscle involvement and inheritance. EMG studies, which may show evidence of myopathy and muscle fiber necrosis and regeneration, is nonspecific in the nonmyotonic muscular dystrophies. Muscle biopsy is usually indicated to demonstrate the appropriate dystrophic changes (Carpenter and Karpati, 1984) and to make alternative diagnoses less likely.

EMG studies demonstrating myotonia can be useful in establishing the diagnosis of mytonic dystrophy. Attention should also be focused on defining the nature of the systemic manifestations of the disease. All of these patients should undergo ophthalmic evaluation for cataracts and an ECG for arrhythmias and signs of conduction block. The latter have the most life-threatening consequences for these patients.

READINGS

Brown WF, Bolton CF (eds): Clinical Electromyography. Butterworth (Publishers), Boston, 1987

Buchthal F: Electrophysiological signs of myopathy as related with muscle biopsy. Acta Neurol 32:1, 1977

Carpenter S, Karpati G: Pathology of Skeletal Muscle. Churchill Livingstone, New York, 1984

Demedts M, Beckers J, Rochette F, Bulcke J: Pulmonary function in moderate neuromuscular disease without respiratory complaints. Eur J Respir Dis 63:62, 1982

DiMauro S, Bonilla E, Zeviani M, et al.: Mitochondrial myopathies. Ann Neurol 17:521, 1985

Engel AG, Banker BQ (eds): Myology, McGraw-Hill, New York, 1986

Gibson GJ, Pride NB, Newsom-Davis J, Loh LC: Pulmonary mechanics in patients with respiratory muscle weakness. Am Rev Respir Dis 115:389, 1977

Hoffman EP, Kunkel LM, Angolini C, et al.: Improved diagnosis of Becker muscular dystrophy by dystrophin testing. Neurology 39:1011, 1989

Morgan-Hughes JA: Diseases of striated muscle. p. 227. In Asbury AK, McKhann GK, McDonald IW (eds): Diseases of the Nervous System. Vol. I. WB Saunders, Philadelphia, 1986

Appendix: Abbreviations Used in the Text

ACE	angiotensin-converting enzyme
ACh	acetylcholine
ACTH	adrenocorticotrophic hormone
AFB	acid-fast bacillus
AIDS	acquired immunodeficiency syndrome
ALD	adrenoleukodystrophy
ALS	amyotrophic lateral sclerosis
AVM	arteriovenous malformation
AZT	azidothymidine
BAER	brainstem auditory evoked response
BIPLED	bihemispheric periodic lateralized epileptiform discharges
BSSS	benign small sharp spikes
BUN	blood urea nitrogen
C3, C4	complement factors 3 and 4
Ca	calcium
CBC	complete blood count
cDNA	deoxyribonucleic acid synthesized in vitro that is complementary to mRNA in tissue
CIDPN	chronic inflammatory demyelinating polyneuropathy
CK	creatine kinase
CMAP	compound motor action potential
COPD	chronic obstructive pulmonary disease
CNS	central nervous system
CPK	creatine phosphokinase
Cr	creatinine
CREST	syndrome of calcinosis, Raynaud's phenomenon, esophageal dysmotility, sclerodactyly, and telangiectasia

CSF	cerebrospinal fluid
CT	computed tomography
CVA	cerebrovascular accident
D	distance
dB	decibel
DIC	disseminated intravascular coagulation
DL_{CO}	lung diffusion capacity for carbon monoxide
ds-DNA	double-stranded DNA
ECI	electrocerebral inactivity
ECG	electrocardiogram
EDTA	ethylene-diamine tetra-acetic acid (divalent cation chelating agent)
EEG	electroencephalography
ELISA	enzyme-linked immunosorbent assay
EMG	electromyography
ENA	extractable nuclear antigen
ESR	erythrocyte sedimentation rate
FANA	fluorescent antinuclear antibodies
FTA-ABS	fluorescent treponemal antibody absorption test (for antibodies directed against *Treponema pallidum*)
GI	gastrointestinal
Hemoglobin A_{1c}	glycosylated hemoglobin
HDL	high-density lipoprotein
HIV-1	human immunodeficiency virus-1
HMSN	hereditary motor and sensory neuropathy
HPLC	high performance liquid chromatography
HSV	herpes simplex virus
HTLV-1	human T-cell lymphotropic virus-1
Hz	hertz (s^{-1})
IA-DSA	intra-arterial digital subtraction angiography
ICP	intracranial pressure
IEP	immunoelectrophoresis
Ig	immunoglobulin
IRDA	intermittent rhythmic delta activity
IV-DSA	intravenous digital subtraction angiography

LDL	low-density lipoprotein
LEMS	Lambert-Eaton myasthenic syndrome
LOD	log of the odds
LP	lumbar puncture
m	meter
MCA	middle cerebral artery
MCTD	mixed connective tissue disease
MERRF	myoclonus epilepsy with ragged red fibers
MHC	major histocompatibility complex
MI	myocardial infarction
MM	the isoenzyme of creatine kinase that contains two M subunits
MNCV	motor nerve conduction velocity
MRI	magnetic resonance imaging
MS	multiple sclerosis
MUPD	motor unit potential duration
MVP	mitral valve prolapse
Na	sodium
NCV	nerve conduction velocity
NPH	normal pressure hydrocephalus
NREM	non-REM (sleep stage)
PAN	polyarteritis nodosa
PDA	polymorphic delta activity
PET	positron emission tomography
PLED	periodic lateralized epileptiform discharge
POEMS	syndrome of polyneuropathy, organomegaly, endocrine abnormalities, M-protein, and skin-lesions
POSTS	positive occipital sharp transients of sleep
PT	prothrombin time
PTT	partial thromboplastin time
RBC	red blood cells
REM	rapid eye movement (sleep stage)
RF	radiofrequency
RFLP	restriction fragment length polymorphism
SEP	somatosensory evoked potential
SGOT	serum glutamic-oxaloacetate transaminase
SGPT	serum glutamate-pyruvate transaminase

SIADH	syndrome of inappropriate secretion of antidiuretic hormone
SLE	systemic lupus erythematosus
SMAC	Sequential Multiply Analyzer Computer panel
SNAP	sensory nerve action potential amplitude
SNCV	sensory nerve conduction velocity
SPEP	serum protein electrophoresis
SSPE	subacute sclerosing panencephalitis
T	delay between stimulus pulse and recorded action potential in NCV measurements
T_3	triiodothyronine
T_4	thyroxine
TB	tuberculosis
TIA	transient ischemic attack
TLC	thin layer chromatography
TSH	thyrotropin stimulating hormone
UBOs	unidentified bright objects (in MRI)
US	ultrasound
VDRL	venereal disease research laboratory test
VER	visual evoked response
VLCFA	very long chain fatty acid
WBC	white blood cells

INDEX

Page numbers followed by f indicate figures; those followed by t indicate tables.

C